Holistic Breast Care

For Baillière Tindall:

Commissioning Editor: Sarena Wolfaard
Project Development Manager: Karen Gilmour
Project Manager: Jane Dingwall
Design Direction: George Ajayi

Holistic Breast Care

Edited by

Karen L Burnet MSc BSc RGN ENB 237 A11
Formerly Nurse Practitioner in Breast Care, now Oncology Nurse Manager, Oncology Centre, Addenbrooke's Hospital, Cambridge, UK

Foreword by

Arnie Purushotham MBBS FRCS(Ed) FRCS(Gen,Ed) FRCS(Glas) MD
Consultant Breast Surgeon, Addenbrooke's Hospital, Cambridge, UK

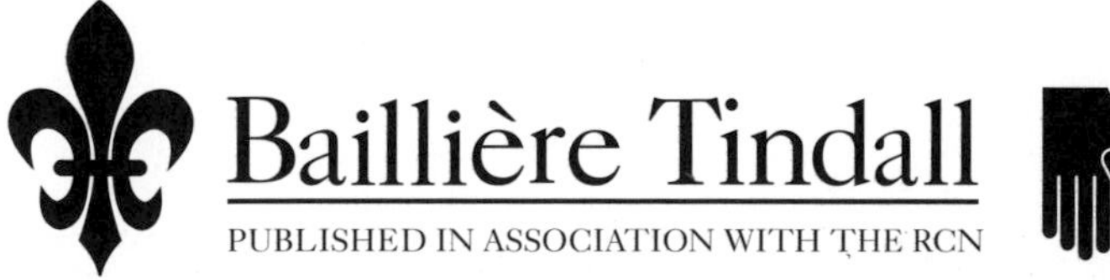

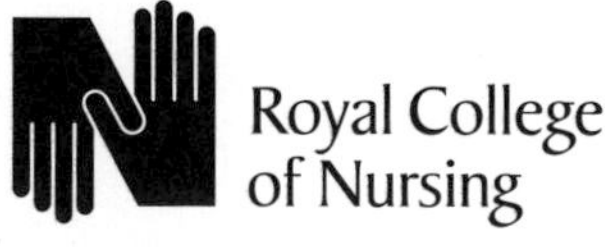

Edinburgh London New York Philadelphia St Louis Sydney Toronto 2001

BAILLIÈRE TINDALL
An imprint of Harcourt Publishers Limited

 is a registered trademark of Harcourt Publishers Limited

First published 2001

ISBN 0 7020 2439 2

British Library Cataloguing in Publication Data
A catalogue record for this book is available from the British Library

Library of Congress Cataloging in Publication Data
A catalog record for this book is available from the Library of Congress

Note
Medical knowledge is constantly changing. As new information becomes available, changes in treatment, procedures, equipment and the use of drugs become necessary. The editors, contributors and the publishers have taken care to ensure that the information given in this text is accurate and up to date. However, readers are strongly advised to confirm that the information, especially with regard to drug usage, complies with the latest legislation and standards of practice.

The publisher's policy is to use **paper manufactured from sustainable forests**

Printed in China

Contents

Contributors

Nikki Burch RGN OncCert A11 ENB 237 998 941
Clinical Nurse Specialist, Breast Diagnostic Unit, Royal Marsden Hospital, London, UK

Karen L Burnet MSc BSc RGN ENB 237 A11
Formerly Nurse Practitioner in Breast Care, now Oncology Nurse Manager, Oncology Centre, Addenbrooke's Hospital, Cambridge, UK

Siobhan Carroll RGN BSc(Hons) Cancer Nursing ENB 998
Breast Care Nurse Specialist, Cork University Hospital, Ireland

Nicki De Zeeuw RGN ENB A11 237 998 941
Oncology Nurse Coordinator (Information and Support), Ruttle Ward, Tallaght Hospital, Dublin, Ireland

Andrea Gamble RGN BSc OncCert ENB A11 DipHE Teaching
Clinical Nurse Specialist – Breast Care/Unit Manager, Churchill Hospital, Oxford, UK

Jill Mitchell RGN BSc(Hons) Health Studies ENB A11 237 N01
Macmillan Breast Care Nurse, The Horton Hospital, Oxford Road, Banbury, UK

Catherine Oakley RGN BSc(Hons)
Operations Manager/Lead Nurse for Cancer, Chartwell Unit, Bromley Hospitals NHS Trust, Farnborough Hospital, Kent, UK

Jan Smith RGN RHV BSc(Hons) MSc PGDE Dip Counselling
Macmillan Holistic Care Manager (Clinical Services and Education), Tapping House Hospice, Snettisham, Kings Lynn; Senior Lecturer Practitioner (Palliative Care), Addenbrooke's NHS Trust, Cambridge, UK

Michelle Taylor RGN BA(Hons) ENB 998 A11
Formerly Clinical Nurse Specialist – Breast Care, Oxford Radcliffe Hospitals, UK

To Neil

Foreword

Breast cancer remains one of the greatest health threats facing women around the world. Only recently are countries demonstrating an improvement in survival. This reduction in mortality is due to several factors: screening; better targeting of therapy; greater understanding of the disease; and the closer working relationship of members of the multidisciplinary team.

There is a wealth of literature available on diseases of the breast. However, this book is unique in its approach: the entire focus is truly holistic. Karen Burnet has gathered a group of highly qualified and experienced nurses and delivered a book that is comprehensive, highly educational, practical and extremely easy to read. The book is uniquely woman-focused which brings out an extraordinary positive dimension, which the contributors should be justly proud of. This book is written primarily for nurses, by nurses and also for women who seek better understanding about disorders of the breast. I would strongly argue the case that in addition to this, it deserves a place on the book shelf of every clinician involved in the management of breast disorders and in particular breast cancer. I personally thoroughly enjoyed *Holistic Breast Care* and found it highly informative and educational. I look forward to the second edition!

Cambridge 2000

Mr AD Purushotham

Preface

As a breast care nurse I have often been made aware that there is no one nursing textbook that covers the range of disciplines that are involved with breast care, although there are many good books available on separate subjects connected with breast care. I have always felt that my practice and the care of my patients have been improved by my understanding the normal breast as well as the abnormal one. This book intends to provide a breadth of information for any woman who wishes to know more about her breasts and for any health care professional who is caring for women who have a breast problem or anxiety about their breasts. Breast care has only recently begun to be recognised outside of pregnancy or cancer screening and treatment, although, as you will read, much health care is involved with regard to this reproductive and sexual organ. By covering both benign and malignant conditions of the breast this book will help the reader understand that breast care is a subtle and complex subject that involves psycho social as well as physical care.

Most women have expectations of what their breasts are like and any unexpected changes can make them worry. With so much written in the media about breasts and breast cancer it is natural that women will seek reassurance from any source they can, including their GP's surgery, well-woman clinics and family planning clinics as well as breast screening centres and hospitals. As a nurse is often the first person a woman will ask for advice, particularly as the breast is such an intimate part of the body, it is important that the nurse has relevant and contemporary information about breast care. With the advent of the Internet many women have access to research data about breast conditions that they may not necessarily understand and will need help to interpret. It is hoped that this book will enable you to be confident of the advice you are giving and will enable you to promote good health practices concerning breast care.

You may find yourself caring for a woman with a breast problem in many different situations, as a practitioner nurse in a GP's practice, as a clinic nurse in a surgical outpatient clinic, as a radiographer in a screening centre or treatment centre, or as a hospital-based nurse in a surgical ward. The advent of more specialised nursing and radiographer roles such as breast care nurses, specialist radiographers and the even newer nurse practitioners means there are more health care professionals whose sole concern is the care of patients with particular breast problems.

A number of highly qualified nurses have contributed to this book and have not only written about their area of expertise factually but have also added their practical expertise, gained from caring for women with breast problems over many years. The chapters intend to lead the reader through the structure and function of the breast, the normal changes the woman's breast will undergo throughout her lifetime and the more common benign conditions of the breast. Care of the normal breast and breast awareness will also be considered. Breast cancer is covered in detail because of the high risk that women in the UK have of developing this cancer and the increasing complexity of the medical and surgical treatments available for treating it. As breast cancer can profoundly affect the life of the sufferer both physically and emotionally, the psychological care and informational support for women who develop this disease is discussed in detail. Finally, the supportive care for the patient with advanced breast cancer is considered. All chapters include relevant, up-to-date references and suggestions for further reading. The Internet has been highlighted in the section on information support and this will not only be useful to the patient/client but to the nurse as well.

The book has used the concept of holistic care throughout, considering the complete person in the context of her environment and specific attention has been paid to the physical, psychological and social dimensions of breast care. The use of complementary therapies has been highlighted and references provided to allow the reader more access to information about such therapies. There are many complementary therapies available that can give real relief from particular breast conditions and, providing that the therapies have been discussed with a medical practitioner, they provide choice and option for the treatment of problems of the breast. Small case studies have been used to illustrate aspects of breast care and to help the reader gain from the experience of other nurses.

There is no nursing text book that covers both the benign and the malignant conditions of the breast in such detail. This book is not the final word on breast care but is written to inform its readers and by using the references provided to enable them to access further detail about a particular breast condition. It is hoped that by being more enlightened about breast care that we can all improve our practice and the care of our patients.

Cambridge 2001 Karen Burnet

ACKNOWLEDGEMENT

I would like to express my thanks to Alison Wetherall without whose support and encouragement this book would not have been completed.

1 The Normal Breast

Nikki Burch

After reading this chapter the reader should understand:

- What breasts can represent
- Structure and function of the normal breast
- Hormonal influences on the breast throughout a woman's life
- Effect of pregnancy and breastfeeding on the breast
- What being 'breast aware' means
- Normal, everyday care of the breasts.

INTRODUCTION

The breast can be a symbol of many things in different cultures:

- Womanhood
- Motherhood
- Sexuality.

In Western society the breast is an important focus for sexual attractiveness and sexual stimulation. We witness, on what seems like a daily basis, how the fashion headlines indicate that cleavage is in, or next, that flat chests are considered more appropriate. Desmond Morris, who has written much on the significance of human behaviour, writes that in some societies breasts are primarily for feeding babies, whilst in other societies the shape of the breast is also an overt sexual signal. Morris posits that breasts in the pubertal child are at the peak of their sexual signalling because of the rounded, firm shape that they display. He goes on to write that for older, sexually active women in their 20s and 30s when the breasts are not as firm, uplifting bras and silicone enhancements are sometimes used to maintain the rounded shape of the breast, and thus to mimic the sexual signalling of a younger breast (Morris 1978). Whether we believe his ideas or not it is true that as a woman gets older the breasts become less firm and her body shape changes. These changes in the shape of the woman's breasts can translate into poor self-image and a lack of self-esteem. The woman often begins to feel less sexually attractive and these feelings are reinforced by the commercial world where well-shaped breasts represent youth, attractiveness, desirability and, as such, are used for successful marketing. Worse still than the shape of the breast changing is the loss of some, or all, of the breast tissue which may be the result of the treatment for a breast condition. For many of us breasts are central to our femininity and self-image and are a very important expression of who we are. This chapter will help the reader to understand how their breasts are formed, the structure and function of their breasts and, finally, how to look after their breasts so that they may make the best of them.

STRUCTURE AND FUNCTION OF THE NORMAL BREAST

This section is designed to provide background detail for the rest of this book. An understanding of the normal breast will facilitate understanding of what is *abnormal* in the breast and this section will frequently be referred to in other chapters. The anatomy and physiology of the breast will be described, focussing on the hormonal influences that affect the breast throughout a woman's lifetime including puberty, pregnancy and the menopause.

Formation of the breast

The breasts, sometimes known as the mammary glands, are present in both sexes although are usually enlarged only in the woman. Breasts begin to develop in the fetus at around 6 weeks' gestation and are formed from the ectodermal ridge, or milk line, which extends bilaterally from the axilla to the groin. At 20 weeks' gestation, 16–20 milk ducts invade the mesoderm of the developing fetus. These ducts continue to penetrate the surrounding tissue forming breast buds, although differentiation of the breast tissue does not occur until triggered by the appropriate hormonal signals later in life. Occasionally, a baby may be born with extra nipples and associated breast tissue along the ectodermal ridge, most commonly, just below the normal breasts. These accessory breasts can be left without surgical intervention unless they are distressing to the individual (Marieb 1989, Reshef et al 1996).

Each breast lies over the pectoralis major and extends beyond the edge of that muscle to lie on the serratus anterior and external oblique muscles. For most people the breast extends from the second to the sixth rib in the midclavicular line.

When describing the breast it is usual to divide it into four quadrants with horizontal and vertical lines dissecting the nipple giving the upper outer and inner and the lower inner and outer quadrants. The axillary tail of Spence, a lateral extension of breast tissue, extends from the upper outer quadrant to the axilla but may not always be present (Fig. 1.1).

Each mammary gland is contained within a rounded, skin-covered breast. In the centre of each breast is the pigmented areola, which surrounds a central protruding nipple. In both the male and the immature female breast the nipple is small but the areola is fully formed. Around the nipple are large sebaceous glands (the glands of Montgomery) which make the area slightly lumpy. These glands produce secretin, which lubricates the areola and nipple, particularly during breastfeeding. The autonomic nervous system controls the smooth muscle fibres in the areola and nipple causing the nipple to become erect when stimulated by tactile or sexual stimuli, or when exposed to the cold.

Each breast is formed by 15–20 lobes that radiate around the nipple. These lobes are padded and separated by fibrous tissue and fat. The interlobular connective tissue forms suspensory ligaments, known as 'Astley Cooper's' or 'Cooper's ligaments,' which attach the breast to the underlying muscle fascia

FIGURE 1.1

Diagnostic divisions of the breast.

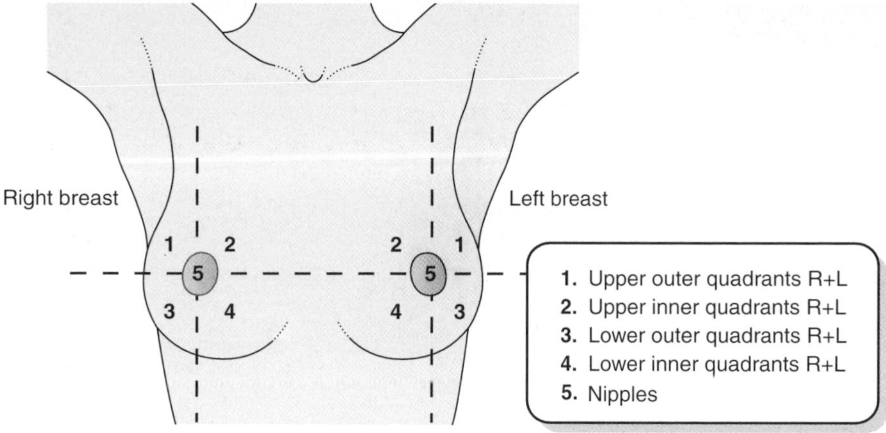

and the overlying dermis. Inside the lobes are chambers called 'lobules,' which are lined by pre-secretory alveolar epithelium. This epithelium is converted into milk-synthesising and milk-releasing glands when a woman is lactating (De Vane 1996). These compound glands pass milk into the lactiferous ducts and sinuses, which lead to the outside of the nipple. Milk accumulates in these sinuses during lactation. The lactiferous ducts are surrounded by myoepithelial cells that contract to eject milk into the nipple in response to the baby's suckling. Many benign breast conditions and almost all malignant conditions occur in the terminal duct lobular unit (Dixon & Mansel 1995) (see Fig. 1.2).

Apart from the lobules and ducts, the breast contains blood vessels, predominantly from the lateral thoracic artery, that curl around the edge of the pectoralis major muscle, and from the internal thoracic artery, that sends branches through the intercostal spaces beside the sternum. Pectoral branches of the acromio-thoracic artery supply the upper part of the breast. Venous return follows the route of the above-mentioned arteries (Last 1978, Blackwell 1996).

The breast is mostly innervated by the intercostal nerves carrying both sensory and autonomic fibres. The nipple and the areola are supplied separately, by the inferior ramus of the fourth intercostal nerve (Blackwell 1996).

The lymph drainage of the immature breast is identical with that of the fully formed organ. Lymph drainage in the breast consists of an interconnecting network of channels that may drain to any point of the compass away from the centre of the breast. However, most of the lymph drains to the pectoralis group of axillary lymph nodes with some lymph draining to the sub-pectoral and apical group of nodes and, via the internal thoracic vein, to the internal mammary or mediastinal nodes (Fig. 1.3).

Hormonal influences on the breast

Puberty

At puberty the pituitary gland in the brain begins to produce the gonadotrophins, follicle-stimulating hormone (FSH) and luteinising hormone (LH). As the levels of these hormones increase, egg follicles within the ovaries are stimulated to release oestrogens. Oestrogens stimulate connective tissue in the breast

FIGURE 1.2

Sagittal section of the female breast.

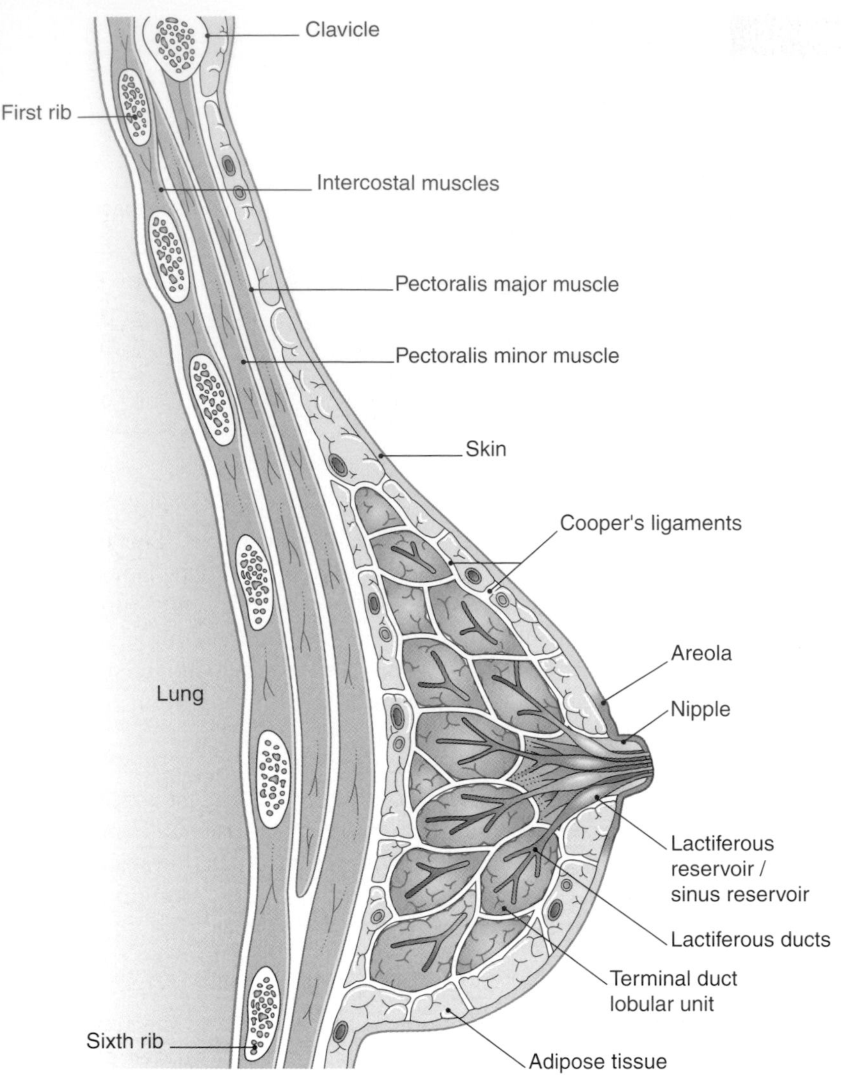

to increase, ducts in the breast to lengthen and the formation of the breast lobules, all resulting in an increase in the size of the breasts. Although oestrogens are primarily involved in ductal proliferation it is thought that various epidermal growth factors are also involved in the process of breast growth (Blackwell 1996). It is not uncommon for breasts to develop slightly asymmetrically (Dixon & Mansel 1995).

Once the breast has developed, it undergoes regular changes in relation to the menstrual cycle. A woman ovulates each month under the influence of FSH and LH. The ovarian follicle, once it has released the ovum, becomes the corpus luteum. The corpus luteum (yellow body) produces the hormone progesterone, which has a secondary function in the growth of the glandular tissue in the breast.

Every month, as the woman approaches menstruation, the size and shape of her breasts change as the breast engorges, secondary to tissue oedema and hyperaemia (Blackwell 1996). If fertilization of the ovum does not occur then

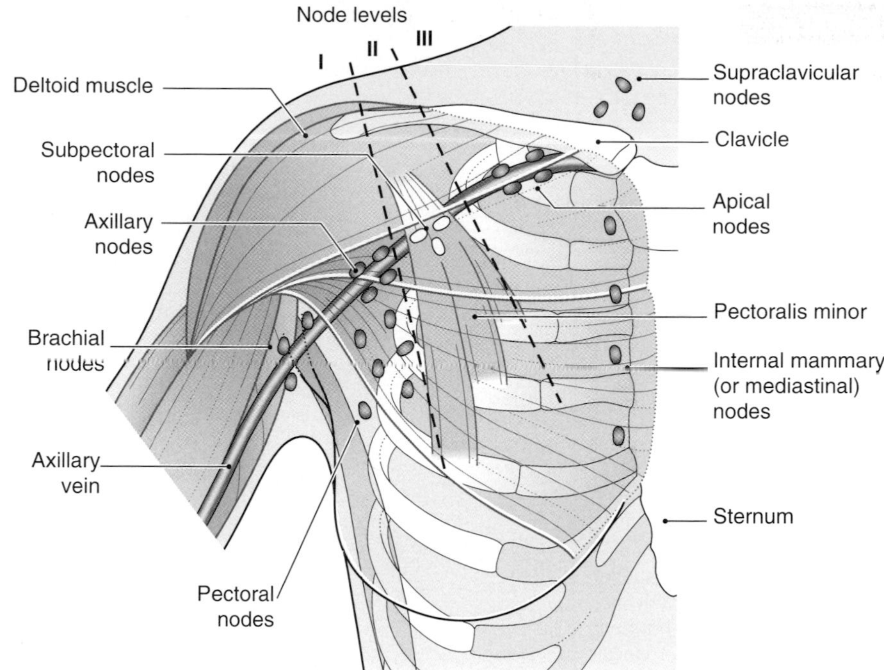

FIGURE 1.3

Location of draining lymph nodes to the breast.

the corpus luteum begins to degenerate, the LH, FSH and progesterone levels decline, the woman has a period and the breasts become less glandular and less swollen (Fig. 1.4).

Pregnancy

If the ovum is fertilized and the woman becomes pregnant the placenta becomes a rich source of hormones. Prolactin and growth hormone cause the breasts to become engorged with blood and, encouraged by increasing levels of progesterone and oestrogen, the areolae darken. As the placenta enlarges it secretes increasing amounts of human placental lactogen, which works with oestrogen and progesterone to stimulate the hypothalamus to release prolactin-releasing hormone (PRH). This then stimulates the anterior pituitary gland to release more prolactin. The breast is capable of producing milk by the second trimester but actual lactation is not initiated until after delivery. Pregnancy can result in doubling of the breast size but it is worth remembering that the size of the breast does not alter its ability to produce milk. Small breasts as well as large ones are just as capable of producing enough milk for the baby. Once the baby is born the breasts produce colostrum for 2 or 3 days before the true breast milk production begins. Colostrum, which is formed from the fifth month of pregnancy onwards, is a yellowish creamy fluid with a lower lactose content than milk and contains very little fat but more vitamin A, protein, and minerals. Colostrum is designed for the transition of the baby feeding from the umbilical cord to feeding from true breastmilk. Like breastmilk, colostrum is rich in IgA antibodies, which may protect the baby's gastrointestinal tract against bacteria and viruses, although it is doubtful that it provides passive immunity for the baby as was once thought (Sweet 1988, Marieb 1989, Hilton & Messenger 1997).

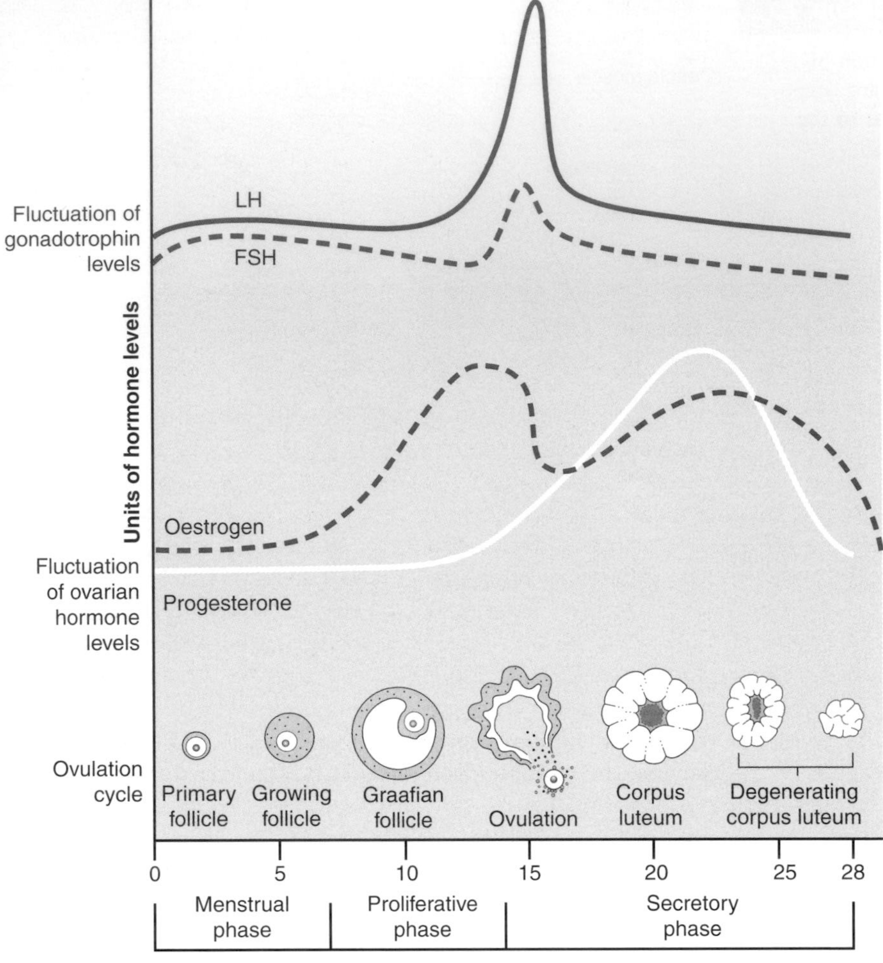

FIGURE 1.4

The monthly hormonal fluctuations.

Colostrum is produced for about 10 days after the birth and begins to mix with true milk after about 3 days. It may seem that the true milk is not as rich as colostrum as the consistency of mature breastmilk is thinner, but this is not the case. Breastmilk consists of lactose, casein and α-lactalbumin. Breastmilk is changed by the mother's diet and health; any medication that the mother needs should only be taken after checking with her GP (De Vane 1996).

Why breast feed?

There is always a great debate about whether breastmilk is best for the baby and the health-care professional will often be asked for their advice on this subject. Following is a comparison of breastmilk with formula feeds and cows' milk:

Thirst quenching

Breastmilk contains large amounts of water, which satisfies babies' thirst, and babies who are breastfed should not need extra drinks as long as they are getting adequate milk from the mother. The water content in formula feeds does not change to suit the baby so bottlefed babies need extra drinks of boiled water, either from a bottle or a sterilised spoon (Hilton & Messenger 1997).

Nourishment

It seems that breastmilk is more nourishing for the baby than other types of milk. The baby's needs are met with breastmilk as they are provided for in two varieties in the one feed: foremilk that has fewer calories and satisfies thirst, and hindmilk, which is richer in calories and satisfies the baby's hunger. Breastmilk should provide enough protein for body growth and in a form that is readily absorbed by the baby's digestive system. Colostrum and early milk have higher levels of protein than later breastmilk and cows' milk. The protein is quickly digested and is vital for a baby's growth. By comparison protein levels in cows' milk are three times higher than in breastmilk, are of a different type and are less digestible. Giving this 'foreign' protein to some babies may cause allergic reactions. The protein level is diluted to acceptable levels in formula feeds, but this will lower the calorie content of the feed (Hilton & Messenger 1997).

Breastmilk contains more fat for energy and growth than cows' milk and is more easily absorbed by the baby. Babies who are breastfed produce different stools (loose, without smell and yellow in colour) than when fed with cows' milk. The baby is not excreting any wasted fats and there is a higher concentration of essential fatty acids in breastmilk compared to cows' milk (Hilton & Messenger 1997).

Carbohydrate, in the form of lactose, is an important source of energy. Breastmilk contains more carbohydrates than cows' milk and vitamins and minerals in the right amounts for a baby's health and development. Vitamins and minerals are present in cows' milk; in fact there are two or three times as much sodium, potassium, calcium and chloride than the baby needs (Hilton & Messenger 1997).

Cows' milk contains everything for a healthy calf but it has to be changed in several ways before it can safely be given to babies under 6 months old and this also applies to goats' milk and sheep's milk.

Advantages and disadvantages of breastfeeding

Breastfeeding can be very emotionally satisfying for the mother and baby and most midwives and obstetricians recommend that mothers breastfeed their babies. Clearly, breastmilk is far more convenient for the mother to provide for night feeds, saves money and can help the mother to return to shape quickly (breastfeeding uses about 500 extra calories per day). The debate seems to favour breastfeeding if the mother can manage it, but for many reasons breastfeeding may not be possible, such as in the case of serious illness or because the child is handicapped in some way. There are good formula alternatives to breastfeeding and the closeness which develops between a mother and her child with breastfeeding can be recreated when a baby is bottlefed. It is important that a mother is not forced to breastfeed if she does not want to or cannot do it. Some mothers do not want to be tied to the baby and want to get their bodies back to being their own as soon as possible. Some babies do not feed well or the mother cannot produce enough milk and the baby may start to lose weight. In this eventuality it is far better that babies are given a set amount of food that can be easily measured with bottlefeeding. Whether the mother chooses to breastfeed or bottlefeed it is important that she is supported in this decision and not made to feel guilty. Providing she has been given all the information about breastfeeding and bottlefeeding the best decision must be the one that makes her a happier and more relaxed mother (Hilton & Messenger 1997).

How does a mother breastfeed?

Once the baby has been born the levels of prolactin diminish and continual milk production relies on the baby sucking at the mother's nipples. Nerve receptors in the nipple send afferent nerve impulses to the hypothalamus, stimulating secretion of PRH. This causes prolactin to be released, which stimulates milk production for the next feed. The same process causes the hypothalamus to release oxytocin, which controls the ejection of the milk from the nipples. Oxytocin stimulates the myoepithelial cells surrounding the breast glands causing milk ejection from both the breasts. The uterus is also targeted by oxytocin causing it to contract to almost its pre-pregnant state following delivery (Sweet 1988, Hilton & Messenger 1997) (see Fig. 1.5).

When breastfeeding stops, the stimulus for prolactin release ends and the milk production stops. When the prolactin levels during breastfeeding are high, the hypothalamic control of the ovaries is not efficient and ovulation does not generally occur. This inhibition of ovarian function was thought to provide natural birth control, although this is not always the case and after a time, most women will start to ovulate even while continuing to breastfeed their babies (Marieb 1989).

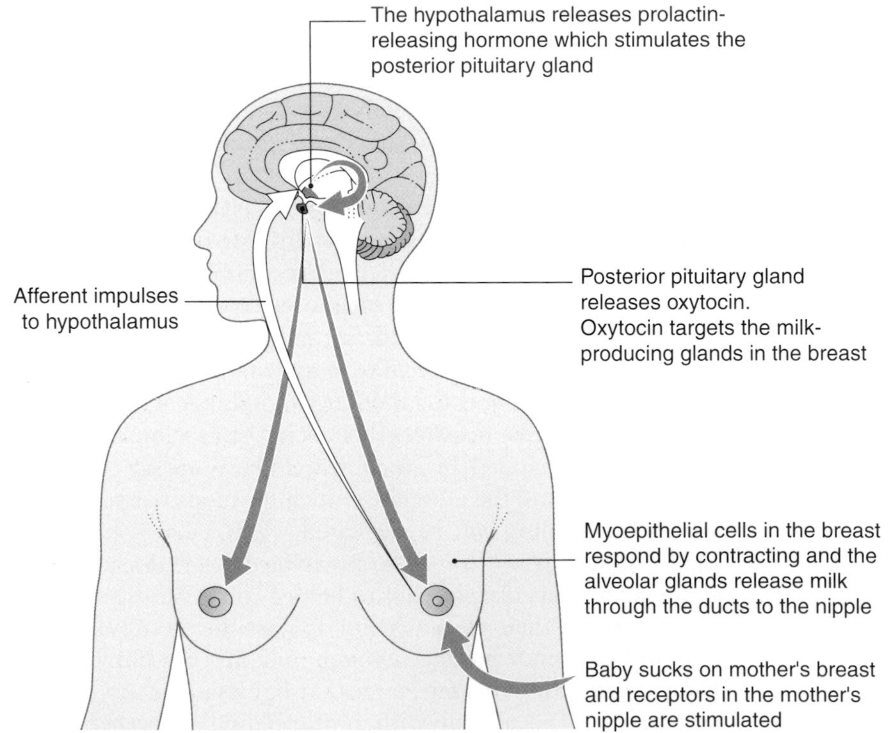

FIGURE 1.5

The physiological influences on milk production and ejection. The positive mechanism of the milk let-down reflex. This continues until the baby stops sucking.

Breastfeeding problems

Sore nipples

The mother can develop sore nipples when she is breastfeeding for a number of different reasons. The baby may be sucking on the nipple instead of the surrounding areolae, or may be removed from the nipple before his suction has been released. The mother may be keeping wet breast pads next to the skin too long or she may be washing the nipples with harsh soaps or detergents. Cracked nipples can follow on from sore nipples and can be a source of infection. Using a nipple shield, a rubber cap that fits over the nipple with a hole to allow the milk through, can help to rest the nipple areolar complex and allow the skin to heal. Mothers should be made aware that sometimes the baby can become so used to the nipple shield that he may reject the healed nipples. Drying the nipples with a hair dryer set to cool rather than rubbing them with a towel can be useful (Hilton & Messenger 1997).

Mastitis

Sometimes whilst breastfeeding the milk ducts can become blocked, causing a tender lump in the breast and a fever in the mother. The baby should be encouraged to keep feeding from the affected breast and the blocked area massaged in the direction of the nipple. Hot or cold compresses can help. Sometimes, if the milk leaks from the milk duct into the surrounding breast tissue the resulting fever and swelling is called 'mastitis'. The treatment for this condition is the same as for blocked milk ducts mentioned above. Infective mastitis can be caused by a germ in the baby's nose and is more serious. The doctor will prescribe antibiotics that are suitable for a breastfeeding mother and the mother may be advised to stop feeding from the infected breast until the infection has cleared, or may be advised to start antibiotics and restart breastfeeding after 24 hours (Dixon 1995). Any painful swelling of the breasts should be reported to the midwife or GP (Hilton & Messenger 1997). For more details on breast infections see Chapter 2.

The menopause

To understand how the menopause affects the breast it is necessary to understand the hormonal influences that occur around the time of the menopause.

In nulliparous women breast involution, or the change from fibrous tissue to fat, begins when the woman is in her 30s. When a woman reaches her 30s ovulation may not occur every 28 days causing her oestrogen levels to fall. As a result the negative feedback system of the pituitary and hypothalamus glands produce more and more FSH in an attempt to stimulate ovarian function. When oestrogen levels fall below a particular level, bleeding stops altogether, and the menopause occurs.

Around the time of the menopause the breasts are affected by the fluctuating hormones. They can become tender and the skin of the breast can become drier and less elastic than before. As the breast stroma is replaced by fat, the breast becomes less dense, softer and ptotic (droopy). This makes the breast much easier to visualise on mammogram, although these changes in a woman's body image can become another external sign that she is getting older.

A woman's breasts change throughout her lifetime and are intimately involved with important life events, such as puberty, childbirth and the menopause. It is no surprise that they are a central part of what it means to be a woman. The following section discusses how a woman may care for her breasts in a more informed way and will enable her to detect any changes and abnormalities in her breast. As nurses we are often asked about general health care, and giving good, clear advice about breast care is an important aspect of this information giving.

BREAST CARE

After reading this section the reader should understand and be able to give advice on:
- The importance of a well-fitted bra
- The importance of good breast and skin care
- The importance of, and the controversy surrounding, breast awareness
- How, when and who should carry out breast examination
- What breast changes to look and feel for.

Breasts consist of fatty and glandular tissue. They are supported by ligaments and large muscles attached to the chest wall. It is important that these muscles and ligaments don't become overstretched, which could cause drooping, or ptosis, of the breasts. One of the best ways to support the breasts is by wearing a well-fitted bra and caring for the skin of each breast.

Brassières

Fashion changes all the time and the ideal shape and size of women's bodies, particularly the breasts, have changed with it. Material used to support the breasts has been worn since the time of the ancient Egyptians at around 3000 BC, when clothing was a status symbol – the higher the rank the more elaborate the clothing. During the 1920s the minimiser bra became very popular. Designed to flatten the breasts and promote the asexual look, this bra was an essential addition to a modern flapper girl's wardrobe. By contrast, in the 1960s at a time of sexual revolution, many women wore no bras at all. Recently, the Wonderbra has been all the rage, promoting a fuller shape, a deep cleavage and sexual attraction. This particular shape was also very popular in the 18th century, when low-cut dresses made a woman's décolletage an essential part of her appearance.

It is important that a bra fits well. Any woman can be measured for a bra at most large department stores and leaflets are also available that explain how to measure for a bra fitting (Fig. 1.6).

It must be remembered that the figures gained by self-measurement are only a guide and the choice of bra should always be tried on. There are many different makes and styles of bra and this can vary the size. When the bra is tried on, normal movements, i.e. bending and stretching, should be carried out to ensure that the bra is comfortable and that it doesn't cut in or ride up.

FIGURE 1.6

How to measure a woman for a bra.

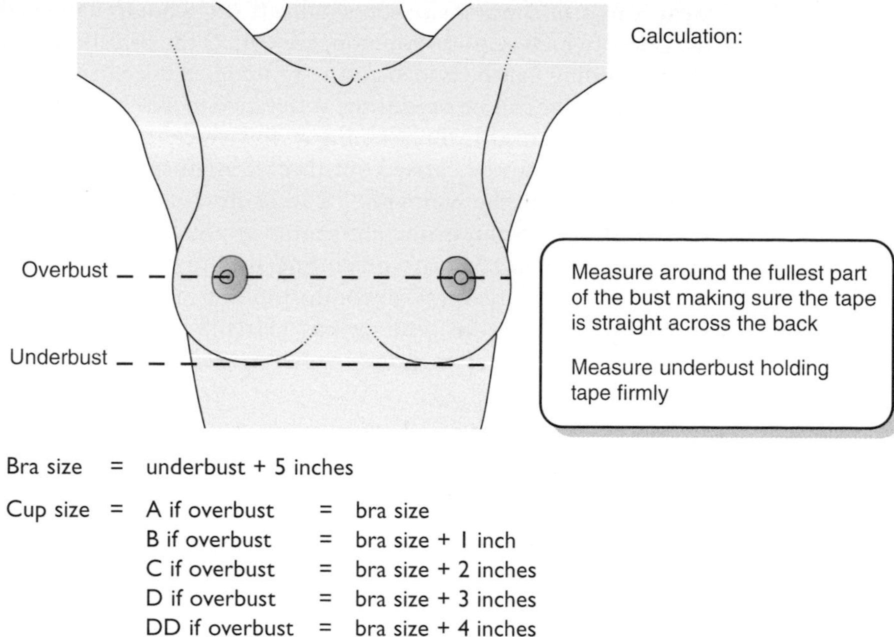

Types of bra and when they should be worn

Underwire bras

It is vitally important that an underwire bra fits correctly; if this is not the case the wires can dig into the breast causing breast pain and bruising. Some of the more expensive underwire bras have softer, more flexible wires, which can be more comfortable and not so harsh on the breast tissue or the ribs. It is inadvisable to wear an underwire bra when pregnant, breast feeding or if there has been recent breast surgery – particularly a mastectomy, as the wires of the bra can cut into the delicate healing tissue. There are instances when, after breast surgery, an underwired bra is requested by the breast surgeon as after care.

Sports bras

When carrying out exercise it is important to have a bra that supports the woman's breasts adequately according to the sport undertaken. High impact sports such as running or aerobics need a bra with more support than a low-impact sport, i.e. walking. Inadequate support can lead to the muscles and ligaments becoming stretched and breast pain. Advice about the sport bras available can be obtained from sports shops and good department stores.

Uncomfortable breasts

Most of us have experienced uncomfortable breasts at some time in our lives. One of the most common reasons for breast discomfort is a badly fitting bra. It is vital to have a bra that fits correctly and doesn't cut in (a woman wouldn't wear a pair of shoes a size too small). If the woman has one breast larger than the other (which is quite common, see Ch. 2) the bra should fit the larger breast. Light padding can be added to the bra cup of the smaller breast and there are prostheses that can be used if the difference in size is obvious and the woman is very conscious of this. Breast surgery to reduce the larger breast or increase the smaller breast can be carried out (breast augmentation) but this should be discussed, first with the woman's GP and subsequently, with a breast surgeon (see Ch. 4). If the woman is uncomfortable at night, a light support cropped top or bra may also help. Many women find that just before and during a period the breasts become larger and uncomfortable. It may be worthwhile to wear a bra specifically to fit at this time such as a stretch bra or a sports bra. More extreme breast pain is covered in detail in Chapter 2.

When to get fitted for a bra

A woman should get fitted for a bra:

- When she has had a gain or loss in weight
- Every year (as bras lose their elasticity)
- If she is pregnant or breastfeeding
- If she is experiencing breast pain
- If she undertakes regular exercise
- After recent breast surgery.

By carrying out good breast care and ensuring adequate support, many common problems can be prevented.

Skin care

The breasts and the surrounding skin should be washed and dried thoroughly, especially underneath the breasts, in the inframammary folds. The Europeans have always been interested in the care of their breasts, rubbing in breast-firming creams and using bracing jets of cold water that is believed to firm up the breast tissue. British women are joining their European counterparts and increasing numbers are using the latest breast cosmetics. There are many special bust-firming products available, which are supposed to maintain the tone and the elasticity of the skin. Some of these cosmetics contain essential oils to firm up the skin of the breasts. These products are not cheap and it is worth shopping around to find a product to suit the individual's needs. Exfoliating the skin with gentle products meant for the face and dousing the breasts with cold water from the shower can also help the circulation, and tighten the skin, and can work out a little less expensive.

Common problems of the breast

Intertrigo

Intertrigo is a rash that can form in the inframammary folds underneath the breasts. It is normally caused by not drying the folds underneath the breasts properly or due to excessive perspiration. This condition is quite common in women with large breasts. The area under the breast should always be dried thoroughly by patting dry after a bath or shower. The woman should be encouraged to wear a cotton bra and *no* talcum powder should be used on the area until the rash has cleared. Hydrocortisone cream, which is now available at chemists without prescription, can be applied to the area. If the rash continues it may be caused by a fungal infection, usually candida. This can be treated with antifungal creams which are also available at the chemist without prescription. Any persistent rash that does not respond to these treatments should be reported to the GP.

Inverted nipples

When the nipple turns inwards rather than standing erect when stimulated by touch or a change in temperature the nipples are said to be inverted. Inverted nipples are normal if they have been present since the breasts developed and can be bilateral or unilateral. They should be kept clean with a cotton wool bud. If there are any changes in the inversion, or if the nipple becomes newly inverted, the woman's GP must be informed.

Unwanted hair

Many women, as they get older, can develop hairs around their nipples. Hair can be removed from the areola by tweezers or by electrolysis. It is better not to use depilatory creams or to shave the hair as the nipple area is very sensitive and can become infected.

Spots

Spots on or around the breast or around the nipple should not be squeezed as this can cause infection or may lead to a breast abscess. If the spot is enlarging then the woman should seek advice from her GP.

Sun care advice

Sunbathing can cause skin damage and increase the risk of developing skin cancer. The skin on the breast is very sensitive and should never be allowed to burn, especially if sunbathing topless. The best advice is that the woman should not sunbathe topless but if she really wants to high factor sun creams (factor 15 or above) should be used, particularly on the nipple area.

Moles

Check moles regularly for any changes. If the mole becomes bigger, browner or it bleeds advice should be sought from the GP. If a mole is in an awkward position such as under a bra strap then it can be removed by a simple surgical procedure.

BREAST AWARENESS

For many years there has been much controversy about the issues of breast self-examination and breast awareness. There are differing opinions as to whether breast self-examination is useful or safe in detecting any changes in the breast. It has been said that self-examination causes anxiety, gives women a false sense of security and doesn't change the course of the disease. Alternatively, it is worth noting that 90% of breast cancers are found by women themselves (DOH 1998) and if women present earlier with smaller tumours, hopefully, less invasive, more effective treatment can be given. A woman who examines her breasts regularly is more likely to notice any changes. It also allows an individual to participate in her own health care and to have more control over her body and her life.

The controversy about breast self-examination has caused much confusion for women and health professionals but the current advice to women is to be 'breast aware'. When comparing breast self-examination and breast awareness there are only subtle differences and both are similar in approach.

What is breast awareness?

Breast awareness is an important activity that woman can carry out themselves in order to maintain their wellbeing. Breast awareness is all about getting to know how the breasts look and feel and what is normal at different times of the month.

The nurse's role is to educate and to facilitate breast awareness and to provide support. It can be helpful to give the woman some information about the basic anatomy of the breast so they can become aware of changes in their breasts at different times of their menstrual cycle. When women become familiar with how their breasts normally look and feel, it becomes easier for them to detect any changes.

It is estimated that nine out of 10 lumps or changes are harmless. However, any changes in the breast appearance or texture detected by the woman should be checked by the woman's GP.

Who should be breast aware?

Every woman, from puberty onwards should become breast aware. Women with very lumpy breasts may find this difficult but they should try to become familiar with any area of lumpiness and report any changes to their GP.

When should you be breast aware?

There is no rigid time – it is up to the woman. Many women find that their breasts become tender and lumpy before a period and soften down afterwards, so it may be easier for the woman to examine her breasts just after a period has finished as this is an easy day to remember. For women who have had a hysterectomy or are postmenopausal they could examine their breasts on the first of each month, an easy date to remember. In pregnancy it is still important to carry out breast checks. There will be changes in the size, and texture of the breasts and some women find that both breasts become swollen, more vascular and tender. All of these changes are quite normal. However, if the woman is concerned about any of the changes she should speak to her GP or midwife.

How often should you check yourself?

There is no point examining the breasts more frequently than once each month as the subtle changes that may occur month to month will not be detected.

How should you carry out breast awareness?

There are two parts to breast awareness:

1. Looking
2. Feeling.

The woman should find a room that makes her feel comfortable and that is also well lit. Some women find that a good time to feel and look at their breasts is in the bathroom when preparing for a bath or a shower (Fig. 1.7).

Looking

Women should stand in front of the mirror and look at their breasts in the following positions:

- With their arms relaxed at their sides, checking the breasts from the front then turning to the left and the right checking the outer sides of each breast
- With their arms extended over their head, checking the front and also checking the outer sides of the breasts
- Then with their hands on their hips and pressing their shoulders and elbows forward, until the chest muscle tightens, look again, turning left and right as before.

By changing the shape of the breasts, abnormalities can be detected in one position rather than another.

What are you looking for?

- An increase or decrease in size (it is very common to have one breast larger than the other)
- Changes in the outline and shape of the breast, causing flattening of the skin
- Dimpling, creasing or puckering of the skin
- A change in direction of the nipple or if it has started to draw in (don't worry about nipples which have always been drawn in)
- Nipple discharge (some women produce a clear or milky discharge that is normal for them)
- New veins which stand out, particularly on one breast and not the other (prominent veins in pregnancy and whilst breastfeeding are very normal)
- Any skin changes on the breast or nipple.

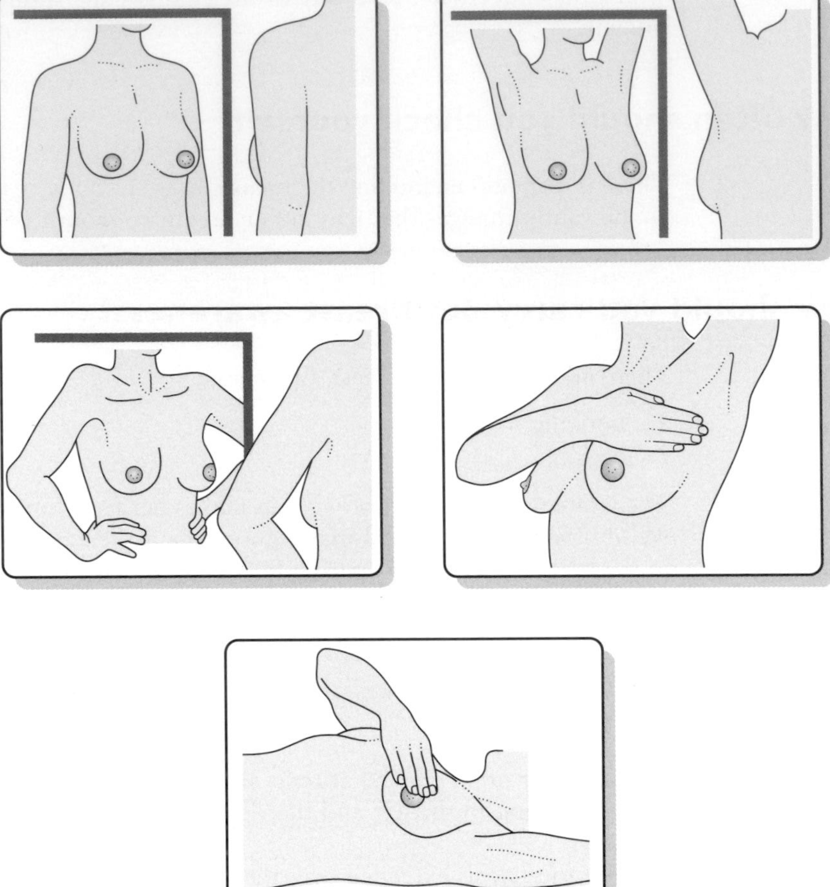

FIGURE 1.7

Breast self-examination.

Feeling

Women can check their breasts while in the bath or shower or when lying on the bed. A soapy hand or one sprinkled with talc or moisturiser will move over the breast easily. A good way to do this is to:

- raise the right arm above the head. With the left hand carefully examine the right breast using the flat part of the fingers – not the finger tips
- cover the whole breast starting from under the armpit, using gentle but firm pressure, examine the breast in ever-decreasing circles to the nipple
- finally push down gently on and around the nipple using one finger.

It is important to make sure that no areas are missed. The whole process should be repeated on the left breast. Women with larger breasts may find it easier to examine the breasts when lying down.

What are you feeling for?

- Any areas of thickening
- Any lumps whatever their shape or form

- Any nodular areas
- New or persistent pain or tenderness within the breast.

Any new changes in the breast or armpit must be checked by the GP.

CASE STUDY 1

Tracey Field, 37, isn't breast aware. Her husband noticed a lumpy area above her left nipple. She went to her GP, who examined her and decided to send her to a breast diagnostic unit for a second opinion. A history was taken and it was noted that her period had finished days ago and she was also taking the oral contraceptive pill, Marvelon. On examination she was found to have general tenderness and lumpiness in both breasts. No suspicious areas or discrete lumps were palpated. A departmental ultrasound was carried out and no abnormalities were seen. She was taught breast awareness and given an information leaflet reinforcing this information before she was discharged.

Breast awareness is an important activity that women can carry out themselves in order to maintain their health and wellbeing. For one reason or another many women are not breast aware. Common reasons for this include: (1) fear – not wanting to find a lump, (2) not being taught how, (3) not having enough time and (4) lack of confidence in their technique. All these can prevent a woman being aware of what is normal for her breasts. With effective health education, teaching and support programme these factors could be alleviated for many women. In the author's opinion this education could be started when young women start to wear bras. Breast awareness could be easily incorporated into adult sex education lectures at school and, if started early, breast awareness doesn't become a frightening experience; it simply becomes a part of a young woman's normal routine.

Guidance about breast awareness should be given by practice nurses, health visitors, well woman clinics and GPs. Leaflets are very useful in teaching breast self-examination, but are not as effective as demonstrative teaching. Leaflets and videos can be obtained from several sources (see section on useful addresses, Ch. 7).

New guidelines on the clinical examination of breasts

In February 1998 the chief medical and nursing officers on behalf of the Department of Health published a paper on clinical examination of the breast. The paper stated that 'the palpation of the breast by either medical or nursing staff should *not* be included as part of routine health screening for women. Examination of the breast in symptomatic women should only be carried out by nurses with specialist training, who include palpation as a significant part of their role and who work within an environment providing immediate onsite access to the full range of facilities necessary for breast cancer diagnosis.' (DOH 1998). The Royal College of Nursing also states that the nurse's role is to educate and facilitate breast awareness, not to diagnose whether a woman has breast cancer or not (RCN 1995). Therefore, breast awareness should be encouraged in women but clinical examination of the breast should not be carried out by health-care professionals in primary care settings.

CONCLUSION

Many women are unsure of their bodies and are ignorant of the changes that occur to their breasts both monthly and over their lifetime. It is only with better health education and increased breast awareness that women will know what is normal and what is abnormal for them and when to see their GP for further advice. There are conditions of the breast that need some form of intervention and the next chapter deals with the abnormalities of the breast in greater detail and the treatments that can be offered.

REFERENCES

Blackwell R E 1996 Breast anatomy, physiology, screening, and self assessment. In: Blackwell R E, Grotting J C (eds) Diagnosis and Management of Breast Disease. Blackwell Science, Cambridge, MA, USA, ch 1, p 5–19

De Vane G W 1996 Breast dysfunction: galactorrhea and mastalgia. In: Blackwell R E, Grotting J C (eds) Diagnosis and Management of Breast Disease. Blackwell Science, Cambridge, MA, USA, ch 2, p 19–77

Department of Health (DOH) 1998 Clinical Examination of the Breast. DOH, Leeds

Dixon J M 1995 Breast infection. In: Dixon J M (ed) ABC of Breast Diseases. BMJ Publishing Group, London, ch 4, p 14–18

Dixon J M, Mansel R E 1995 Congenital problems and aberrations of normal breast development and involution. In: Dixon J M (ed) ABC of Breast Diseases. BMJ Publishing Group, London, ch 2, p 6–11

Hilton T, Messenger M 1997 The Great Ormond Street New Baby and Child Care Book. The essential guide for parents of children aged 0–5. Vermilion, London

Last R J 1978 Anatomy: regional and applied, 6th edn. Churchill Livingstone, London

Marieb E N 1989 Human Anatomy and Physiology. Benjamin Cummings Publishing Company Inc., California, USA

Morris D 1978 Manwatching: A field guide to human behaviour. Triad/Panther Books, St Albans

Reshef E, Sanfilippo J S, Levine N 1996 Breast dysfunction: congenital anomalies of the breast. In: Blackwell R E, Grotting J C (eds) Diagnosis and Management of Breast Disease. Blackwell Science, Cambridge, MA, USA ch 3, 77–93

Royal College of Nursing 1995 Breast Palpation and Breast Awareness: Guidelines For Practice. Issues in Nursing and Health, 35 RCN, London

Sweet B R 1988 Mayes' Midwifery. A Textbook for Midwives, 11th edn. Baillière Tindall, London

FURTHER READING

Blackwell R E, Grotting J C (eds) 1996 Diagnosis and Management of Breast Disease. Blackwell Science, Cambridge, MA USA

Dixon J M (ed) 1995 ABC of Breast Diseases. BMJ Publishing Group, London

2 Benign Disorders of the Breast

Nikki Burch and Karen Burnet

After reading this chapter the reader should be able to:

- Recognise some of the developmental problems of the breast
- Have an understanding of the variety of different benign breast diseases
- Be able to give advice about breast pain and breast infections
- Know the basic nursing care of the more common benign breast problems.

INTRODUCTION

The breast is affected by different hormonal influences throughout a woman's lifetime. Breast tissue develops at puberty and is altered by the menstrual cycle, pregnancy and ageing. Most benign problems of the breast occur during one of these episodes and are so common that they can be termed as 'aberrations of the breast' rather than breast disease (Hughes 1992, Dixon & Mansel 1995).

At some time most women will visit their GP with a breast problem. Some develop a lump or a lumpy area in their breast, and others have symptoms including breast pain, nipple retraction or discharge. Other breast disorders can be congenital or a result of later abnormal development. It is estimated that around 80% of breast lumps are benign (Baum & Schipper 1999); this chapter has been written so that the reader may better understand the range of non-malignant conditions of the breast and recognise that a problem of the breast does not always indicate malignant disease.

ABERRATIONS OF BREAST DEVELOPMENT

Polythelia

About 1% of men and 5% of women are born with one or more extra nipples (polythelia). These extra nipples usually develop whilst the fetus is in the womb and the most common site for them is just below the normal breast, along the milk line or the ectodermal ridge. Extra breasts (polymastia) can also develop and often occur in the lower axilla. Extra nipples are usually unilateral and should not be treated surgically unless they are unsightly or are embarrassing to the patient. Accessory breast tissue can develop the same problems as the normal breast and needs to be cared for in the same way

FIGURE 2.1

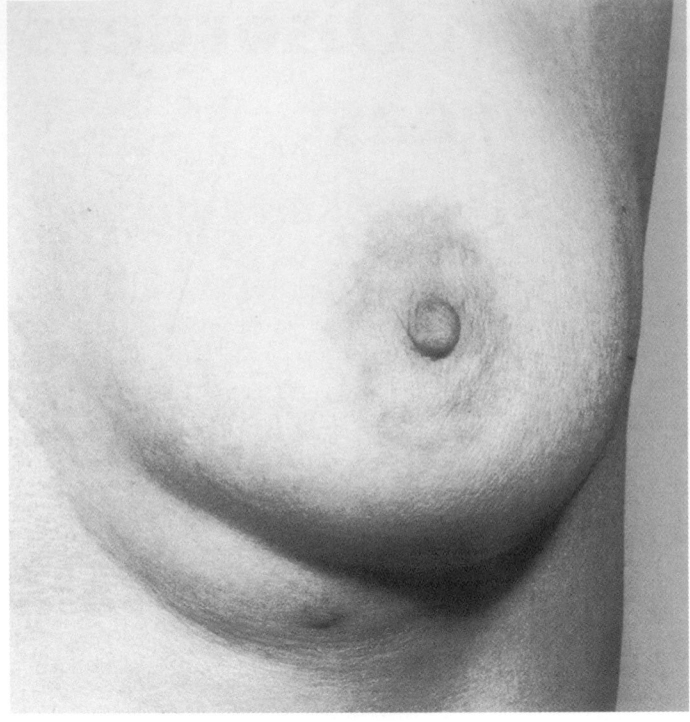

An accessory nipple. Reproduced with kind permission from the Royal Marsden Hospital Photographic Department and Breast Diagnostic Unit.

(Dixon & Mansel 1995, Reshef et al 1996). Figure 2.1 is a photograph of an accessory nipple.

Gynaecomastia

Growth of breast tissue in males (gynaecomastia) is benign and, for most men, is usually reversible. It can be extremely embarrassing for young and old men alike because of the obvious association with femininity. Senescent gynaecomastia affects men between 50 and 80 years of age and is not usually associated with a detectable hormonal imbalance. The usual form of gynaecomastia is seen in 30–60% of boys aged 10–16 years and is often associated with a hormonal imbalance that reverses with no treatment (Dixon & Mansel 1995).

The cause of gynaecomastia should be investigated in every individual. Causes can include conditions that promote the production of oestrogen or the under production of testosterone such as puberty, cirrhosis of the liver, malnutrition, primary hypogonadism, testicular tumours, secondary hypogonadism, hyperthyroidism and renal disease, e.g. in Klinefelter's syndrome. Gynaecomastia can also be drug related with cimetidine, digoxin, spironolactone, and any androgens or anti-oestrogens being the most likely causes. Some body builders who take anabolic steroids have developed breasts, but have reversed this effect by taking the anti-oestrogen drug tamoxifen. If gynaecomastia is caused by drugs then withdrawal of the treatment or changing to an alternative treatment is recommended. Hormone levels should be measured if no clear cause is found; a mammogram may differentiate between breast enlargement due to fat or true gynaecomastia, and will help confirm the diagnosis if a malignancy is suspected.

A biopsy or fine-needle aspiration should be performed if there is any suspicion of breast cancer (Dixon & Mansel 1995). Where gynaecomastia is due to the oversecretion of oestrogen, the drug danazol can produce a symptomatic improvement in some patients by inhibiting the pituitary gonadotrophins (Dixon & Mansel 1995). Surgery is not usually recommended for gynaecomastia if medical interventions do not improve the condition, unless the patient is embarrassed or the breasts continue to enlarge.

Nursing care

Breasts are considered to be a female characteristic and the overdevelopment of breast tissue in a man may cause a profound altered body image and emotional distress. Some men who develop gynaecomastia believe they are losing their masculinity and may experience anxiety and depression as a result. Gynaecomastia may be particularly hard to bear in the young or adolescent male at a time when they are trying to define their sexuality. These emotions should be explored by the nurse and a clear explanation of why the breast tissue has developed and the action and side-effects of any treatment given is essential. More formalised psychological support should be offered if appropriate.

Breast asymmetry

Most women have some breast asymmetry with the left breast often larger than the right. However, some women develop only one breast (amastia) or have an underdeveloped (hypoplastic) breast, sometimes with one or both nipples missing. Occasionally women are born with Poland's syndrome, a congenital abnormality of the pectoral muscles, associated with an absence or hypoplasia of the breast, an upper limb defect and chest wall anomalies. In this condition usually only one of the breasts is missing. Amastia may be caused by insufficient production of oestrogen, which can occur in such diseases as Turner's or Kalman's syndrome. Abnormalities of the chest wall, such as pectus excavatum, and defects of the thoracic spine can also make the breasts seem asymmetrical (Dixon & Mansel 1995, Reshef et al 1996).

Juvenile or virginal hypertrophy

Pre-pubertal breast enlargement occurs quite often and only requires further investigation and treatment if it is associated with other signs of sexual maturation such as premature menstruation. Unchecked growth of the breasts occurs in adolescent girls whose breasts develop normally and then continue to grow. Referral to a surgical outpatient clinic is appropriate, although the routine investigations that are carried out often reveal no endocrine or other abnormality. These women can suffer discomfort, sometimes pain, and often find the enlarged breasts prevent them from living a normal life because of social embarrassment. Surgical intervention such as a reduction mammoplasty can considerably improve their quality of life and, although not always readily available, can be asked for by the woman (Dixon & Mansel 1995, Reshef et al 1996). Figure 2.2 is a photograph of a patient with juvenile hypertrophy.

FIGURE 2.2

Juvenile hypertrophy. Reproduced with kind permission from Dixon J M and Mansel R E, 1995 ABC of Breast Diseases, BMJ Publishing Group.

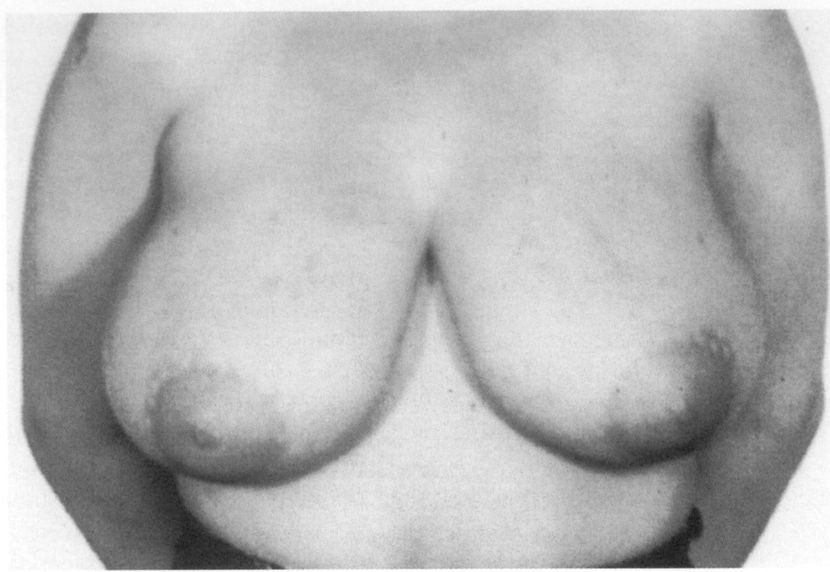

Nursing care

Breast asymmetry can be treated with augmentation of the smaller breast, a reduction or elevation of the larger breast, or a combination of the two procedures. Treatment for Poland's syndrome would include the surgical repair of the chest and shoulder abnormalities. Breast augmentation or reduction should be undertaken very carefully, ensuring that the eventual contour and size of the contralateral breast has been taken into account. The woman must be properly prepared for such an operation as her body image will be altered by the surgery and she will have some scarring. The introduction of the tissue expander prosthesis has helped the plastic surgeon achieve a more satisfactory shape in the augmented breast (see Ch. 5 for more detail on breast augmentation and reconstruction).

For a woman who does not have the ideal feminine shape, the consideration of breast reduction or augmentation can be traumatic. The nursing staff have a responsibility to explore these feelings with the woman and to ensure that she understands what is involved with the surgery, where the scars will be (however discrete they may be) and what sort of rehabilitation she will need. Advice about a supportive bra and when to resume activities such as sports and lifting will be crucial to her recovery.

BENIGN BREAST DISEASE

A GP will see a large number of women with breast pain and lumpiness. It is worth remembering that many breast lumps are caused by benign conditions and not a malignancy, but a woman should report to her GP any new changes in either of her breasts. A recent study from the Sheffield Institute of General Practice and Primary Care showed that the mean number of consultations about breast problems per GP (n = 248) over a 4-week recording period was 2.05. At their first consultation, 40% of the women presented with a breast lump and 40% with breast pain. Of the women with breast lumps, 58% were referred for specialist care and after the first or subsequent evaluation, 17% of the women with breast pain were referred for specialist care. Women were most likely to be referred if they had a breast lump. The conclusion from this local study was that the GPs in the study refer about one-third of their patients with breast problems to secondary care (Newton et al 1999). When a woman presents with a breast problem, the GP has to decide whether or not the problem necessitates referral to a specialist breast clinic. They have to balance the risk of missing a possible breast cancer with an inappropriate referral of a woman with an easily treatable breast problem. Dixon and Mansel (1995), who have written a lot about benign breast conditions, have designed criteria that may guide the GPs in deciding which women with breast problems should be referred. These referral guidelines are:

- All patients with a discrete mass or a recently changed area of nodularity
- Nipple discharge in patients over 50 years of age and blood-stained nipple discharge in any patient
- Any recent change in the shape of the nipple, particularly retraction or eczema
- Mastalgia that interferes with a patient's lifestyle or sleep and that has not responded well to simple measures
- Ulcers in the breast
- Request for assessment by a patient with a strong family history of breast cancer
- Asymmetrical nodularity that persists after menstruation.

Benign breast disease can be grouped into several categories. The largest category includes a number of conditions that are as a result of anomalies of normal development and involution or ANDI (Saunders & Baum 1998).

ANOMALIES OF NORMAL DEVELOPMENT AND INVOLUTION

Fibrocystic disease

This is an ill-defined condition of the breast where palpable lumps can be felt and is usually associated with pain and tenderness that fluctuates with the menstrual cycle. Fibrocystic disease can define a variety of different conditions including chronic cystic mastitis, cystic disease, cystic hyperplasia and epithelial dysplasia. On histological examination lesions of fibrocystic disease are of epithelial origin. A woman's breasts are subjected to hormonal fluctuations and, in response to these fluctuations, the glandular breast tissue can develop areas of fibrosis, the formation of small or large cysts, and an increase in the number of glandular elements (adenosis). These aberrations are thought to be caused by the incomplete involution of breast tissue during each menstrual cycle, causing an increase in the number of cells lining the terminal duct lobular unit. These different causes of breast lumpiness are described in greater detail later.

Breast cysts

Breast cysts rarely occur before the woman is 35 years old and develop most frequently in peri-menopausal women. Cysts will usually disappear around the

FIGURE 2.3

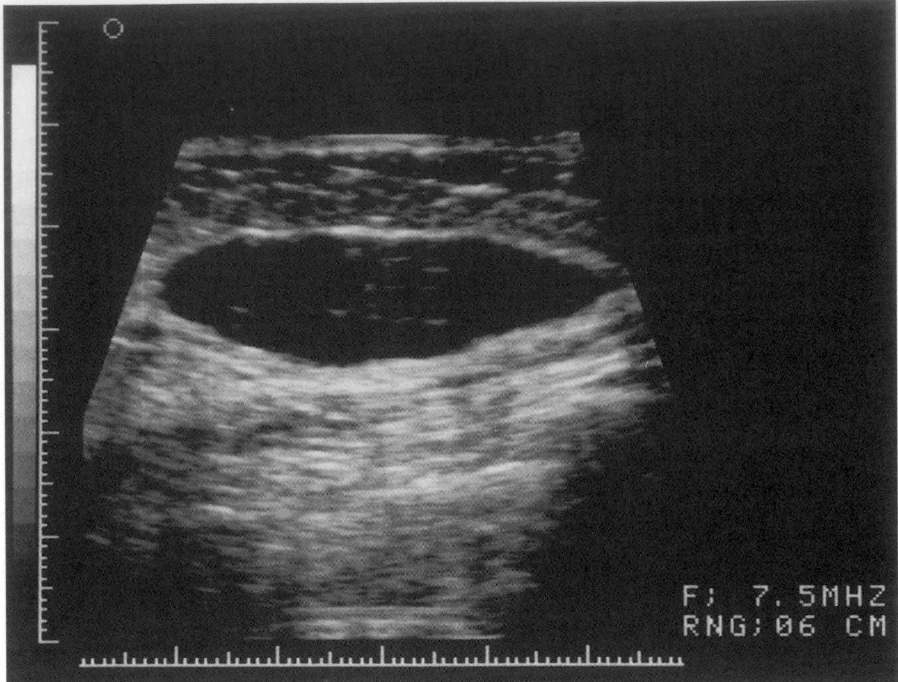

Cyst as seen on ultrasound. Reproduced with kind permission from Addenbrooke's NHS Trust Photography Department and Dr P Britten of The Addenbrooke's Breast Unit.

menopause unless the woman is taking hormone replacement therapy. Cystic disease affects around 7% of women in western countries, and cysts constitute around 15% of all breast masses. Patients who have many cysts may be at a slightly increased risk of developing breast cancer, although this risk is not thought to be significant (Dixon & Mansel 1995).

Cystic disease can present with pre-menstrual tenderness coinciding with an increased nodularity of the breast. The woman may have a smooth and discrete breast lump, which can be tender and fluctuant on clinical examination. When examined with ultrasound, cysts are shown to be fluid-filled, and when seen on a mammogram, have a characteristic luscent halo (Fig. 2.3).

Cysts may increase in size, stay the same size or sometimes disperse by themselves. Treatment can include monitoring the cyst's development by regular breast examination, and periodic mammography. Fluid can be aspirated from the cyst with a small-grade needle, sometimes under ultrasound control, but the fluid often re-accumulates. The withdrawn fluid can be grey, brown, clear, straw-coloured or a greenish colour. If the fluid is bloodstained, it should be sent for cytology as there is the small possibility that this may indicate malignancy. After aspiration of the cyst the breast should be clinically examined again to see if the palpable mass has disappeared. Rarely, a cyst can mask an underlying tumour and, if there is an underlying mass, then further cells should be acquired by fine needle aspiration and sent to cytology for analysis. Because there is often associated breast pain with these lesions, treatment is also directed at minimalising the pain (Dixon & Mansel 1995, Curling & Tierney 1997).

Nursing care

The monitoring of cystic disease may take place in a designated breast clinic under the supervision of a breast surgeon. This sort of problem is also suited to the care of the nurse practitioner or clinical nurse specialist who, if appropriately trained, can examine breasts and aspirate cysts under ultrasound control (Curling & Tierney 1997).

When caring for such women the nurse can take the opportunity to promote breast health by discussing breast screening and breast awareness. Cysts can fill very rapidly with fluid, frightening the woman and perhaps making her fearful that she has a cancer, so reassurance and explanation are essential. It may be appropriate to discuss how breast comfort can be enhanced by a correctly fitting bra. Women who have pre-menstrual breast discomfort associated with their cystic disease may find that reducing salt and saturated fats or omitting caffeine from their diet is helpful. Others find a course of evening primrose oil brings relief (Curling & Tierney 1997). For persistent cysts the breast surgeon may decide that surgical removal is the best solution. For more detail please refer to Chapter 5.

Epithelial hyperplasia

Hyperplasia is defined as an increased number of cells relative to the basement membrane of the terminal duct lobular unit. Breast hyperplasias range from mild hyperplasia, constituting three or more cells above the basement membrane, to moderate or florid hyperplasia with a larger number of cells above the basement membrane. Hyperplastic cells can show cellular atypia, called 'atypical hyperplasia' and this condition is associated with an absolute risk of carcinoma of 8% at 10 years but rises to 20–25% for a woman with a first-degree relative with breast cancer (Dixon & Mansel 1995, Baum & Schipper 1999). In this case regular screening may be advised. The woman may present with areas of diffuse nodularity or thickening of the breast tissue, which may contain single or multiple cysts. Commonly, it is bilateral, although it may occur in only one breast.

Adenosis

Adenosis occurs when there are increased numbers of acini (glands) within the lobular unit of the breast. There are several types of adenosis: sclerosing, radial scars and complex sclerosing lesions. These lesions can cause diagnostic problems when they are detected on screening as it is not clear whether they represent a cancer or not. Thought to be caused by a disturbance of the normal stromal involution, sclerosing adenosis is associated with a slightly increased risk of malignancy and does cause a marked disturbance of the normal breast cell architecture. On clinical examination large areas of sclerosing adenosis can resemble carcinoma, although it often feels more rubbery to the touch. Adenosis is more common in younger women, especially in their 30s and 40s, and is rarely seen after the menopause. Surgical excision is usually the only way to get a definitive diagnosis and to exclude a malignancy (Schindler 1993, Dixon & Mansel 1995, Blackwell 1996).

Duct ectasia

Duct ectasia occurs during the involution of the breast when the major subareolar ducts dilate and shorten. Although usually a disease of women nearing

FIGURE 2.4

Duct ectasia of the left breast. Reproduced with kind permission from Dixon J M and Mansel R E, 1995 ABC of Breast Diseases, BMJ Publishing Group.

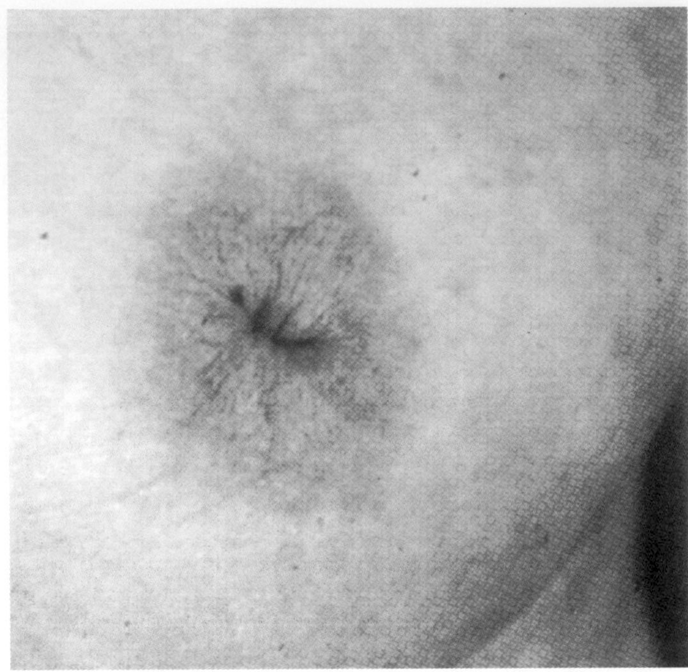

the menopause, it occasionally occurs in younger women (Schindler 1993). Duct ectasia presents as lumpiness in the breast tissue beneath the areola with or without nipple discharge. Normal breast secretions are retained behind these blocked ducts and the substance can become cheese-like in consistency. Nipple inversion and periductal inflammation will also be seen. Fissures and fistulas of the nipple may develop over time if the condition is not treated. Antibiotics and warm compresses applied to the affected area may help and surgery is indicated if the discharge becomes a problem (Schindler 1993, Curling & Tierney 1997). Figure 2.4 shows a duct ectasia of the left breast.

Fibroadenomas

Often termed as benign neoplasms, fibroadenomas are more accurately considered aberrations of normal growth and are composed of both structural (fibro) and glandular (adenoma) breast tissue (Haagensen 1983, Robbins et al, 1984, Schindler 1993). Under the same hormonal influences as the rest of the breast, a fibroadenoma grows as a centrifugal small nodule that is usually well circumscribed and freely movable from the surrounding breast tissue. They are very common, accounting for 13% of all palpable breast lesions, and in women aged 20 years or younger, they account for 60% of palpable breast lesions (Dixon & Mansel 1995).

Most fibroadenomas occur in the upper outer quadrant of the breast and can vary in size up to 10 cm. There are three types of fibroadenoma:

- Common
- Giant – measuring over 5 cm

- Juvenile – occurring in adolescent girls, can grow rapidly but are managed the same as usual fibroadenomas.

A definitive diagnosis of a fibroadenoma can be made using ultrasound, fine-needle aspiration (FNA) and clinical examination. Although fibroadenomas do not become malignant, they can enlarge with pregnancy and breastfeeding (Schindler 1993). In an older woman a fibroadenoma will shrink with age and can be clearly seen on mammogram as it calcifies. Fibroadenomas are usually surgically removed in women over 40 years of age but in women younger than 40 they are only removed if requested by the woman or there is some doubt as to their true diagnosis (Dixon & Mansel 1995). Figure 2.5 shows a fibroadenoma as seen on ultrasound and Figure 2.6 shows a calcified fibroadenoma.

CASE STUDY

Emma Green, 24, regularly attends a diagnostic unit. Her mother developed breast cancer at the age of 38 and her sister at 23. She has been breast aware for many years. Emma came for her yearly screening appointment with a 1-week history of a lump in her right upper outer quadrant, which she discovered by feeling her breasts just after her period. She was obviously very anxious. On examination a firm, regular, mobile 2 cm nodule was palpated. Because of her family history, a mammogram was carried out, which revealed no abnormalities. She was sent for an ultrasound, which revealed a 1.8 cm solid, regular nodular mass in the right upper outer quadrant of her breast, with the characteristics of a fibroadenoma. Aspiration cytology was performed on the lump. The cytology report was C2 and a diagnosis of a fibroadenoma was made, to everyone's relief. A 3-month follow-up appointment was made to re-check the size of the fibroadenoma. If, at that appointment, the fibroadenoma was found to be bigger and was troubling Emma, it could be removed surgically.

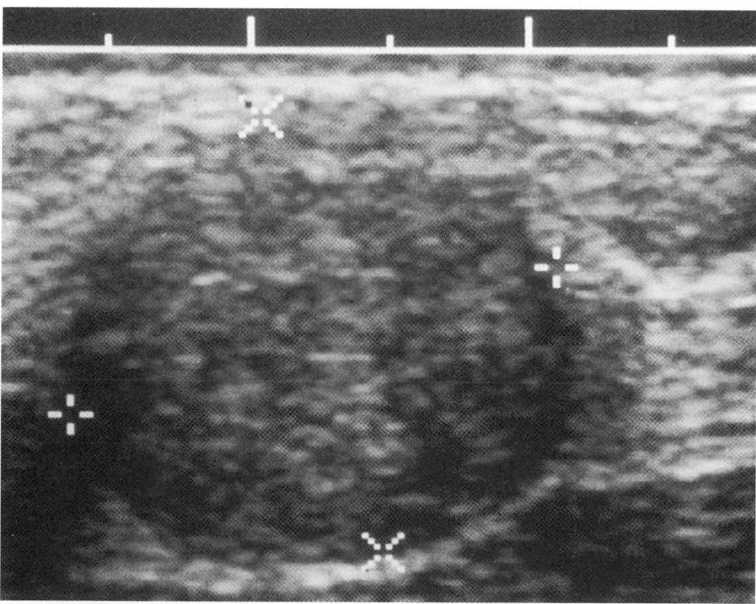

FIGURE 2.5

Fibroadenoma as seen on ultrasound. Note the well circumscribed edge of the lesion. Published with kind permission of the Royal Marsden Hospital Photographic Department and Breast Diagnostic Unit.

FIGURE 2.6

A calcified fibroadenoma as seen on ultrasound. Published with kind permission of the Royal Marsden Hospital Photographic Department and Breast Diagnostic Unit.

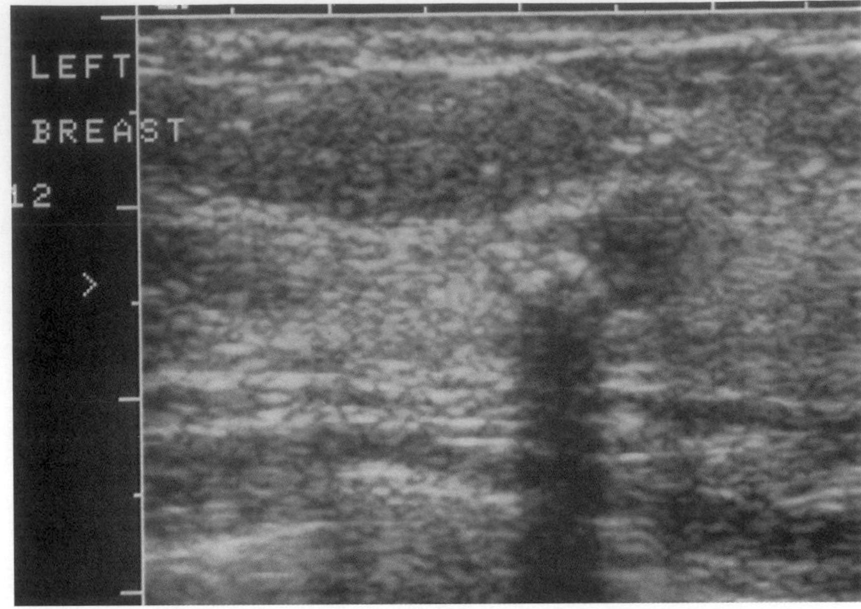

Phyllodes tumours

These lesions are most common in middle-age women and present as painless masses, ranging from 1 cm to occupying the whole of the breast. They can be cystic or lobulated and are identified by their proliferating stromal involvement; they are also sharply demarcated from the surrounding breast tissue. Phyllodes tumours can be grouped into three main categories: benign, borderline and malignant. Treatment would be by complete surgical removal. Benign phyllodes tend not to re-occur after complete local dissection. If the lesion is found to be malignant then it usually re-occurs within 3 years (Crowe & Lampejo 1996).

Lipomas

When clinically examined these fatty lumps can be mistaken for cysts within the breast tissue. They do not cause major problems and diagnosis by ultrasound and cytology should be all the treatment that is needed.

Intraduct papillomas

These are benign wart-like lesions of the lactiferous duct wall and occur centrally, beneath the areola, in 75% of all cases. The woman often presents with pain or a bloody nipple discharge with a palpable, soft lesion that may be difficult to locate. These lesions are not pre-cancerous and are best treated by surgical excision. Intraduct papillomas usually occur in women who are in their late child bearing years, although they have been reported in adolescents (Schindler 1993, Blackwell 1996). See Figure 2.7 for an ultrasound of a papilloma.

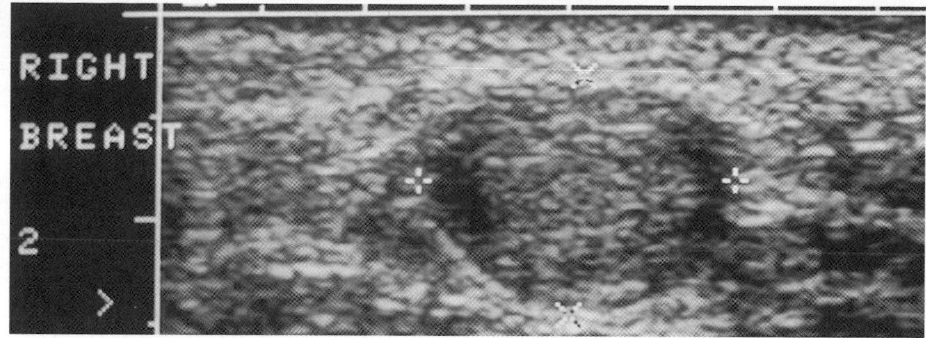

FIGURE 2.7

Ultrasound of an intraduct papilloma. Published with kind permission of the Royal Marsden Hospital Photographic Department and Breast Diagnostic Unit.

Other benign breast diseases

Nipple discharge

Spontaneous nipple discharge can be considered abnormal, although in most cases it is not problematic. Discharge can be of bloody, sero-sanguineous, serous, clear or greenish grey fluid and is often located to a single duct. Nipple discharge can represent intraductal papilloma, duct ectasia and, rarely, carcinoma and, as such, needs to be investigated until the cause is diagnosed. A small amount of nipple discharge in women younger than 50 years old may be as a result of recent breast feeding and needs no intervention unless it becomes profuse (Dixon & Mansel 1995, Saunders & Baum 1998). Reassurance and explanation about such a discharge for the woman is necessary and important for her wellbeing.

Galactorrhoea

Galactorrhoea is the inappropriate secretion of milk from the breasts and can occur in men and women. It may occur as an isolated finding or in association with amenorrhoea, oligomenorrhoea, and infertility. The milk that is secreted is usually persistent and variable in colour. A range of clinical investigations may be necessary as galactorrhoea can represent abnormal levels of prolactin perhaps caused by pituitary or hypothalamic disease, Addison's disease or Cushing's syndrome (De Vane 1996). A magnetic resonance (MR) scan or a computerised axial tomography (CT) scan may be carried out to exclude a pituitary tumour.

Mondor's disease

Caused by a superficial thrombosis of a vein in the breast, this condition is usually very painful. On examination the area of thrombosis can be represented by a crease on the skin and when palpated can feel like a piece of string or cord in the breast. Malignancy should always be excluded, but no other treatment should be necessary and the condition usually resolves in about 6 months (Curling & Tierney 1997). Figure 2.8 is a photograph of Mondor's disease of the right breast.

FIGURE 2.8

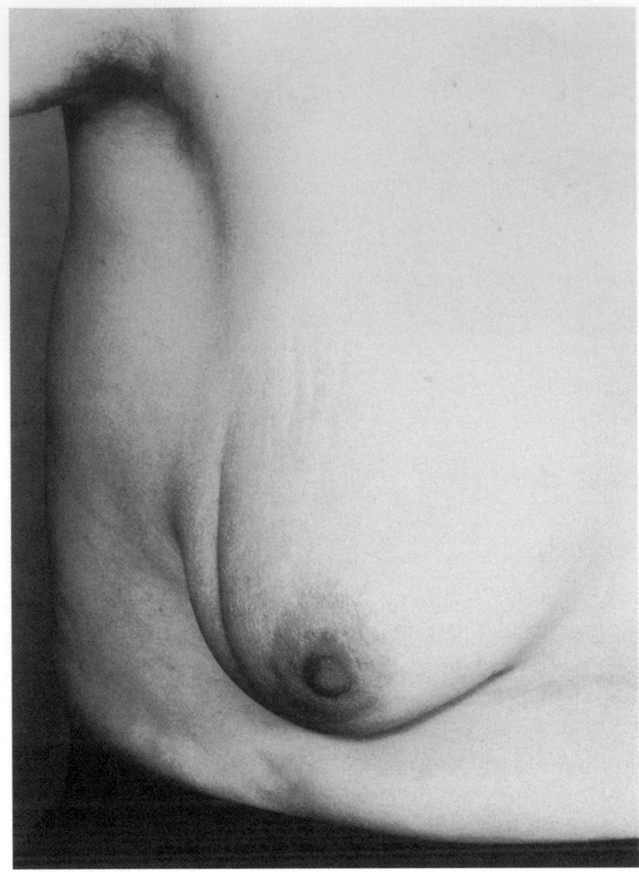

Mondor's disease of the right breast. Note creasing of the skin. Published with kind permission of the Royal Marsden Hospital Photographic Department and Breast Diagnostic Unit.

Galactocoele

This is a cystic lesion containing milk that occurs in the breasts of pregnant or lactating women. Once diagnosed, treatment is by aspiration. This may have to be performed on several occasions to allow the walls of the cyst to adhere together (Curling & Tierney 1997).

Fat necrosis

Fat necrosis often occurs as a painless, round and firm lump formed by damaged and disintegrating fatty tissues (Schindler 1993). The woman may present with a history of trauma to the breast and subsequent pain or may just present with a hard lump that may be tender. The clinical signs are very similar to that of a carcinoma and can be very disturbing to both the woman and the clinician who examines her until the true diagnosis is known. Skin retraction can sometimes be seen and some irregularity is often felt at the edges of the lump. Because of the difficulty of telling whether this lesion is malignant or not, the usual screening investigations are carried out. Fine micro-calcifications may be seen on mammogram. Excisional biopsy is the treatment of choice and, afterwards, the histology often shows a collagenous scar that surrounds an oily cyst. Haemorrhage may also be seen in the fatty tissue.

BREAST PAIN

Breast pain (mastalgia) has been reported in over 50% of women who attend benign breast clinics (Mansel 1995). A study by Preece et al (1976) determined the pattern of breast pain and discovered that there are three types of mastalgia: cyclical breast pain, non-cyclical breast pain and non-breast pain.

Cyclical breast pain

For most women some breast discomfort is accepted as a part of the normal changes that their breasts go through each month. However, some women suffer more intense pain (usually from mid-cycle onwards) that affects their quality of life and is often relieved by menstruation. The pain can differ from cycle to cycle and can continue for many years. Such women are usually in their early 30s and often do not get complete relief from the pain until they reach the menopause. The pain varies in intensity, can be increased by physical activity, is sometimes described as making the breasts feel heavy and tender, and is not affected by pregnancy, oral contraceptives or parity. The pain can be unilateral or bilateral and is often not well localised. Cyclical mastalgia often radiates to the ipsilateral arm and axilla.

Non-cyclical breast pain

Non-cyclical breast pain is usually experienced in women over 40 years old and is thought to be caused by benign lesions of the breast such as macrocysts, fibroadenomas and duct ectasia. This type of pain can occur in pre- and post-menopausal women and is not connected with cyclical ovarian function (Hughes et al 1989). Non cyclical breast pain tends to be well localised in the breast and is often described as 'drawing' or 'burning' (Hughes et al 1989).

Non-breast pain

This type of pain does not originate from the breast but can be referred pain to the breast from the chest wall, e.g. in Tietze's syndrome (costochondritis), or from outside the chest, e.g. in cervical and thoracic spondylosis, and lung disease. This non-breast pain can also arise from physical exertion with subsequent soreness of the pectoral muscle. On clinical examination, chest wall pain must be differentiated from referred breast pain or true breast pain so that appropriate treatment can be given (Mansel 1995).

Treatment for mastalgia would include a clinical history and a careful clinical examination to exclude a malignancy. Often organised breast clinics will ask the woman to complete a pain chart for several months to record the number of days the breasts are painful within each menstrual cycle. Although no direct link has been found between the levels of hormones and mastalgia there does seem to be a link between low fatty acid levels and mastalgia. Evening primrose (Efamast), a perennial herb, is rich in the essential fatty acid gamolenic acid and has been found to provide some relief with minimal side-effects (De Vane 1996). Star flower oil has similar concentrations of gamolenic acid to evening primrose oil and has also been used to relieve pain. Many women present with mastalgia and are convinced that it is linked to breast cancer. Once they are reassured that breast pain is a very rare presenting symptom of breast cancer most women find they are happy to manage their breast pain.

To mediate the hormonal influence on breast pain the oral contraceptive pill and in some cases danazol, which inhibits the pituitary gonadotrophins, or bromocriptine or buserelin have all been found to benefit some patients. Such drug interventions should be medically supervised at a benign breast disease clinic, where the clinicians are used to dealing with breast pain. The woman will be asked to try one of these drugs at a time and unless she is taking the contraceptive pill she will need to use a mechanical form of contraception. Each drug will be taken for 3–6 months to assess if there is going to be a response (Blackwell 1996).

Sometimes the breast pain originates from a trigger spot in the breast and an injection of local anaesthetic and a steroid will help. True diffuse breast pain can be helped by giving the woman a non-steroidal inflammatory drug. For both cyclical and non-cyclical mastalgia, wearing a firm and well-fitted bra can help. Diuretics, to relieve pre-menstrual bloating have no role to play in the treatment of mastalgia, although they have been prescribed (Mansel 1995). Persistent chest wall pain can be helped by infiltrating the painful area with a local anaesthetic and a steroid injection.

Nursing care

Most of the care for breast pain takes place in an outpatient clinic. The nurse can do much to help with practical advice on bra fitting and dietary modifications to include the reduction of caffeine and saturated fats in the diet. The problem of breast pain can cause great distress and anxiety for some women and should be taken seriously. However, a small group of women with intractable breast pain that does not respond to conventional treatment may have an underlying depressive disorder. In a few cases their breast pain can be so severe that they request bilateral mastectomies as the ultimate treatment. It is now becoming routine to refer these women for a psychiatric assessment to ensure that their pain merits such drastic surgical intervention. It is only through gentle questioning about the nature of their breast pain and the treatments they have received that such women can be helped.

BREAST INFECTIONS

Infections of the breast are a relatively common problem and mostly affect women between the ages of 18 and 50, although newborn babies can occasionally be affected. The infection can be in the structure of the breast or it can occur secondary to a lesion in the skin, such as a sebaceous cyst.

Lactating infection

Infection that occurs when the woman is breastfeeding is termed 'lactating infection'. Better maternal hygiene and education has reduced the incidence of infection and abscess formation during lactation, but it can still be problematic. Infection mostly occurs within the first few months of breastfeeding and there is often a history of an abrasion or a cracked nipple prior to the infection starting. *Staphylococcus aureus* is the most common organism responsible, but *S. epidermis* and streptococci are occasionally isolated. Breastfeeding is encouraged, despite the infection, to drain the infected quadrant of the breast of milk. The antibiotics flucloxacillin 500 mg and erythromycin 500 mg are recommended as first-line treatment. If the infection does not respond to these co-amoxiclav is the next choice. Tetracycline, ciprofloxacin, and chloramphenicol should all be avoided as they can enter the mother's milk and harm the baby. If the inflammation persists, the possibility of an inflammatory cancer should be excluded. A defined collection of pus should be treated by surgical excision and drainage (Dixon 1995).

Non-lactating infection

All other breast infections are termed as non-lactating and may have many causes. The infection may start from the peri-areolar region, originating from the non-dilated sub-areolar breast ducts – a condition termed 'periductal mastitis'. This condition is similar to duct ectasia but is not the same. Smoking is strongly related to periductal mastitis and it is thought the substances in the smoke damage the wall of the sub-areolar duct, allowing infection to take hold. Symptoms of peri-areolar infection are: central breast pain, nipple retraction at the site of the diseased duct, and nipple discharge. Treatment includes antibiotics and excision of the abscessed area. About one third of patients develop a mammary duct fistula after drainage and this is best treated with surgical excision of the infected duct with antibiotic cover.

Mammary duct fistula

Fistulas can develop between the skin and the major sub-areolar ducts. Treatment is by surgical excision with appropriate antibiotic cover. The rate of recurrence is high but is reduced by the surgery being performed in a specialist breast unit.

Breast abscesses

Peripheral non-lactating breast abscesses are far less common than peri-areolar breast abscesses and are associated with underlying conditions such as diabetes, rheumatoid arthritis, steroid treatment, granulomatous lobular mastitis, and trauma. In young, parous women, large areas of infection may develop with multiple simultaneous abscesses. There is a high chance that, despite surgery, this condition will recur and large surgical excision is to be avoided because of the disfiguring and scarring effect it may have. Peripheral breast abscesses should be treated with recurrent aspiration or surgical incision and drainage. Primary infection of the breast can present with cellulitis or an abscess. These infections are most common in women who are overweight, have large breasts, or poor personal hygiene. Cellulitis is most often seen after radiotherapy and is most often caused by the organism *S. aureus*.

Large areas of breast infection can be very alarming to the patient and breast surgeon alike. Figure 2.9 shows an ultrasound of a large breast abscess. Note the loculated areas of pus. Large abscesses can mimic the symptoms of an inflammatory breast cancer and if the infection does not respond to antibiotics other more sinister causes of the inflammation need to be considered quickly.

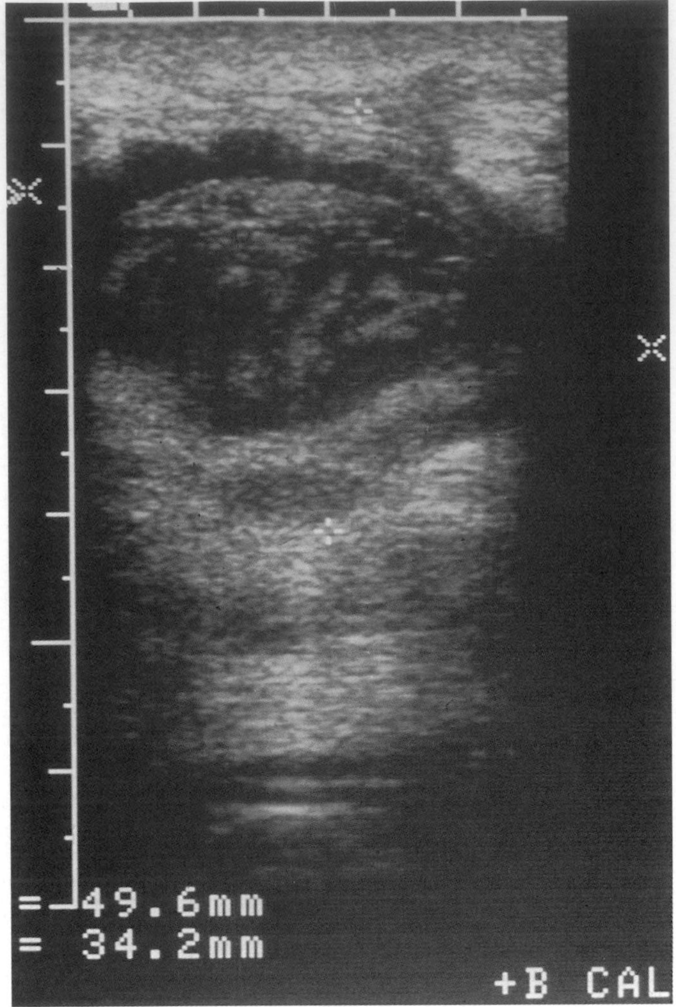

FIGURE 2.9

Ultrasound of a large breast abscess. Published with kind permission of the Royal Marsden Hospital Photographic Department and Breast Diagnostic Unit.

Nursing care

The general treatment of acute bacterial infection of the breast is with antibiotics and the drainage or aspiration of the pus. Where surgical excision of the abscess is required, nursing management will be similar to that for a woman undergoing an excision biopsy (see Ch. 5). The nurse should be aware that a postoperative wound infection is a possibility.

Women should be advised to keep the area under their breasts as clean and dry as possible. Wearing natural materials next to the breast will help, such as a cotton bra or a cotton T-shirt inside a bra. Avoiding pore-clogging skin creams and talcum powder will also help and gentle washing with an unperfumed soap and patting the skin dry will help to maintain the integrity of the skin. A breast infection can cause discomfort and pain, which are usually the most distressing features of the condition. A supportive bra, the application of a cold pack and padding to protect a sore nipple may all reduce discomfort, but mild to moderate analgesics are usually necessary to ease the pain.

RISK FACTORS FOR BENIGN BREAST DISEASE

Nulliparity and a late menopause may increase the risk of fibrocystic disease, whilst a high parity is thought to decrease the risk (Goerhing & Morabia 1997). The risk of an aberration of normal breast development is increased by any physiological process that increases cellular proliferation such as the second part of the ovulatory cycle. Most benign breast conditions do not increase the risk of breast cancer, and it is only hyperplasias that are significantly associated with malignancy (Goerhing & Morabia 1997).

CONCLUSION

Many things can happen to the breast that cause problems but are not breast cancer. For both men and women most benign breast problems are treatable and are often quite common. It is always worth checking with the GP any changes that do occur in a patient's breasts and every women should be encouraged to be breast aware.

REFERENCES

Baum M, Schipper H 1999 Fast Facts – Breast Cancer. Health Press Ltd. Oxford

Blackwell R E 1996 Breast anatomy, physiology, screening, and self assessment. In: Blackwell R E, Grotting J C (eds) Diagnosis and Management of Breast Disease. Blackwell Science. Cambridge, MA USA, ch 1, p 5–19

Crowe D R, Lampejo O T 1996 Malignant tumours of the breast. In: Blackwell R E, Grotting J C (eds) Diagnosis and Management of Breast Disease. Blackwell Science. Cambridge, MA USA, ch 5, p 103–135

Curling G, Tierney K 1997 Breast screening and breast disorders. In: Andrews G (ed) Women's Sexual Health. Baillière Tindall, London, ch 10, p 221–257

De Vane G W 1996 Breast dysfunction: galactorrhea and mastalgia. In: Blackwell R E, Grotting J C (eds) Diagnosis and Management of Breast Disease. Blackwell Science, Cambridge, MA USA, ch 2, p 19–77

Dixon D J 1995 Breast Infection. In: Dixon J M (ed) ABC of Breast Diseases. BMJ Publishing Group, London ch 4, p 14–18

Dixon J M, Mansel R E 1995 Congenital problems and aberrations of normal breast development and involution. In: Dixon J M (ed) ABC of Breast Diseases. BMJ Publishing Group, London ch 1, p 6–11

Goerhing C, Morabia A 1997 Epidemiology of benign breast disease, with special attention to histologic types. Epidemiologic Reviews 19, 2

Haagensen C D 1983 Diseases of the breast. WB Saunders Company, Philadelphia

Hughes L E, Mansel R E, Webster D J T 1989 Breast Pain and Nodularity. Baillière Tindall, London

Hughes L E 1992 Benign Breast Disorders: The clinician's view. Cancer Detection and Prevention 16: 1–5

Mansel R E 1995 Breast Pain. In: Dixon J M (ed) ABC of Breast Diseases. BMJ Publishing Group, London p 11–14

Newton P, Hannay D R, Laver R 1999 The presentation and management of female breast symptoms in general practice in Sheffield. Family Practitioner 16(4): 360–365

Preece R, Mansel R E, Bolton P et al 1976 Clinical Syndromes of Mastalgia. Lancet, p 670

Reshef E, Sanfilippo J S, Levine N 1996 Breast dysfunction: congenital anomalies of the breast. In: Blackwell R E, Grotting J C (eds) Diagnosis and Management of Breast Disease. Blackwell Science. Cambridge, MA, USA, ch 3, 77–93

Robbins S L, Cotran R S, Kumar V 1984 Pathologic Basis of Disease. WB Saunders Company, Philadelphia

Saunders C, Baum M 1998 Breast disease: refer or reassure? Practitioner 242 (1584): 216–219

Schindler L W 1993 Understanding breast changes: a health guide for all women. United State Institutes of Health, National Cancer Institute

FURTHER READING

Baum M, Schipper H 1999 Fast Facts – Breast Cancer. Health Press Ltd, Oxford
Blackwell R E, Grotting J C (eds) 1996 Diagnosis and Management of Breast Disease. Blackwell Science, Cambridge, MA, USA
Dixon J M (ed) 1995 ABC of Breast Diseases. BMJ Publishing Group, London

3 Breast Screening

Michele Taylor and Karen Burnet

It is intended that after reading this chapter the reader should understand:

- How the breast screening programme in the UK works
- The proposed benefits of breast screening
- Why a woman would be recalled for further investigations of her breast and what those investigations might be
- The arguments for and against breast screening
- Future plans for the screening programme in the UK.

INTRODUCTION

Need for a breast screening programme

Breast cancer is a serious disease that affects many women in the UK. It is responsible for the highest number of female deaths than any other cancer and will affect one woman in 12 at some time of their lives (CRC 1996). Because of these alarming statistics, in the mid-1980s, the government commissioned a report into the advisability of a breast screening programme. Led by Sir Patrick Forrest, the report examined evidence from several major screening trials including The Swedish Two Counties Trial, two Dutch studies from Nijmegen and Utrecht and the Health Insurance Plan of New York Trial in the USA.

BREAST SCREENING TRIALS

The Swedish Two Counties Trial studied the effectiveness of a single view mammogram every 2 years for women in their 40s and every 3 years for women in their 50s. The study showed an overall reduction in mortality of 29% during the 12 years of follow up in women over 50. There was a small reduction in the number of deaths in women younger than 40 years, although this was not thought to be significant. The take-up rate by women for a screening mammogram in this trial was considered to be unusually high at 89% of those invited (Tabar et al 1985). The Health Insurance Plan of New York was a very large study, conducted over a period of 20 years to examine the effects of mammographic screening. A group of 31 000 women aged between 40 and 64 years old were selected for yearly mammograms and physical examinations for 4 years. The mortality rate was reduced by up to 30% at 10 years in those women who were screened. Interestingly, only 65% of the women in this study attended for their mammogram and physical examination (Shapiro et al 1988). Two Dutch studies carried out in Nijmegen and Utrecht provided further evidence supporting the use of a screening programme to reduce mortality from breast cancer (Verbeek et al 1984).

Recommendations of the Forrest report

From these studies it was calculated that screening by mammography could reduce mortality by up to 25% amongst those screened. Sir Patrick Forrest presented his report to the government in 1986.

The report (Forrest 1986) concluded that:

> 'The information that is already available from the principal overseas studies demonstrates that screening by mammography can lead to prolongation of life for women aged 50 or over with breast cancer. There is a convincing case on clinical grounds for a change in UK policy on the provision of mammographic facilities and the screening of symptomless women. Screening programmes should be easy to apply, cheap, easy and unambiguous to interpret, and able to identify women with disease and exclude those without disease.'

And also that:

> 'The preliminary view of the Working Group is that it would not be sensible to introduce mammographic screening on a UK basis without providing the necessary back up services to assess the abnormalities that would be detected.'

The NHS breast screening programme (NHSBSP) was established by the Government in 1988, following the recommendations of the Forrest report. The problems facing the Government were to organise a sophisticated screening programme across the country and to ensure that the service being provided was of a high quality. The NHSBSP is a free national service that co-ordinates the UK breast screening service by calling and recalling women aged 50–64 years every 3 years, for a mammogram. There are 77 screening units in England organised to screen women with the intention of reducing the number of deaths from breast cancer. The screening mammogram aims to detect breast cancer when it is small and before it has had the chance to spread. In addition, microcalcifications, small white flecks of calcium in the breast, may be seen. Microcalcification can be local or widespread and particular patterns of microcalcification may be the only indication of ductal carcinoma in situ (DCIS) (Blamey et al 1995, Curling & Tierney 1997). See Chapter 4 for more detail on DCIS.

The success of the national screening programme depends on women attending for their mammogram when they are invited. An uptake rate of 70% will have to be achieved in the UK if the hoped-for 25% reduction in mortality is to be realised. If fewer women participate in the programme the cost of implementing the programme per lives saved increases and, although some women will clearly benefit, the cost effectiveness of the programme will be called into question.

Monitoring and evaluation

The national programme is organised into 17 UK regions (NHSBSP 1997). Each region has several local breast screening centres that work to establish initiatives to achieve the standards that are set nationally by the NHSBSP. These national standards for patient care are monitored through a network of people covering each region in the NHS. The National Coordinating Office and National Advisory Committee oversee the programme and report to the Department of Health. The programme provides an expert service that is constantly looking for ways to improve itself and each region has established a Quality Assurance Reference Centre. To this end health care purchasers have a particular responsibility to ensure that the local screening unit complies with the regional quality assurance service and participates in national quality assurance initiatives (DOH 1994).

Role of the primary health care team

For the NHSBSP to continue to be successful it relies on the contribution and cooperation of the primary health care team (PHCT). The PHCT can influence the screening programme in three areas:

1. Quality of the programme
2. Uptake by women
3. Information and counselling (Austoker 1990).

Quality of the programme

For the PHCT to be most effective it relies on good communication with the regional screening office. Each GPs practice should be visited by representatives from the screening office so that current information for local screening is exchanged, i.e. the time schedule and organisation of screening. Prior consent from the GP for automatic referral of all women with abnormal mammograms to the specialist screening team should be established.

Uptake of the women

Uptake from breast screening has ranged from 81% in East Anglia to 58% in the North East Thames region (Chamberlain et al 1993) and these differences have, rightly, caused some concern. The most common reasons for women not attending for their screening mammogram appointment are:

- Fear of an abnormality being detected that will indicate cancer
- Belief that the test is painful and may be damaging (Arö et al 1999)
- Belief that if they have no symptoms they will not have cancer.

The uptake of the programme by women can be improved by certain methods. Ensuring the prior notification lists are checked for accuracy and completeness is vital to avoid missing invitations. Eligible women should be encouraged to attend by GPs and practice nurses. There has been some suggestion that women's attendance for breast screening may be increased by raising the GP's perception of the threat of breast cancer, addressing their concerns about the breast screening programme and enhancing their views of the importance of the role of primary care in the NHSBSP (Bekker et al 1999).

Information and counselling

Practical advice should be available for women who are invited to attend for a screening mammogram concerning the site of the mobile screening vans, availability of public transport, parking, provision for the disabled, and practical clothing to wear when attending for a mammogram. Practice nurses can also assist in the dissemination of information by promoting screening with notice board displays and discussing screening issues in their well-woman clinics. Clearly, breast screening needs to be explained carefully and women should be educated about what a screening mammogram is and why it is important that they attend if they are invited.

The breast screening service should take into account the needs of ethnic minorities by ensuring that the service provided meets the cultural and linguistic needs of the population of a particular area. Ethnic minority status is thought to be one of the factors affecting uptake and GP receptionists who speak an Indian language appear to improve attendance (Atri et al 1997). The Leeds Health Promotion Unit have taken this one step further by developing a training pack to involve lay people from minority ethnic communities in promoting the breast screening message (Fong 1994). Concepts of health and illness, perceived susceptibility to certain diseases and attitudes towards combating disease all have an influence on breast screening uptake. GPs in particular should take opportunities to ask about breast screening attendance at patient consultations. GPs should also feel confident about discussing the implications of recall to the screening centre, biopsies of suspicious breast tissue and the range of diagnostic tests that may be used (DOH 1994).

Who is involved in the screening unit?

A highly skilled multidisciplinary team is involved in providing the screening service including a programme manager, a radiologist, radiographers, a pathologist, an oncologist, a breast surgeon and nurses (sometimes a specialist breast care nurse). The programme manager is responsible for the day-to-day running of the service. The manager has a team of clerical staff who will aim to provide a friendly reception service, collect data for computer analysis and store and retrieve women's records. The screening unit is led by a director who is often a medical professional, usually the most experienced radiologist. The radiologist's clinical role is to provide a highly skilled service detecting cancers using mammography, ultrasound and biopsy methods. The radiologist is responsible for ensuring that the appropriate levels of sensitivity (the ability to detect a disease) and specificity (excluding those who do not have the disease) are reached by the screening service offered (Cotton 1996, CRC 1997). The diagnostic radiographers provide a specialist X-ray service within the context of the screening unit, whether it is the mobile van or in the static unit. The first mammogram will be carried out by a radiographer and it may be that the woman will not see a radiologist if she has a normal mammogram, although it is usual for two radiologists to review her films. If the woman has a lesion that looks worrying she will be recalled to an assessment clinic where tissue samples may be taken from the suspicious area. A histopathologist with an interest in breast disease will be involved in the histological diagnosis. If a larger area of breast tissue is needed to confirm a diagnosis, the breast surgeon will be involved. The Royal College of Surgeons have endorsed standards of care produced by surgeons working within the NHSBSP. If the woman is diagnosed with a breast cancer then the oncologist will be a valuable member of the team, contributing their knowledge about the need for radiotherapy and chemotherapy treatments. If possible, a breast care nurse should be available to give emotional support and to explain the breast screening procedure to women who attend for breast screening.

Screening procedure

The screening procedure can be divided into three stages:

1. Identification and invitation
2. Mammography
3. Further investigation.

Identification and invitation

Every woman aged 50–64 who is registered with a GP will be sent an invitation for breast screening every 3 years. Although the screening starts for women over 50 years of age, a woman may not be called until she is 53 years old. Whole general practice areas are targeted in turn with the aim of improving cooperation and uptake. This aids dissemination of information and improved publicity in one area at a time. The first stage of the programme is carried out by the clerical staff in the breast screening service. The screening office identifies a group of eligible women in one practice surgery and a list (prior notification list) is compiled for the GP and sent to the GP to be checked and corrected. Once the list is returned to the screening office women are invited by letter to attend for mammography. Women are encouraged to change their screening appointment if the date is inconvenient (Cotton 1996).

Mammography

This takes place at either a mobile screening van that parks in any large municipal car park such as the local supermarket or a static screening unit at the local hospital. The aim is to provide a convenient service for women local to their home in order to increase uptake of the service. Each X-ray area in the van or unit is designed to respect dignity and privacy with private changing cubicles and cloth tabards to wear once the woman has removed her top and bra. The screening unit is meant to provide modern waiting areas that are light, well decorated and warm and have refreshments available.

Although mammography is expensive and requires high-technology machinery, special film processing, and highly dedicated radiologists to interpret the films, it is still the best tool available to detect breast cancer and the only screening method that has been evaluated in trials (Blamey et al 1995). The aim of breast cancer screening by means of mammography is to detect breast cancer at an earlier stage than is possible by clinical examination or breast self-examination, i.e. before a lump is palpable in the breast. In particular, it is hoped that more women will be detected with pre-invasive (in situ) cancer before the cancer cells have shown any evidence of spreading. With good technique and reading, mammography should pick up 85–90% of all breast cancers in the breasts examined. It is most effective in postmenopausal women in whom involution has taken place and the breast tissue is largely replaced by fat, which is easy to X-ray (Blamey et al 1995). Figure 3.1 shows the two types of views of screening mammograms.

FIGURE 3.1

Mammograms. (A) Oblique views and (B) cranio-caudal views Reproduced with kind permission from Addenbrooke's NHS Trust Photography Department and Dr P Britten of The Breast Unit, Addenbrooke's NHS Trust.

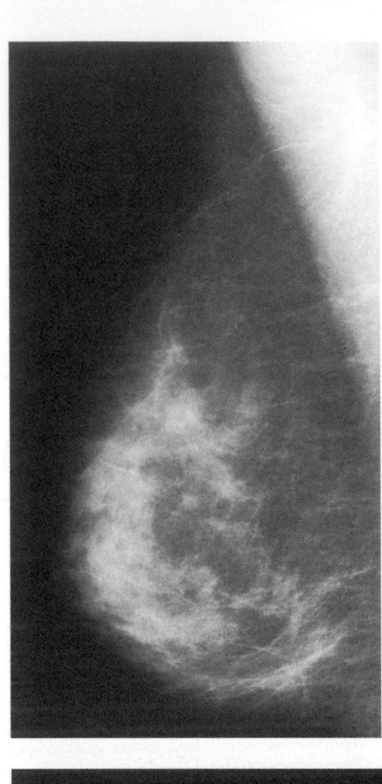

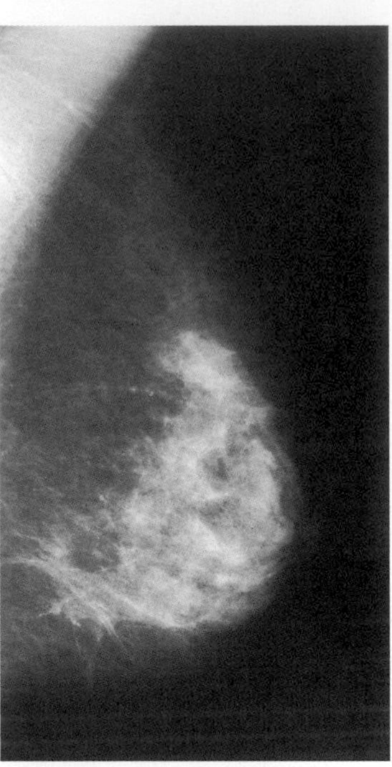

A

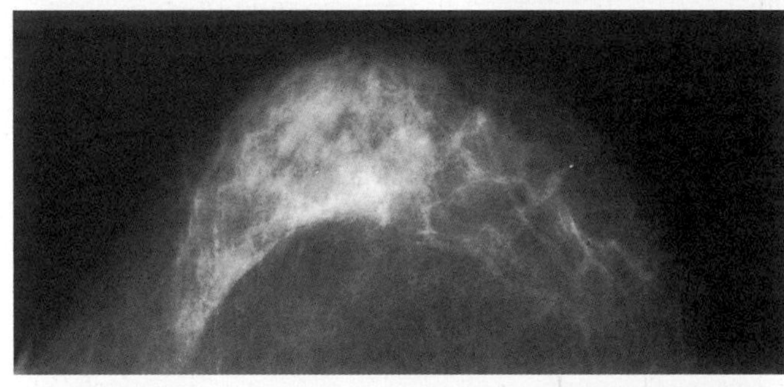

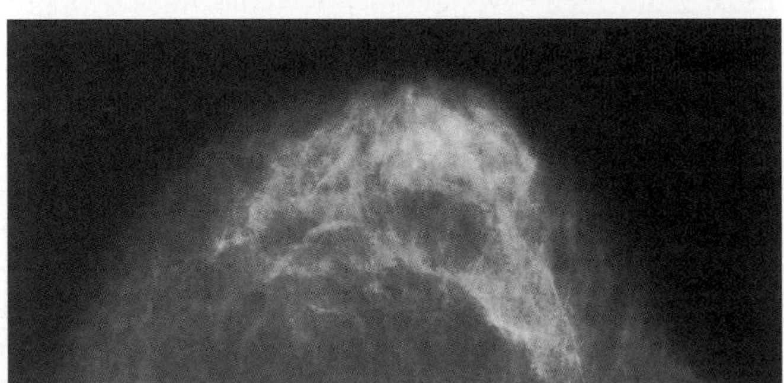

B

The first screen involves two mammographic views: an oblique view, which visualises the axillary tail, pectoral muscle and inferior portion of the breast and a cranio-caudal view, which can demonstrate whether the lesion is medial, central or lateral to the nipple (Yeowell 1993). Most breast lesions are in the upper, outer quadrant and the oblique view clearly demonstrates this area. The breast is compressed between two plates prior to the X-ray exposure. This can be an uncomfortable experience and the woman needs to be prepared for the increase in pressure.

For women aged 50–64 years, at least 50 cancers should be detected for every 10 000 screened women. At the subsequent screens, 35 cancers should be identified for every 10 000 attenders, which reflects the national incidence of cancer (Blamey et al 1995). Women are informed by letter whether they have a normal or abnormal mammogram. An abnormal mammogram will result in a cancer in about 1 out of 10 cases and may cause a great deal of anxiety for the woman involved. An appointment at the assessment centre for further investigations will be made, usually within 2 weeks, to help to reduce anxiety. Figure 3.2 shows mammograms of suspicious microcalcifications in the breast.

Further investigation

Re-screening involves further assessment using mammography, clinical examination, ultrasound (high frequency soundwaves) and fine needle aspiration cytology (FNAC) or a core biopsy of the suspicious area. This is sometimes known as triple assessment.

Women recalled for these investigations will attend a clinic where radiographers, radiologists and nurses will aim to provide an effective service for anxious women. Most of the women seen will not have a serious problem and, after investigation,

FIGURE 3.2

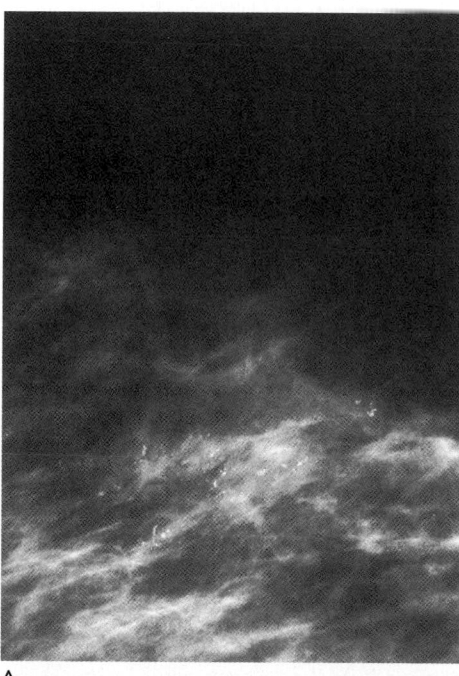

A

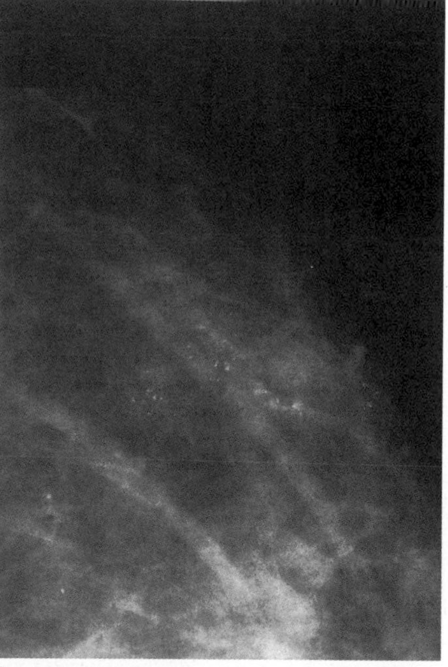

B

Mammograms showing suspicious flecks of microcalcification. Reproduced with kind permission from Addenbrooke's NHS Trust Photography Department and Dr P Britten of The Breast Unit, Addenbrooke's NHS Trust.

rejoin the routine, 3-yearly recall system. However, some women will undergo a series of diagnostic tests that can often be confusing and threatening. These tests will now be described.

Diagnostic tests

Breast examination

Breast examination is carried out by the medical staff to assess the woman for palpable abnormalities. Each of the four quadrants of the breast will be examined with the woman lying down and sitting up. The loco-regional lymph nodes will also be palpated and a clinical history will be taken. Breast awareness can be reinforced by the nurses and radiographers working in the the assessment clinic.

For further information regarding breast palpation in asymptomatic women and breast awareness, see Chapter 2.

FNAC

Simple FNAC is a quick and effective way of obtaining cells from a suspicious area. The advantages of the test are that it is quick, relatively painless and can, in some units, provide a result whilst the patient waits. The needle, usually a 22 gauge, attached to a 5 ml or 10 ml syringe, can be pushed through the skin of the breast and into the lesion. Once the operator is confident that the needle is located in the right place the plunger of the syringe is withdrawn several times and the needle is rotated before the needle and syringe are removed from the breast. The content of the syringe is spread onto glass slides and fixed or air-dried before being sent to the pathology laboratory for analysis (Cotton 1996, Curling & Tierney 1997). The possible complications of FNAC are uncommon but can include haematoma and, very rarely, pneumothorax. Bruising can be avoided by applying adequate pressure to the FNAC area. A pneumothorax is indicated if the woman has sharp pain and coughing develops shortly after the procedure and should be reported immediately to the medical staff if they are not already aware.

Ultrasound

This technique uses high frequency soundwaves that are beamed through the breast using a 12–14 MHz transducer held by the practitioner. Images from within the breast are built up on a screen and can be frozen so that the practitioner can take a better look at the breast and print a picture for future reference. On ultrasound, cysts and benign lesions tend to have well-defined edges and often look hollow whilst cancers tend to have a more ragged edge and appear to be solid, although this may not always be the case.

Ultrasound can also be used for obtaining cells from an impalpable lesion by allowing the radiologist to see the needle pass through the breast tissue and into the lesion. This is not a particularly painful procedure and usually takes only a few minutes in the hands of a skilful practitioner (Curling & Tierney 1997).

Stereotactic FNAC

Stereotactic FNAC (stereo FNAC) is a technique using stereo X-rays to detect the position of an impalpable lesion or an area of microcalcification. Once the position of the lesion has been identified, local anaesthetic is injected into the skin prior to passing a needle into the lesion to aspirate cells for cytology. This procedure is carried out while the woman is sitting in a chair and her breast is compressed under a mammographic plate. This can be a difficult test for women to endure and good radiographer or nursing support is vital. This procedure is not available in all screening centres and has been largely superseded by core biopsy (Curling & Tierney 1997).

Core biopsy

Today many screening units are using the biopsy gun to obtain a core of tissue from the breast instead of aspirating cells with a needle. A radiologist will make an incision in the skin of the breast, allowing the narrow-bore biopsy needle to be pushed to the area of tissue being sampled. This has the advantage of reducing the number of passes to obtain an adequate specimen and can provide a high-quality core specimen for histopathology analysis (Hopper et al 1991). The gun releases a spring-like mechanism that is attached to the needle, pushing the needle into the tissue to be sampled. The noise as the spring is being released can be quite alarming and the woman should be warned about this. If the lesion is malignant this procedure can often differentiate between invasive or pre-invasive disease and so alter the treatment options available to the woman.

If the result is malignant and the lesion remains impalpable, the woman will have a wire inserted into the breast under X-ray control, marking the area (mammographic localisation) before the definitive breast surgery. See Chapter 5 for more detail on surgery.

In order to explain the range of diagnostic tests further, three case histories of different experiences have been identified. These also illustrate the possible pathways through the screening process.

CASE STUDY 1

June Brown, a 53-year-old, attended the assessment clinic with her husband. It is her second screening visit; she was recalled after her first visit. Her previous mammogram, 3 years ago, was normal.

June is anxious to find out the reason for her recall. At the clinic she meets the radiographers, who explain that she has some small opacities on the right side of her mammogram that need to be investigated. June is shown the mammogram and the opacities are pointed out to her. At this screening visit, different mammographic views are taken. The consultant radiologist reviews her X-rays and explains to her that the opacities are very likely to be small cysts but that an ultrasound is required to confirm this diagnosis.

The ultrasound confirmed that June had three small microcysts, thought to be too small to aspirate. Her clinical examination was normal. The radiologist told June and her husband the result and said that no further treatment was indicated. June continued to be quite anxious and had been shocked at her recall. Contact was established with the breast care nurse attached to the screening unit and June was encouraged to call the nurse if she continued to feel ill at ease. The breast care nurse emphasised the importance of breast awareness to June, taught her how to look and feel for any changes in her breasts, and told her to report any new changes to her GP. June was discharged and informed that she would be invited for screening in 3 years' time.

CASE STUDY 2

Mary Baker, a 50-year-old, attended the recall breast assessment clinic alone. She was told that there was an area of microcalcification on the left side of her mammogram that needed to be investigated. Her husband had recently been diagnosed with bowel cancer and was too frightened to attend with her. This was Mary's first screening in the NHSBSP and she felt very anxious.

At the assessment clinic Mary was noticeably agitated. The breast care nurse was asked to see Mary and to explain why she had been recalled. Mary insisted her breasts felt normal and the breast care nurse explained that the breasts often do feel normal but the X-ray had detected a small area that needed to be investigated further.

The radiologist requested magnification X-rays of this area and a physical examination took place. No palpable lesion was found but the radiologist was suspicious and performed a FNAC to confirm the diagnosis.

As the lesion in question could not be palpated this had to be undertaken using a special method called a 'stereotactic FNAC'. The investigation revealed DCIS (pre-invasive disease) and Mary was referred to a breast surgeon for advice on surgical treatment with the support of a breast care nurse. Mary discussed her treatment with her breast care nurse and decided to have a wide local excision of the lesion.

CASE STUDY 3

Mary Dodds is a 62-year-old. Her screening mammogram showed a new opacity in her right breast. Mary was recalled by the radiologist and was given a repeat mammogram and physically examined. As the breast lump was impalpable the radiologist was able to carry out an ultrasound-guided core biopsy. Mary was supported by the breast care nurse and the radiologist whilst she underwent this procedure and a clear explanation was given of what to expect. The radiologist shared his concerns about the lesion with Mary and prepared her for the fact that it might be a cancer and that surgery could be the next step. Mary was, understandably, very shocked and chatted to the breast care nurse after the core biopsy for some time. The breast care nurse reiterated what the radiologist had said to Mary. Mary was given a contact number and asked to bring a member of her family or a friend next time she came to clinic, in 3 days' time, to get the results of her biopsy. Mary attended the clinic with her sister and the diagnosis of breast cancer was confirmed by the radiologist. The breast surgeon was also present at this appointment and he explained that the proposed surgery would be a wide local excision of the lump and the removal of some axillary lymph nodes. The breast care nurse was present for the whole consultation and was able to sit down afterwards with Mary and her sister, to re-explain what had been said by the radiologist and surgeon. Mary was also given more practical details about her admission to hospital. Mary said that she felt well supported and expressed her thanks to her breast care nurse.

The nurse's role in the screening unit

The Forrest report (1986) recommended that trained nurses should be available to support women who are undergoing screening. The report stressed the importance of specialist nurses with an in-depth knowledge of breast disease and its treatment and some training in counselling to give support to women recalled to assessment centres following the detection of an apparent abnormality. Any woman who attends for screening may have a need for more information regarding the (1) mammogram or any other procedure, (2) degree of discomfort she may experience, which can be considerable in some instances (McIlwaine 1993), (3) time to receive the results, and (4) implication of the results. The nurse is well placed to offer clear explanations of what the woman is to expect. When the woman is going through any procedure the nurse, along with other members of the screening team, has a responsibility to maintain the woman's dignity, ensure that she is comfortable and warm, has an opportunity to express her anxieties and, above all, to treat her like an individual.

All nurses have a role in health education and should take every appropriate opportunity to raise women's awareness of the availability and benefits of screening programmes. Breast care nurses have an additional health promotion role within the screening programme. They can provide information and advice to other health professionals who want to promote breast awareness in their practice, e.g. health visitors and practice nurses, or can provide a direct service to the public by giving informational talks to women's groups. Community nurses in particular can encourage women to attend for screening, and can answer queries or discuss worries about breast screening as part of their general health promotion on an individual basis, or through group discussion, e.g. in well-woman clinics. Most women who present for breast screening are asymptomatic, apparently healthy people, who on the whole, come to be reassured that all is well. Inevitably, however, screening reminds the individual that breast cancer is a potential threat. It is therefore important that within the screening programme efforts are made to reduce anxiety where possible. It is particularly important that results are sent quickly. If the first screening is a positive experience the woman will be more likely to attend 3 years later, and may urge her friends to do the same.

Breast palpation and breast awareness

It is important to clarify the role of breast examination within the screening programme as much confusion often exists. The effectiveness of breast examination in reducing mortality from breast cancer has never been consistently demonstrated (DOH 1997) therefore breast self-examination has not been chosen as a screening procedure. However, it is believed that 90% of breast cancers are found by women themselves and, as of 1991, breast awareness has been promoted as a positive health behaviour. Within the screening programme breast awareness is encouraged from the initial screen by radiographers and nurses. These health-care professionals are available to discuss the concept and provide information leaflets to all well women who attend for screening and those who might drop in to the mobile van or static unit who are interested.

Screening issues

Despite the establishment of the screening programme in this country there continues to be some debate about its effectiveness. Since the original Forrest report (1986), a new report, *Breast Cancer Screening: Evidence and Experience* has been published by the Department of Health Advisory Committee (Vessey 1991). Examining the results of various screening trials including updates on the Swedish Two Counties Trial, the New York study and the Edinburgh randomized trial, the report acknowledged that the results were not encouraging. As an example, the Edinburgh trial showed that mortality for those women screened was reduced but this was not significant. These results were tempered by the fact that there was only a 47% attendance and that the attendance was particularly poor in the lower socio-economic classes. To this end the report concluded that 'if 70% of the population accept the invitation to screening, the reduction in mortality will be about 25%' (Vessey 1991).

This certainly emphasises the need for health promotion and encouragement for all women who are eligible for screening to attend for their mammogram or the programme will not be at all cost effective.

The Swedish mammographic screening programme continues to be evaluated and one of the most recent studies shows that the observed number of deaths was only 55 (0.8%) less than would have been expected for the same population of women had they not been screened, so calling into question the high cost of implementing breast screening in Sweden (Sjonell & Stahle 1999). However, this research has been heavily criticised by Rosen & Rehnqvist (1999) who thought that the data analysis was flawed and stated that they think the Swedish screening programme should continue. A smaller study from Norway of 60 147 women aged 50–69 attending for 2-yearly mammograms drew different conclusions from their results. Of the women that had been screened, 337 cancers were discovered. The use of breast conserving surgery had gone up by 17% as cancers were being discovered when tumours were smaller; the breast cancer mortality was reduced by 30% and the number of life-years saved per breast-cancer-prevented death was calculated as 15 years. The study concluded that mammography screening in Norway looks to be cost effective and generally screening programmes should be encouraged (Norum 1999).

The debate continues up to the present day. Gøtzsche & Olsen (2000) of the Nordic Cochrane Centre re-examined the evidence of eight major screening trials. In six of these trials (Edinburgh, New York, and areas of Sweden) they concluded that randomisation was inadequate and the groups of women were not strictly comparable because of substantial differences in age and other risk factors. In reply to these criticisms Dr Gray, Director of the UK National Screening Committee, said he could see no reason to change the screening programme in Britain as, although the study was important, it had been rushed and had not been adequately peer reviewed.

In contrast, Baum, a leading UK breast cancer expert, has heavily criticised the breast-screening programme in this country and wonders if the money would be better spent on symptomatic women (Baum 1999). Diagnosing a cancer before it becomes symptomatic may not alter the outcome of the disease for that individual but may increase their morbidity once they know they have cancer (CRC 1997).

Sometimes, even after a mammogram, a cancer can be missed. The woman may have been reassured by her false-negative result and, despite symptoms may not seek medical advice. Equally, women who are recalled for what turns out to be a benign lesion or a radiological artefact can suffer severe anxiety from their false-positive test until the true diagnosis is found (CRC 1997).

The frequency and age range of the screening programme is often being called into question. A recent meta-analysis of the important research studies conducted on the efficacy of mammographic screening by age showed that mammographic screening significantly reduced breast cancer mortality for women aged 50–70 years (not 64). There is much less evidence to support the screening of women aged 40–49 years, which is why for now, the screening programme will only screen women over the age of 50 (Kerlikowske et al 1995). Reducing the screening interval to 2 years is thought to decrease the interval cancer rate as a proportion of the underlying incidence by 30% (Woodman et al 1995). Further research is underway in this country to assess the optimum screening interval. A total of 50 000 randomly selected women are being screened annually for 3 years before returning to the 3-yearly screening programme. A record will be kept of the timing and incidence of any breast cancers that are picked up and the results may well change the organisation of the screening programme (NHSBSP 1997).

Two-view mammography has been studied closely because of the cost and service implications. It is thought that it may detect 20% more breast cancers than one-view mammography and this policy has been adopted by most screening centres across the UK and Europe (Thurfjell 1990, Van Dijck et al 1992).

The use of hormone replacement therapy (HRT) in women below the age of 60 years continues to increase. HRT is thought to reduce the sensitivity of the mammogram X-ray as the density of the breast tissue increases, but it is thought that the advantages of protection against heart disease and osteoporosis outweigh the disadvantages. The general consensus is that women who are in the screening programme should continue to take HRT if they wish to do so (Litherland et al 1999).

CONCLUSION

At present there is little chance for control of breast cancer through primary prevention as the definitive cause of the disease is unknown. Genetic factors may result in some families having a higher risk than others but this is an uncommon cause of breast cancer (see Ch. 4). Control of breast cancer has more recently focused on secondary prevention, i.e. screening, as a means of early detection and therefore improved survival; on the data available so far this does appear to make a difference on the mortality rates from breast cancer. It will only be through continual surveillance of the NHSBSP and attention given to priority setting, quality assurance and collection of survival and outcome data, that the true value of breast screening will be known.

REFERENCES

Arö A R, de Konig H J, Absetz P, Schreck M 1999 Psychosocial predictors of first attendance for organised mammography screening. Journal of Medical Screening 6(2): 82–88

Atri J, Falshaw M, Gregg R, Robson J, Omar R, Dixon S 1997 Improving uptake of breast screening in multiethnic populations: a randomised controlled trial using practice reception staff to contact non attenders. British Medical Journal 315: 1356–1359

Austoker J 1990 Breast cancer screening and the primary care team. British Medical Journal 300: 1631–1634

Baum M 1999 NHS breast screening programme. Money would be better spent on symptomatic women. British Medical Journal 6; 3318(7180): 398

Bekker H, Morrison L, Marteau TM 1999 Breast screening: GPs' beliefs, attitudes and practices. Family Practitioner 16(1): 60–65

Blamey R W, Wilson A R M, Patnick J 1995 Screening for breast cancer. In: Dixon J M (ed) ABC of Breast Diseases. BMJ Publishing Group, London, Ch 6, p 22–26

Cancer Research Campaign (CRC) 1996 Breast Cancer Fact Sheet 6.1–6.6. CRC, London

Cancer Research Campaign (CRC) 1997 Breast Cancer Screening Fact Sheet 7.1–7.5. CRC, London

Chamberlain J, Moss S M, Kirkpatrick A E, Michell M, Johns L 1993 National Health Service Breast Screening Programme results for 1991–1992. British Medical Journal 307: 353–356

Cotton T 1996 Screening for breast cancer. In: Denton S (ed) Breast Cancer Nursing. Chapman and Hall, London

Curling G, Tierney K 1997 Breast screening and breast disorders. In: Andrews G (ed) Women's Sexual Health. Baillière Tindall, London, Ch 10, p 221–257

Department of Health (DOH) 1994 The Health of the Nation. Breast Cancer. Health Publication Unit, Lancashire

Department of Health (DOH) 1997 Statistical bulletin: Breast Screening programme, England 1995–1996. Department of Health, London

Fong C 1994 Keeping abreast of the issues. Healthlines June: p 8–9

Forrest A 1986 Breast Cancer Screening, Report to the Health Ministers of England, Scotland and Northern Ireland. HMSO, London

Gøtzsche P C, Olsen O 2000 Is screening for breast cancer with mammography justifiable? Lancet 355(9198): 129–134

Hopper K, Parker S, Yakes W 1991 The biopsy gun. Hospital Medica. November: 52–55

Kerlikowske K, Grady D, Rubin S M, Sandrook C I, Ernster V L 1995 Efficacy of screening mammography. A meta-analysis. Journal of the American Medical Association 273: 149–154

Litherland J C, Stallard S, Hole D, Cordinor C 1999 The effect of hormone replacement therapy on the sensitivity of screening mammograms. Clinical Radiology 54(5): 285–288

McIlwaine G 1993 Satisfaction with the NHS Breast Screening Programme: Women's views. In: Austoker J, Patnick J (eds) Breast Screening and Acceptability: research and practice. NHSBSP Publications 28: p 14–16

Norum J 1999 Breast cancer screening by mammography in Norway. Is it more cost effective? Annals of Oncology 10(2): 197–203

National Health Service Breast Screening Programmme (NHSBSP) Review 1997. NHSBSP, Clear Communication, Sheffield

Rosen M, Rehnqvist N 1999 Breast screening. No need to reconsider breast screening: programme on basis of results from defective study. British Medical Journal 318(7186): 809–810

Shapiro S, Venet W, Strax P, Venet L 1988 Periodic Screening for Breast Cancer: the Health Insurance Plan Project and its sequelae 1963–1986. Johns Hopkins University Press, USA

Sjonell G, Stahle L 1999 Scientific foundation of mammographic screening is based on inconclusive research in Sweden. British Medical Journal 319(7201): 55

Thurfjell E L 1990 One versus two view mammographic screening. A prospective trial. Svenska Lakaresaliskapets Handlinger Hygiea 99: 220

Woodman C B, Threlfall A G, Boggis C R, Prior P 1995 Is the three year breast screening interval too long? Occurrence of interval cancers in NHS breast screening programme's North Western Region. British Medical Journal 310: 224–226

Van Dijck J A, Verbeek A L, Hendrix J H, Holland R 1992 One view versus two view mammography in baseline screening for breast cancer: a review. British Journal of Radiology 65: 971–976

Verbeek A et al 1984 Reduction of breast cancer mortality through mass screening with modern mammography. First Results of the Nijmegen project. Lancet 1: 1222–1224

Vessey M 1991 Breast Cancer screening: Evidence and experience since the Forrest Report. NHS Breast Screening Programme Publication

Yeowell M 1993 Mammography positioning technique. In: Tucker A K (ed) Textbook of Mammography. Churchill Livingstone, Edinburgh, Ch 3, p 28–54

4 Cancer of the Breast

Karen Burnet

By the end of this chapter the reader should be able to:

- Understand the significance of breast cancer in the UK
- Understand the risk factors for breast cancer
- Have an understanding of the different types of breast cancer
- Know something about breast cancer and pregnancy
- Know about the breast cancer pre-disposing genes.

INTRODUCTION

The possibility of having breast cancer is an emotive and frightening prospect for any patient who undergoes investigations for a breast problem. To achieve a definitive diagnosis of malignancy the patient will have already undergone a variety of tests and investigations including mammogram, ultrasound and, usually, a biopsy of the suspicious tissue. Once diagnosed, the woman (for it is mostly a disease that effects women) may have a bewildering amount of treatment offered to her including surgery, radiotherapy, chemotherapy and some form of hormone therapy. She may find she is swamped with information that she is expected to understand and then asked to make a decision based on this information. This situation can cause extreme stress and is not a good start for someone who is about to embark on a potentially complicated course of treatment. Many people are involved in caring for women with breast cancer, both in the community and hospital, and can include nurse practitioners, practice nurses, district nurses, Macmillan nurses and Marie Curie nurses. In the course of being diagnosed the woman may well come into contact with a specialist breast care nurse, diagnostic radiographers, surgical nurses on the ward, treatment radiographers in the radiotherapy department and chemotherapy nurses in the oncology outpatient department. All these health care professionals will need to know about their own area of expertise but also something about the other treatments and care the woman will be offered so that a coordinated care plan can be implemented. Much of this book has been dedicated to understanding what breast cancer *is* and the range of investigations and treatments that can be used to treat it. This first section highlights the different types of breast cancer, the risk factors, the staging, and the usual presenting symptoms of a breast cancer. The following chapters will concentrate on screening for breast cancer, surgical treatments, medical treatments, the psychological care of the patient with breast cancer and, if the disease returns, the medical and nursing care for control of the disease, including good symptom management and palliation.

INCIDENCE AND MORTALITY

In the UK breast cancer is one of the most common malignancies in women, accounting for 20% of female cancers; approximately one out of every 12 women in the UK will develop breast cancer at some time in their lives (CRC 1996). Breast cancer is the highest cause of death in women aged 40–50, although 90% of these deaths occur in women over 50 (McPherson et al 1995). There are 29 000 new cases of breast cancer and 12 500 deaths due to breast cancer each year (Office for National Statistics 1996). The 5-year survival rate for the UK appears lower than other European Countries and this survival rate varies in different parts of the UK (CRC 1996). However, recent figures show that the survival rate is improving and this improvement is thought to be due to the screening programme and widespread use of tamoxifen in the treatment of breast cancer.

These statistics emphasise what an enormous health problem breast cancer is in this country. Most nurses, at some point in their careers, are likely to care for a patient with breast cancer and should have some understanding of this disease and the way it is treated.

MALE BREAST CANCER

Although breast cancer is predominantly a female disease, approximately 1% of all breast cancers occur in men (Baum et al 1994). It is important for nurses to be aware of the particular problems that men experience when they are diagnosed with breast cancer. It is thought that men present later with their breast cancer as they are less aware that a breast lump may represent something as sinister as a malignancy and so do not seek help promptly. Men are often ignorant that the treatments for breast cancer in women also apply to themselves. Men usually undergo some form of hormone therapy treatment, usually with tamoxifen, which can cause feminising effects. This can, in turn, threaten a man's sexuality and will require particular support from the nurses who care for him. It is unlikely that a man who has breast cancer will encounter anyone else in the same situation and this may emphasise the rarity of his condition and make him feel isolated. Nurses should offer support to the man as they would if he were female but should also take into account the particular needs he has as a man (Denton 1996).

RISK FACTORS FOR BREAST CANCER

The main risk factors associated with breast cancer are described as follows. Of these, only sex and increasing age are known to be of any substantial significance.

Sex

Breast cancer is mainly a female disease, although it does affect males. There are approximately 175 cases of male breast cancer and 90 deaths in the UK per year, which is about 1% of all the diagnosed breast cancers per year (CRC 1996).

Increasing age

Breast cancer is predominantly a disease of older women. It is very rare in women below the age of 35 years, but incidence rates increase steadily from then, reaching over 300 per 100 000 of the population by the time women are 85 years old. The greatest number of women are diagnosed between the ages of 45 and 75 years. Breast cancer in men is almost always seen beyond the age of 65 years (CRC 1996).

Benign breast disease

There is some evidence that several forms of benign breast disease can predispose to breast cancer. Atypical hyperplasias or atypical forms of fibrocystic change can result in the individual having a 4–5 times higher risk of developing breast cancer. Women who have complex fibroadenomas, duct papillomas, sclerosis, and moderate or florid epithelial hyperplasia have a slightly increased risk of breast cancer but this increase is not thought to be significant (McPherson et al 1995, Crowe & Lampejo 1996). Women who develop benign breast disease such as cysts, papillomas, and fibroadenomas often experience a great deal of anxiety concerning the malignant potential of these conditions and should be reassured that the increased risk is very small. Women who have previously diagnosed benign breast disease are often followed up by a benign breast disease clinic and are taught how to be breast aware so they may take some control over their health care (see Ch. 1).

Previous breast cancer

If a woman develops breast cancer in one breast she is more likely to develop a cancer in the contralateral breast. The risk of developing a secondary primary breast cancer after the first is up to five times the general risk and is often a cause of great concern to women who attend follow-up breast cancer clinics (Blackwell 1996).

Exposure to hormones

It is known that women who have their first child after the age of 35 or who are nulliparous, those who experience early menarche, and those who have a late menopause are all found to have a slightly increased rate of breast cancer. It has also been found that there is a 70% reduction of breast cancer in women who undergo an oophorectomy before the age of 35 (Blackwell 1996). These observations have led to the belief that unopposed oestrogen may make breast tissue more susceptible to the other risk factors associated with breast cancer and, therefore increases that individual's chances of developing the disease (McPherson et al 1995, Blackwell 1996).

In recent years there has been much speculation as to the effects of the contraceptive pill and hormone replacement therapy on the incidence of breast cancer. The oral contraceptive pill only raises the relative risk of having breast cancer diagnosed to 1.24 in current users and there is no increase in risk after 10 years of stopping the pill (Collaborative Group on Hormonal Factors in Breast Cancer 1997). There is thought to be an increased risk in women who have taken the oral contraceptive pill for more than 4 years before their first full-term pregnancy (McPherson et al 1995). It seems that more research is needed to show clearly that whether or not taking the contraceptive pill is a risk to be avoided.

The use of hormone replacement therapy (HRT) for reducing menopausal symptoms is thought to increase the risk of getting breast cancer if taken for 10–15 years and women who use combination HRT with oestrogen and progesterone face a greater risk than those taking oestrogen alone (Schairer et al 2000). Some studies have suggested that the users of HRT who develop breast cancer have slightly more favourable pathological features (Stallard et al 2000) and the benefits of taking HRT for the first 10 years, by reducing ischaemic heart disease and osteoporosis, are thought to outweigh the increased risk of breast cancer (McPherson et al 1995). The use of HRT has made the breast increasingly difficult to screen as the breast tissue remains dense rather than involuting to fat, which is easier to see clearly on mammogram. Because of the advantages and disadvantages of HRT, research is ongoing to get a definitive answer about the circumstances under which, and for how long, HRT should be taken.

For the present, menopausal symptoms and the risks of HRT should always be discussed with the woman before she commences on a course of treatment and alternative help for such symptoms should be offered as the first intervention (see Ch. 7 on hormone therapies).

For postmenopausal women who are diagnosed and treated for breast cancer it is usual to advise them to stop taking HRT. However, some women feel that they cannot return to the distressing symptoms of the menopause as well as cope with breast cancer. These women may benefit from a referral to an oncology clinic where a discussion of the benefits and risks of HRT can take place (Howell et al 1995).

Pregnancy

Having an early pregnancy appears to give a protective effect against breast cancer and women who become pregnant after pre-menopausal stage I or II breast cancer show no increase in mortality compared to women who do not go on to become pregnant (Kroman et al 1997, Velentgas 1999).

Ionising radiation

It is known that a high dose of radiation can increase the risk of breast cancer. This has been established for women who were exposed to high levels of radiation during treatment for mastitis and tuberculosis and those women who were exposed to the atomic fallout during the Second World War. This knowledge has raised public anxieties concerning the safety of mammography as a screening procedure, although it is estimated that the increased risk of getting a radiation-induced breast cancer is minute and is far outweighed by the benefits of screening.

Stress

Many women believe that stressful life events such as the death of a husband or close friend are related to breast disease. In a recent American meta-analysis examining the relationship between psycho-social factors and the development of breast cancer, it was shown that there is little evidence to support the premise that personality and stress influence the development of breast cancer (McKenna et al 1999). In a British case-control study determining the relationship between stressful life events and the onset of breast cancer, no relationship was found (Protheroe et al 1999). However, for the sufferer of breast cancer there is often the inevitable question of 'why have I got this cancer'? The sudden appearance of a cancer (particularly in asymptomatic screen detected cancer patients) produces the need to rationalise its presence by the attribution of a tangible and understandable cause. Fallowfield (1991) called this 'effort after meaning' and for many women the attribution of stress as a causal factor helps them to make sense of their situation and regain some control. As Fallowfield (1991) suggests, it is important for health professionals to listen to and appreciate lay understandings and rationalisations and not dismiss them as irrational or implausible. If rationalisation of the cause of breast cancer is the way that a woman copes with her disease, then this should be respected and only challenged if it starts to have a negative effect on the woman or her significant others.

Diet

Populations with a high rate of breast cancer generally have a diet high in fat. Obesity has also been found to be associated with a slightly increased risk of breast cancer in postmenopausal women. However, a clear link between diet and the risk of breast cancer has not been established (McPherson et al 1995, Blackwell 1996).

Alcohol

There is some evidence to suggest that excess alcohol intake increases a woman's long-term risk of developing breast cancer although evaluation of this particular risk factor is ongoing (CRC 1996).

Geography

England and Wales have the highest mortality figures for breast cancer in the world, followed by Scotland, Northern Ireland, the Netherlands and the USA (McPherson et al 1995). Generally, incidence in western Europe, North America and Australia is about five times higher than in Asia and Africa. Japanese women have low rates of breast cancer, but incidence rates are seen to rise by the second generation among Japanese-Americans. This suggests that environmental and social risk factors may contribute to the development of a breast cancer (Miller 1995).

Familial breast cancer

Breast cancer is a common disease and there could be more than one individual in a family affected by the disease. Most cases of breast cancer are sporadic, which means that there is no identifiable cancer predisposing gene within the breast cells (Eeles 1996). However, about 5–10% of breast cancers are inherited (Rahman 1999) meaning that the individual has an identifiable breast-cancer-causing gene. Genes are made up of deoxyribonucleic acid (DNA) which itself consists of amino acids. Each cell has about 50 000 genes that are found in the 23 pairs of chromosomes within a cell and determine such characteristics as eye colour, hair colour and the growth mechanisms of that particular cell. Having a breast-cancer-causing gene does not mean that the individual will automatically develop breast cancer but that they are at a much higher risk than the general population of developing the disease and carriers of such genes have a 50% chance of passing the faulty gene to their offspring (Eeles 1996). Two of the genes involved in familial breast cancer have been identified as *BRCA1* and *BRCA2*. Both of these genes are constructed of long chains of amino acids and mutations can occur anywhere along their length. *BRCA1*, which predisposes the carrier to breast and ovarian cancer, was mapped on chromosome 17q. *BRCA2* was mapped on chromosome 13q and predisposes the carrier to early onset breast cancer and a low risk of ovarian cancer (MacDonald 1997). It is likely that there are other breast cancer predisposition genes that have yet to be identified (Rahman 1999).

Increasing awareness of inherited factors fuelled by the publicity surrounding the discovery of the breast cancer genes *BRCA1* and *BRCA2* has led many women to seek advice about their familial risk. This in turn has led to a demand for counselling, screening, genetic testing and prophylactic treatments (chemoprevention and surgery). The GP may well be the first port of call for a woman (or man) who is worried that they have a familial disposition to breast cancer. The general guidelines for referral onto a specialised genetic clinic are:

- There are several cases of breast cancer in a single family
- The relatives in that family have an early onset of cancer
- There is a combination of ovarian and breast cancer in a family (Page et al 1995).

A specialised genetics clinic is often led by a consultant clinical geneticist who is usually supported by one or several clinical nurse specialists. In families that are suspected of having a cancer-causing gene, it is important that the geneticist or specialist nurse gets an accurate family history or pedigree, going back several generations, to assess who developed cancer and the type of cancer they had. These details will allow the geneticist and clinical nurse specialist to calculate the chances that a cancer gene is present and to estimate the likelihood that any member of the family has the gene (White & Mackay 1997). Family histories are very often difficult to recall and sometimes it is necessary to extend and verify such details by using public records of births, deaths and marriages, pathology reports and hospital records. The individual will be told if they have a moderate or high chance of carrying a breast cancer gene. A women is considered to be at moderate risk if she has:

- A first-degree relative (parents, siblings and children) under the age of 40 with breast cancer

- Two first- or second-degree relatives (aunts, uncles, nieces and nephews) on the same side of the family under 60 years of age with breast or ovarian cancer
- Three first- or second-degree relatives on the same side of the family with breast or ovarian cancer
- A first-degree relative with breast cancer in both breasts
- A first-degree male relative with breast cancer.

(CRC 1997)

If the individual has four close relatives with breast or ovarian cancer, it may be possible to offer them a genetic test to identify the faulty gene. The breast cancer predisposing genes *BRCA1* and *BRCA2* can be identified by genetic linkage analysis. This involves taking tissue or blood samples from affected family members and using specialised genetic techniques to search for the problematic gene. Women who are at an increased risk of developing cancer because of a genetic predisposition will be offered genetic counselling and psychological support by the geneticist and specialist nurses that work in the clinic. Individuals who know that they have a breast-cancer-causing gene can experience feelings of denial, low self-esteem, guilt and anxiety (RCN 1997). Guilt may be felt within the family by the carriers of the gene and by those who have not inherited the gene and it is important that clear and accurate information is given and that these family members have an opportunity to express their feelings.

Many women find reassurance from genetic counselling/testing particularly if some form of preventative treatment can be offered (Watson 1994). If the chances of developing cancer are very high, this will be discussed with the woman and her future care will be considered. There are various ethical details involved in genetic screening, such as ensuring the confidentiality of family history details, the disclosure of information to other members of the family and gaining written informed consent to test for the gene. It is one thing to know that an individual has a breast-cancer-causing gene, but what they do with this information and who they should tell are separate issues that have to be addressed with tact and understanding. Clinical nurse specialists are involved in counselling women about their level of risk of developing a cancer, ensuring that they understand the meaning of risk and any advice and interventions that may be offered. Such options include:

- Screening
- Chemo-prevention
- Prophylactic surgery.

Interventions are very much under evaluation at the moment because this is a new area of cancer care. Instituting regular mammographic screening 5–10 years younger than the youngest relative to have already developed the disease is a current recommendation. Studies in the UK using the oestrogen-blocking agent tamoxifen for women at risk are ongoing (Powles 1998) but there are drawbacks as tamoxifen cannot be given to women of childbearing age (Eeles 1996) and the results of these chemoprevention trials will not be be available for 10–15 years. Finally, some women will have the *BRCA1* or *BRCA2* gene confirmed by DNA analysis and may be offered bilateral subcutaneous mastectomy as a preventative treatment although this is clearly a serious undertaking.

Bilateral mastectomy does not remove all the remaining breast tissue (even with the most radical operation) and the risk from the remaining tissue, in which each cell retains the defective gene, is unknown (Eeles 1996). Research into this area of cancer care will continue far into this century. The implications for breast care are potentially very exciting as women who are likely to develop breast cancer could be identified and treated prophylactically (McPherson et al 1995, Page et al 1995).

HISTOPATHOLOGY OF BREAST CANCER

The breast is a modified gland consisting of a group of branching ducts and lobules that connect the smallest secretory gland, the acinus, to the excretion point or the nipple-areolar complex. These ducts and lobules comprise the terminal duct lobular unit, which is lined with epithelial cells and is separated by denser extralobular collagenous stroma and fat. Malignant cancers, that is, cells that are growing uncontrollably, occur both in the epithelial cells and the stroma but it is the epithelial tumours that are the most prevalent (Crowe & Lampejo 1996).

Breast cancers may be classified according to the type of tissue from which they arise and their appearance under the microscope. The histological type of a cancer is often relevant to the choice of treatment as different breast cancers behave in different ways, with some being more aggressive and more likely to metastasise than others.

Ductal and lobular carcinomas

Ductal or lobular carcinomas are the most common types of breast cancers and both are thought to arise from the epithelial cells of the terminal duct lobular unit. Infiltrating ductal carcinomas account for 75% of all breast cancers (Stuart Goodman 1987). Lobular carcinomas account for around 15% of breast cancers and are more commonly multifocal and bilateral than ductal carcinomas (Crowe & Lampejo 1996). Infiltrating carcinoma cells have the ability to invade the basement membrane of the duct or lobule of the breast and to spread elsewhere in the body. This ability to invade and to metastasise will determine the type of surgery and follow-up medical treatment the patient is offered.

In situ disease

Cancer cells that remain within the terminal duct lobular unit are termed 'non-invasive' or 'in situ' disease and can be either lobular or ductal carcinoma in situ. Ductal carcinoma in situ (DCIS) is more prevalent than lobular carcinoma in situ (LCIS) (Crowe & Lampejo 1996). In situ disease is not always palpable and is often detected on mammogram by the small calcium deposits called microcalcifications (see Fig. 3.2) and the screening programme has been able to detect in situ disease at a much earlier stage than before (see Ch. 3). Ductal carcinoma in situ represents a very early stage of breast cancer and with adequate surgical excision plus or minus radiotherapy, can be cured (Crowe & Lampejo 1996). It cannot be predicted when, or if, a non-invasive breast cancer will become invasive. The woman undergoing treatment for in situ disease should not be reassured that her condition has been cured unless the suspicious area of tissue has been completely removed and the full histology of the excised tissue, including the margin status, is known.

Medullary, mucinous (colloidal) and tubular carcinomas are all types of breast cancers arising from ductal tissue. Mostly these cancers arise in one area of the breast but can be multifocal although are rarely bilateral, and carry a much better prognosis than other cancers of no special type. Surgery is often the treatment of choice. The cells of a medullary carcinoma are characteristically surrounded by lymphoid infiltrate. Mucinous carcinoma accounts for 2% of all cancers and occurs mostly in older women (Crowe & Lampejo 1996). Tubular carcinoma is a very well-differentiated type of infiltrating ductal carcinoma.

Inflammatory carcinoma

Around 4% of all breast carcinomas are described as inflammatory. Such cancers are poorly differentiated (unlike the tissue of origin) ductal carcinomas that have invaded the lymphatic channels of the breast. An inflammatory breast cancer may also infiltrate the Cooper's ligaments of the breast, causing a characteristic skin dimpling also known as peau d'orange. Often the woman presents with an inflamed and swollen breast; to the GP this may look like an acute breast infection except that it will not respond to antibiotics. Referral to a breast unit will lead to diagnosis by cytology, mammogram and ultrasound. The prognosis is poor with the median survival of these patients at about 2–2.5 years (Rodger et al 1995). Surgery may not be the most appropriate treatment in the first instance and hormone therapy or chemotherapy may be a better choice. Surgery can be used at a later date if the tumour responds well to medical treatment by shrinking down sufficiently so that a good surgical clearance can be achieved. The operation should be followed by radiotherapy for further local control (Rodger et al 1995, Denton 1996, Curling & Tierney 1997). These cancers can ulcerate through the skin, causing bleeding, necrosis and can become infected. This lesion is called a 'fungating lesion' and requires very specific nursing care, which is covered in detail in Chapter 8.

Paget's disease

Paget's disease of the nipple is a highly specialised form of ductal carcinoma. Malignant cells are found in the epidermis of the nipple and are usually associated with small multifocal areas of ductal cancer behind the nipple and deep in the breast. The incidence of this type of breast cancer is very low at around 0.5–3.2% of all breast cancers (Fowble et al 1991, Crowe & Lampejo 1996). The woman usually presents to her GP with a nipple discharge, eczema-like skin changes, nipple retraction and sometimes an underlying thickening of the breast tissue. Treatment depends on the woman's choice but would usually involve complete surgical excision of the affected area.

Phyllodes tumours

These tumours often present in middle-aged women as a painless mass; they can be grouped into three categories: benign, borderline and malignant. Benign phyllodes tumours do not recur after surgical resection but malignant phyllodes tumours usually recur within 3 years of the original surgery. Metastatic spread is via the blood vessels and survival from malignant phyllodes tumours is around 5 years (Crowe & Lampejo 1996).

Angiosarcomas

These tumours make up only a small percentage of all breast tumours and usually affect 30–40-year-old women. These tumours spread via the blood vessels and are graded as I, II and III. Angiosarcomas may arise in a breast that has been exposed to radiation given as a previous therapy.

Lymphomas

Primary lymphomas of the breast make up less than 1% of breast malignancies and can occur in any age group. They often present as fast-growing, circumscribed masses and are often thought to be a more prevalent type of breast cancer until the full histology is known.

Other breast cancers forming in the stroma of the breast are less common and secondary cancers in the breast are rare.

Once the diagnosis of breast cancer has been confirmed by mammogram, ultrasound and cytology, the surgical removal of the tumour is the most likely treatment unless the tumour is large and the patient has been offered medical treatment (see Ch. 6). The removed breast tissue will be sent to the laboratory for analysis and this information will define the stage of the cancer and therefore, the prognosis for the patient.

STAGING BREAST CANCERS

After the initial surgery the breast cancer is given a histological diagnosis and various other factors such as the size of the tumour, the lymph node status and the presence of metastases are taken into account to stage the disease. The staging of a breast cancer will enable the clinicians to select the optimum treatment for the patient, will allow comparisons of different treatments between similar groups of patients with breast cancer and finally, will improve our understanding of breast cancer, perhaps helping the development of new treatment strategies (Miller 1995).

Tumour size

The size of the primary tumour can predict the survival of the patient. Those who have a smaller tumour are likely to have a better survival than those with a bigger tumour.

Cellular differentiation

Cellular differentiation, i.e. the degree to which cancer cells resemble their tissue of origin, is another important histological factor in determining prognosis. Cells are described as well, moderate or poorly differentiated, or grades I, II or III. Poorly differentiated cancers tend to be more aggressive, with the ability to metastasise at an earlier stage and so carry a poorer prognosis.

Lymph node status

The axillary lymph node status, i.e. the number of lymph nodes involved with cancer cells, determines the chances of survival for that individual. The surgeon will aim to remove a substantial number of lymph nodes from a level I to a level III clearance (see Ch. 5). The presence of cancer cells in the blood vessels or lymphatic channels indicates a more aggressive cancer, and patients who demonstrate this are at greater risk of developing a local or systemic cancer recurrence. The presence of metastases, where the cancer has spread beyond the axillary or the internal mammary lymph nodes, means a much worse survival rate than in patients in whom the disease is apparently localised. This will mean that there is a need for systemic treatment.

Composition of tumour

A component of in situ lobular or ductal disease that is greater than 25% of the whole malignant tumour is not a good prognostic feature. Such patients are more likely to develop locally recurrent disease after breast-conserving treatment (Crowe & Lampejo 1996).

Receptor status

Another prognostic factor is the presence of oestrogen or progesterone receptors on the surface of the breast cancer cells. The presence of these steroid receptors means that any hormone therapy is likely to be more effective and that the cancer cell itself is more differentiated and therefore less aggressive (Crowe & Lampejo 1996).

Oncogenes

The formation of a cancer cell involves the activation of oncogenes that cause the cell to divide without control, or the inactivation of tumour suppression genes, which prevent the cell from dividing uncontrollably (Gutierrez et al 1992). The proto-oncogene *erb*B-2 is over expressed in 15–30% of all invasive breast cancers and 80% of non-invasive breast cancers. Tumours that express *erb*B-2 are more likely to be resistant to chemotherapy and hormone therapy (Miller 1995).

Classification of stage

To order all this information and to provide continuity between the surgical and oncological teams there are three recognised grading systems used to select the appropriate treatment to manage a patient with breast cancer. The two staging classifications in current use are the tumour node metastases (TNM) (Table 4.1) and the Union Internationale Contre Cancer (UICC) (Table 4.2) which stages cancers as I, II, III and IV and is combined with the TNM. In order to clarify the TNM classification a further grading system, the Nottingham Prognostic Index,

TABLE 4.1 ***TNM clinical classification***

Stage	Characteristics
TX	Primary tumour cannot be assessed
T0	No evidence of primary tumour
Tis	Carcinoma in situ: intraductal carcinoma, or lobular carcinoma in situ, or Paget's disease of the nipple with no tumour*
T1	Tumour 2 cm or less in greatest dimension
T1a	0.5 cm or less in greatest dimension
T1b	More than 0.5 cm but not more than 1 cm in greatest dimension
T1c	More than 1 cm but not more than 2 cm in greatest dimension
T2	Tumour more than 2 cm but not more than 5 cm in greatest dimension
T3	Tumour more than 5 cm in greatest dimension
T4	Tumour of any size with direct extension to chest wall† or skin
T4a	Extension to chest wall
T4b	Oedema (including peau d'orange), or ulceration of the skin of the breast, or satellite skin nodules confined to the same breast
T4c	Both 4a and 4b, above
T4d	Inflammatory carcinoma‡
N – Regional lymph nodes	
NX	Regional lymph nodes cannot be assessed (e.g. previously removed)
N0	No regional lymph node metastasis
N1	Metastasis to movable ipsilateral axillary (same side) node(s)
N2	Metastasis to ipsilateral axillary node(s) fixed to one another or to other structures
N3	Metastasis to ipsilateral internal mammary lymph node(s)
M – Distant metastasis	
MX	Presence of distant metastasis cannot be assessed
M0	No distant metastasis
M1	Distant metastasis (includes metastasis to supraclavicular lymph nodes)§

* Paget's disease associated with a tumour is classified according to the size of the tumour.

† Chest wall includes ribs, intercostal muscles and serratus anterior muscle but not pectoral muscle.

‡ Inflammatory carcinoma of the breast is characterised by diffuse, brawny induration of the skin with an erysipeloid edge, usually with no underlying palpable mass. If the skin biopsy is negative and there is no localised, measurable primary cancer, the T category is pTX, when pathologically staging a clinical inflammatory carcinoma (T4d). When classifying pT, the tumour size is a measurement of the *invasive* component. If there is a large in situ component (e.g. 4 cm) and a small invasive component (e.g. 0.5 cm) the tumour is coded pT1a. Dimpling of the skin, nipple retraction or other skin changes, except those in T4, may occur in T1, T2 or T3 without affecting the classification.

§ The category M1 may be further specified according to the following notation: BRA: brain, HEP: hepatic, LYM: lymph nodes, MAR: bone marrow, OSS: osseous, OTH: other, PER: peritoneum PLE: pleura, PUL: pulmonary, SKI: skin.

Pathological classification not listed. (UICC 1987)

TABLE 4.2 *Union Internationale Contre Cancer staging system combining the TNM classification*

UICC Stage	TNM CLASSIFICATION
I	T1, N0, M0
II	T1, N1, M0; T2, N0–1, M0
III	Any T, N2–3, M0; T3, any N, M0; T4 any N, M0
IV	Any T, any N, M1

(Baum & Schipper 1999)

may be used; this system combines the three independent prognostic factors of tumour size, axillary nodal status and the histological grade. Each of the prognostic factors is assigned a number (from 1–3) which are added together to give a prognostic index (from 3–9). The higher the prognostic index, the worse the prognosis for the patient (Sainsbury et al 1995, Miller 1995, Baum & Schipper 1999).

COMMON PRESENTING SYMPTOMS

Often it is the woman herself or her partner that discovers she has a breast lump or a change in her breast size or shape. The nipple may have become newly inverted or dimpling or creasing of the skin of the breast may develop. When felt, a palpable breast cancer is usually painless, is often irregular to the touch or may be an area of thickened breast tissue. Signs of inflammation and tissue oedema may also be present, and superficial veins may dilate and become more visible if partially obstructed by a tumour. Pain is rarely a presenting feature, but sometimes a sharp, pricking pain is the first symptom experienced.

Increasingly, cancers are being diagnosed during routine breast screening and are seen as a defined mass, or a collection of irregular calcification, on the mammogram.

In extreme cases the tumour may be advanced at the time of presentation. The tumour may be fixed to the muscles beneath the breast. There may also be large palpable axillary lymph nodes, or ulceration of the tumour through the skin causing an infected, bleeding, malodorous wound. Oedema of the arm will result if the cancer in the axillary lymph nodes are involved with tumour and this blocks the drainage of lymph fluid from the arm.

BREAST CANCER AND PREGNANCY

About 200 patients annually will develop gestational breast cancer. The traditional belief was that women should abort their pregnancy if they developed a breast cancer; however the recent research strongly suggests that, although gestational breast cancers present at a later stage than cancers in non-pregnant women, the age and stage-matched outcome is the same (Saunders & Baum 1993). The diagnostic delay is probably because the breast is engorged and lumps are thought to be a normal part of the pregnant breast, and any lump that is detected is attributed to the effects of pregnancy (Saunders & Baum 1993).

Any woman who has the signs and symptoms of a breast cancer should be investigated as soon as possible. There are problems if the woman is pregnant such as engorged breasts, making the breasts difficult to examine. Mammograms are possible if the fetus is shielded in some way, although the breasts are often too dense to reveal any abnormality and ultrasound is probably the best way of visualising the breast. Cytology can be difficult to obtain from a swollen breast but every effort should be made to get a definitive diagnosis.

The management will probably include a mastectomy because often the tumour is discovered when it is quite large and this procedure will mean that the woman has a good chance of avoiding radiotherapy. Radiotherapy is not usually given because of the risk to the fetus, although it can be delayed and given once the baby is born. As a rule, hormone therapy is not given during the pregnancy, although milk production is suppressed with bromocriptine to reduce the size and vascularity of the breasts pre-operatively and to lessen the risk of infection and the formation of galactocoeles in the healing breast.

Chemotherapy is not given in the first trimester of pregnancy but is not thought to cause any problems to the developing fetus after that.

Nursing care

The care of a woman who is pregnant and has breast cancer is best handled with great sensitivity and by a multidisciplinary team with some prior experience of handling patients with this problem. The social and psychological support required by the woman and her partner will be considerable and referral on to the breast care nurse and/or other forms of psychological support will be invaluable. The care of the baby after it is born will be crucial so that the mother can recover from her surgery and cope with any adjuvant chemotherapy or radiotherapy treatment that she is recommended. Organising this support may need some ingenuity involving her local social services as well as any family or friends who are willing to help.

PREVENTION IN THE PRESENT

Over the last 30 years advances in treatments for breast cancer have begun to reduce the UK mortality rate. Research has been unable to identify clear causative factors that would enable the implementation of a primary prevention programme, but we know that if women are diagnosed at an early stage in their disease, treatment is likely to be more effective. Taking measures to detect breast cancer earlier appears to be one way of reducing breast cancer deaths and the breast cancer screening programme has been set up in the UK to this end. Only constant review of the screening programme will tell us if this is an effective strategy. Much research is ongoing into all areas of breast cancer treatment and the causes of breast cancer, in an attempt to reduce the mortality, morbidity and prevalence of this disease.

The physical and psychological nursing care of the woman with breast cancer will be covered in detail, in the following chapters.

REFERENCES

Baum M, Saunders C, Meredith S 1994 Breast Cancer, A guide for every woman. Oxford University Press, Oxford

Baum M, Schipper H 1999 Fast Facts – Breast Cancer. Health Press Ltd, Oxford

Blackwell R E 1996 Benign tumours of the breast. In Blackwell R E, Grotting J C (eds) Diagnosis and Management of Breast Disease. Blackwell Science, MA, USA, ch 1, p 5–19

Cancer Research Campaign 1996 Breast Cancer UK, Fact sheet 6.1–6.5, Cancer Research Campaign, London

Cancer Research Campaign 1997 Cancer Genetics Fact Sheet. Cancer Research Campaign, London

Collaborative Group on Hormonal Factors in Breast Cancer 1997 Breast cancer and hormone replacement therapy: Collaborative reanalyses of data from 51 epidemiological studies of 52 705 women with breast cancer and 108 411 without breast cancer. Lancet 350: 1047–1059

Crowe D R, Lampejo O T 1996 Malignant tumours of the breast. In: Blackwell R E, Grotting J C (eds) Diagnosis and Management of Breast Disease. Blackwell Science, MA, USA, ch 5, p 103–135

Curling G, Tierney K L 1997 Breast screening and breast disorders. In: Andrews G (ed) Women's Sexual Health. Baillière Tindall, London, ch 10, p 221–257

Denton S 1996 Breast Cancer Nursing. Chapman and Hall, London

Eeles R 1996 Testing for the breast cancer predisposition gene, BRCA1. Editorial, British Journal of Medicine 313: p 572

Fallowfield L 1991 Breast Cancer. Routledge, London

Fowble B, Goodman L R, Glick J H, Rosato E F 1991 Breast Cancer Treatment – A comprehensive guide to management. Mosby, St Louis

Gutierrez A A, Lemoine N R, Sikora K 1992 Gene therapy for breast cancer. Lancet 339: 715–721

Howell A, Baildam A, Bundred N, Evans G, Anderson E 1995 Should I take HRT, doctor? Hormone replacement therapy in women at increased risk of breast cancer and in survivors of the disease. Journal of the British Menopause Society 9–17

Kroman N, Jensen M-B, Melbye M, Wohlfahrt J, Mouridsen H 1997 Should women be advised against pregnancy after breast cancer treatment? Lancet 350: 319–322

MacDonald D J 1997 Cancer Genetics. Seminars in Oncology Nursing 13: 123–128

McKenna M C, Zevon M A, Corn B, Rounds J 1999 Psychosocial factors and the development of breast cancer: a meta-analysis. Health Psychology 18(5): 520–531

McPherson K, Steel C M, Dixon J M 1995 Breast cancer. Epidemiology, risk factors, and genetics. In: Dixon J M (ed) ABC of Breast Diseases. BMJ Publishing Group, London, ch 5, p 18–22

Office for National Statistics 1996 ONS MONITER MBI 96/1. Registrations of cancer diagnosed in 1991, England and Wales

Miller W R 1995 Prognostic factors. In Dixon J M (ed) ABC of Breast Diseases. BMJ Publishing Group, London, ch 13, p 49–53

Page D L, Steel C M, Dixon J M 1995 Carcinoma in situ and patients at high risk of breast cancer. In: Dixon J (ed) ABC of Breast Diseases. BMJ Publishing Group, London, ch 16, p 61–65

Powles T, Eeles R, Ashley S et al 1998 Interim analysis of breast cancer in the Royal Marsden Hospital tamoxifen chemoprevention trial. Lancet 352: 98–101

Protheroe D, Turvey K, Horgan K, Benson E, Bowers D, House A 1999 Stressful life events and difficulties and the onset of breast cancer: a case control study. British Journal of Medicine 319, 1027–1030

Rahman N 1999 Genetics for Oncologists: Genetic Predisposition to Breast Cancer. CME Oncology, Rila Publications Ltd. 1(3): 76–80

Rodger A, Leonard R C F, Dixon J M 1995 Locally advanced breast cancer. In: Dixon J M (ed) ABC of Breast Diseases. BMJ Publishing Group, London. ch 11, p 42–45

Royal College of Nursing (RCN) 1997 Genetic Screening and Confidentiality. Issues in nursing and health 44. Royal College of Nursing, London

Sainsbury J R, Anderson T J, Morgan D A 1995 Breast cancer. In: Dixon J M (ed) ABC of Breast Diseases. BMJ Publishing Group, London, ch 7, p 26–30

Saunders C M, Baum M 1993 Breast Cancer and Pregnancy: a review. Journal of the Royal Society of Medicine, 86: 162–165

Schairer C, Lubin J, Troisi R, Sturgeon S, Brinton L, Hoover R 2000 Menopausal estrogen and estrogen-progestin replacement therapy and breast cancer risk. JAMA 283(4): 485–491

Stallard S, Litherland J C, Cordiner C M et al 2000 Effect of hormone replacement therapy on the pathological stage of breast cancer: population based, cross sectional study. British Medical Journal 320: 348–349

Stuart Goodman M 1987 Breast Malignancies, in Cancer Nursing Principles and Practice. Jones and Barlett, Boston, USA

UICC 1987 TNM Classification of Malignant Tumours. Springer Verlag, Berlin

Watson M 1994 Psychological aspects. In: Eng C et al (eds) Familial Cancer Syndromes. Lancet 343: 709–713

Velentgas P, Daling J R, Malone K E et al 1999 Pregnancy after breast carcinoma: outcomes and influence on mortality. Cancer 85(11): 2424–2432
White E, Mackay J 1997 Genetic Screening: risk factors for breast cancer. Nursing Times 93(41): 57–59

FURTHER READING

Baum M, Saunders C, Meredith S 1994 Breast Cancer, A guide for every woman. Oxford University Press, Oxford
Denton S 1996 Breast Cancer Nursing. Chapman and Hall, London
Dixon J M, Sainsbury R 1993 Diseases of the Breast. Churchill Livingstone, London
Dixon J M 1995 (ed) ABC of Breast Diseases. BMJ Publishing Group, London

5 Surgical Interventions for Disorders of the Breast

Jill Mitchell and Andrea Gamble

By the end of this chapter the reader should be able to understand more about:

- Surgical excision for benign breast problems
- Breast cosmetic surgery
- Wide local excision for the treatment of breast cancer
- Mastectomy for the treatment of breast cancer
- Breast reconstruction
- Postoperative complications.

INTRODUCTION

Surgery for breast disorders is continually evolving due to changes in surgical techniques and because women are becoming more active participants in their care. This shift in practice has resulted in less radical and mutilating surgery for women with breast cancer, with a move towards breast conservation in the majority of cases.

Surgery remains the commonest form of treatment for both benign and malignant breast conditions.

SURGERY FOR BENIGN BREAST DISORDERS

Surgical excision

There are a range of significant benign breast conditions that are most effectively treated by surgical excision. These conditions are:

- Fibroadenoma
- Benign phyllodes
- Duct ectasia
- Duct papilloma
- Lipoma
- Some aberrations of breast development.

See Chapter 2 for more detail on these conditions.

Breast cysts that have required aspiration on more than two occasions or whose aspirate has been bloodstained may also be treated by this method.

Prior to undergoing an operation the majority of patients will have attended a specialist breast clinic and received a diagnosis following triple assessment. The triple assessment process involves a clinical examination followed by a mammogram or ultrasound and fine-needle aspiration. This process ensures the lump is examined clinically, radiologically and cytologically so that a clear diagnosis can be made. In some centres these investigations and results are all available at the one visit. In other hospitals patients may have to return on separate days to undergo these investigations. Patients are actively encouraged to bring a friend, relative or partner to their hospital visits for support.

During the outpatient consultation a description of the scar and likely cosmetic result are discussed.

Pre- and postoperative care

Pre-operative assessment

Standard pre-operative assessment is usually undertaken prior to surgery and includes:

- Pulse and blood pressure
- Weight
- Urinalysis
- Blood tests
- Electrocardiogram (ECG) depending on patient's age and health
- Chest X-ray (CXR) depending on patient's age and health
- Consent form
- Pain relief information
- Anaesthetic assessment.

A standard pre-operative preparation should include the following steps:

- Gain informed consent
- Provide written and verbal information on the operative procedure
- Ensure the patient has the contact number for the breast care nurse should they have any queries
- Ensure a pre-operative nursing assessment is completed
- Provide the patient with a name band with their identity number on it
- Ensure the patient is nil by mouth for 4–6 hours
- Ensure all make up, jewellery and prosthetics are removed
- Check for allergies
- Carry out an anaesthetic assessment
- Give pre-medication if prescribed
- Escort the patient to theatre.

In addition, the woman (or man) may have been seen by the breast care nurse – a specialist nurse who concentrates on the care of women who have a problem, more specifically cancer, with their breasts. It is generally accepted that a breast care nurse is an important and essential member of the multidisciplinary team in caring for a woman with a breast condition.

On admission to the ward or day case unit, the ward nurse should check that the patient:

- has a full understanding of the operation they are about to undergo
- has an idea of the probable size and position of the scar and cosmetic result
- is aware that there may be some numbness around the scar.

Immediately prior to surgery the patient should see the surgeon, who will indicate the operation site with a marker pen.

Postoperative care

Standard postoperative care should be undertaken to include:

- Checking level of consciousness
- ½-hourly observations: checking pulse and blood pressure, increase to 1-hourly and 2-hourly when stable
- 1-hourly temperature checks
- Providing adequate pain relief
- At each observation checking and observing wound site and drains for oozing, swelling, and haematoma formation
- Keeping an accurate check on fluid input and output.

Some breast surgeons recommend that women should wear a comfortable bra to help alleviate postoperative discomfort.

Breast asymmetry

There are many reasons why breast size varies from person to person (see Ch. 2 on aberrations of normal breast development). In addition, changes are apparent during puberty with the initial development of breast tissue, during pregnancy and when breastfeeding. As a woman gets older, the breasts naturally begin to droop (ptosis). Also, breast shape and size alters with large losses of weight. Although breasts are naturally different in size (asymmetrical) some women have noticeable differences with one breast much larger than the other. Surgery to treat breast asymmetry involves either augmentation of the smaller breast, reduction or elevation of the larger breast or a combination of approaches.

Breast cosmetic surgery

Breast augmentation

Throughout the centuries there have been a variety of surgical techniques aimed at enhancing the appearance of the breast. Oberle & Allen (1994) mention implantation procedures using ivory, stainless steel and rubber, which failed to achieve the desired results! During the early 1900s, injection of a mixture of petroleum jelly, paraffin and olive oil into the breast failed to show improvements on initial efforts made. Later attempts to use injections of free fat from the buttocks were disastrous and left women with scarred, nodular and encysted breasts (Riddle 1986). Other approaches included use of injected silicone and sponge implants but high rates of complications led to their demise (Oberle & Allen 1994). Cronin and Gerow started using a capsule filled with silicone during the early 1960s (Oberle & Allen 1994) which has led to the wide use of implants today. Until recently the use of oil-based implants provided an alternative to saline- or silicone-filled implants. Their use was recently banned by the Government due to reports of local complications in a small number of women, including localised swelling caused by the rupture of implants (Independent Review Group 1998).

Breast surgery to correct asymmetry involves placement of an implant either under breast tissue or behind the muscle on which the breast lies (the pectoralis major muscle). An incision is made either along the inframammary fold, around the areola, or in the axilla. The implant of choice for this procedure is a saline-filled tissue expander. As an alternative a reduction of the opposite breast can be performed.

Mastopexy and reduction mammoplasty

Breast shape and size can be adjusted to achieve a more symmetrical appearance either following surgery for breast cancer or breast augmentation. Surgery involves either reducing the size of the natural breast or lifting it to reduce the natural droop of the breast.

Mastopexy involves removing skin from the breast, the breast being made to look tighter and more cone-like by lifting the breast tissue. The nipple/areola complex is invariably repositioned, resulting in a peri-areolar incision with some potential for loss of nipple sensation.

Reduction mammoplasty is offered to patients where there is a significant difference in size between the normal and reconstructed breast, or both breasts are overenlarged as with juvenile hypertrophy. This is an option for women who have undergone mastectomy and may wish to have the option of wearing a smaller and lighter prosthesis. This is not a minor operation and therefore has disadvantages and risks including substantial scars that may spread, loss of or changes in nipple sensation, delayed skin healing, skin and nipple necrosis and a possible inability to breastfeed. However, some women may be prepared to accept these risks for their breast shape and size to look more balanced.

Excision biopsy

If a patient has abnormal, but inconclusive histology results from a suspicious breast lesion they may require a formal excision biopsy.

On admission to the ward the woman may be both anxious and distressed due to the uncertainty of her diagnosis. Routine pre-operative preparation should be undertaken. The ward nurse should be sensitive to the fact that this patient's outcome is less certain and that, ultimately, a diagnosis of cancer may be made. Postoperative care should be routine, although the ward nurse should be aware of the possibility that the patient is likely to remain anxious until the final pathology results are available.

Wire localisation biopsy

For a woman who presents via the National Breast Screening Programme (see Ch. 3) with a lesion that is both impalpable and suspicious, the abnormal area of breast tissue needs to be biopsied using a needle positioned under mammographic or ultrasound control. The procedure can be both anxiety-provoking and stressful as the woman will be aware of the possibility that she may have breast cancer. Once a diagnosis has been made the area should be surgically removed.

Prior to undergoing the localisation and surgical excision the woman should have ample opportunity to meet the breast care nurse, who can provide a full and detailed explanation of the procedure. Written information can be provided to support explanations.

Following admission to the ward, the woman is normally accompanied to the breast screening unit by a ward nurse. During the diagnostic test a standard baseline mammogram or ultrasound is performed. The area of abnormality is identified by this procedure, and a local anaesthetic injected to numb the area. A small incision is then made into the overlying skin and under further mammographic control, a needle or guidewire is placed in the centre of the abnormal tissue. The area is then X-rayed again with the wire in place to confirm the lesion has been localised. The wire is then covered by a dressing and taped into position to prevent movement prior to its excision. Following the procedure the woman is escorted back to the ward and prepared for theatre.

Regular analgesia can be offered pre-operatively but this is usually unnecessary because the local anaesthetic remains effective for the duration of the pre-operative phase. In a number of centres the localisation may take place the day before. In this instance the woman is likely to be admitted 24 hours before the operation. She may also require analgesia and possibly sedation to aid sleep during the pre-operative night. Patients are normally admitted as a day case but in some instances may need to stay in hospital overnight. Routine postoperative care should be performed. Depending on the formal histology results, more extensive surgery may be required.

Role of the breast care nurse specialist

Faced with a diagnosis of breast cancer, a woman may feel an array of strong emotions. These may disrupt her normal way of coping and make thinking about information and considering complex treatment options difficult. At the end of this process it is often difficult to make decisions. Indeed, the timing of decisions is often fraught due to the need to have surgery relatively quickly. Whilst it is important to involve a woman in the decision-making process, this can feel overwhelming. The breast care nurse specialist plays a key role in ensuring there is adequate time to talk about treatment options and to fully explore feelings in relation to the patient's breast surgery and diagnosis of breast cancer.

SURGICAL MANAGEMENT OF BREAST CANCER

Until the 1970s the surgical management of breast cancer was straightforward. Women routinely underwent a Halsted radical mastectomy. Today the surgical management of breast cancer varies as both breast conservation and mastectomy are considered appropriate treatments: the ratio being 3:1 (Sainsbury et al 1995). The aims of breast surgery are to minimise the risk of local recurrence whilst considering the ultimate cosmetic result.

Breast conservation is becoming an increasingly popular option as it usually offers a more acceptable cosmetic result. The extent of surgery is dependent upon one or more of the following factors:

- Size of lump in proportion to size of breast
- Position of the lump in the breast
- Multifocality of disease (whether there is more than one area in the breast that is diseased)
- Involvement of the nipple
- Involvement of subcutaneous tissues
- Patient choice
- Whether previous breast surgery has been undertaken and, if so, to what extent.

The surgical management of early breast cancer may involve one or more of the following operations:

- Breast conservation – either wide local excision, segmental excision, or quadrantectomy
- mastectomy
- lymph node sampling
- lymph node clearance.

Breast conservation

Breast conservation, also known as a wide local excision, segmental excision or quadrantectomy involves the removal of the lump with a clear margin of normal breast tissue from around the edge of the tumour. As the three terms suggest, each describes the removal of slightly more breast tissue than the last.

Breast cancers suitable for breast conservation include:

- Unifocal disease (single tumours)
- Tumours smaller than or equal to 4 cm
- Tumours larger than 4 cm in a large breast
- No locally advanced disease, no extensive spread to the loco-regional nodes or metastases.

(Sainsbury et al 1995, Baum & Schipper 1999)

Various studies have reviewed the thickness of the surgical excision margin required to safely reduce the risk of local disease recurrence. Opinions differ; Dixon & Sainsbury (1993) suggest a circumference of 1 cm of normal breast tissue. Most surgeons aim to remove 1 cm macroscopically with the knowledge that the tumour may be closer to the excision margin microscopically.

The operation is seen as a minor physical procedure. In some instances it is performed as a day case, in others cases a stay of between 3–5 days in hospital is involved. Nonetheless the mental adjustment to a diagnosis of breast cancer should not be underestimated. This surgery is usually combined with a secondary procedure to remove some or all (known as axillary sampling or axillary clearance) of the loco-regional lymph nodes. This will be discussed in more detail later.

On admission to the ward the patient should be given adequate time and understanding. They may feel anxious and tearful as they are likely to have only recently received their diagnosis.

As for the previous breast operations, standard pre-operative preparation should be undertaken. In addition, the patient normally has an opportunity to meet the consultant breast surgeon and the breast care nurse in clinic, who should discuss the following:

- The diagnosis and its implications
- Treatment options
- Position and likely appearance of the scar
- Support that is available locally and nationally.

At the operation one or two surgical incisions will have been made depending on the position of the tumour, to remove both the tumour itself and a sample or clearance of lymph nodes. None, one or two drains may be inserted at this time and are usually left in place until they drain less than approximately 30 ml in 24 hours. The wounds are sutured with either interrupted, continuous or dispersible sutures. (If the sutures need to be removed this is normally done either in clinic, at home by the district nurse, or at the doctor's surgery by the practice nurse between 7–10 days postoperatively.) Surgical wounds are covered by a dressing, the choice of which is usually dependent on the surgeon's preference. This is normally left in place until the sutures have been removed, when the patient feels able to cope with the wound being left exposed, or when patient comfort allows.

Mastectomy

A mastectomy usually involves the removal of all breast tissue, the covering skin, and the nipple and areola.

Breast cancers that are more suitably treated by a mastectomy include:

- Widespread pre-invasive breast disease
- Tumours ≥5 cm
- Clinical or mammographic evidence of more than one area of disease
- Tumours that occur within the central portion of the breast and that are close to or involve the nipple
- Relapsed local disease previously treated by breast conservation
- Patient preference.

Halsted radical mastectomy

Whilst the radical mastectomy is not performed today, it was the most commonly performed operation, even for a small breast cancer, until the early 1970s. Both the pectoralis major and minor muscles were removed in addition to all of the breast tissue. The operation was mutilating as it left a hollowed chest and an exposed rib cage covered only by skin as well as a number of long-term postoperative complications such as lymphoedema, nerve damage, and restricted arm movement.

Today the most commonly performed mastectomy procedures are: (1) modified radical (Patey) mastectomy and (b) simple mastectomy.

Modified radical/Patey mastectomy

In the modified radical or Patey mastectomy procedure, all of the breast tissue, the covering skin, nipple, areola and pectoralis minor muscle are removed. The removal of the muscle allows for easy access to the axilla so that a full level 3 axillary clearance and the surrounding pad of fat can be removed.

Simple/total mastectomy

A simple/total mastectomy involves removal of all of the breast tissue, the covering skin, nipple, areola, and axillary tail with or without a sample of axillary lymph nodes. Cosmesis for both of these two procedures is similar.

According to Sainsbury et al (1995), one in three breast tumours are unsuitable for breast conservation but are treatable by a mastectomy. The operation is seen as a more major procedure than breast conservation surgery and usually involves a hospital inpatient stay of between 2–7 days.

On admission to the ward the patient should be given adequate time and understanding. They may be both anxious and tearful as they are likely to have only recently received their diagnosis.

As for the previous breast operations standard pre-operative preparation should be undertaken. In addition the patient normally has an opportunity to meet the consultant breast surgeon and the breast care nurse in clinic, who should discuss the following:

- The diagnosis and its implications
- Treatment options
- Position and likely appearance of the scar
- Discuss and show a photo of a scar
- Discuss and show a temporary and permanent breast form
- Support that is available locally and nationally.

One surgical incision is usually made transversely across the chest wall so that both the breast and the axillary surgery can be performed at the same time. One or two drains are inserted and usually remain in situ for several days or until they drain less than 30 ml in 24 hours. As for breast conservation the wound is usually sutured with continuous, interrupted or dispersible sutures that remain in situ for 7–10 days. The wound is then covered by a dressing, which is usually left intact for as long as the patient wishes.

Axillary surgery

Whilst the management of primary breast tumours is important, research indicates that death occurs as a result of metastatic disease (i.e. breast cancer that spreads to other parts of the body). As breast cancer is spread via either the

CASE STUDY 1

Caroline is a 48-year-old woman whose partner has discovered a small lump in the upper outer quadrant of her left breast. Following referral to her local consultant breast surgeon, triple assessment has confirmed that this lump is malignant. Caroline and her partner are devastated by the news and are offered immediate support, information and advice from a breast care nurse.

During their consultation with the surgeon and the breast care nurse, Caroline is offered a choice in relation to treatment options.

As the lump is small and mobile, and in the outer quadrant of her breast, Caroline is offered a wide local excision and axillary sampling followed by radiotherapy, or a mastectomy and axillary sampling plus or minus radiotherapy depending on the histology results. The advantages and disadvantages of both procedures as seen by Caroline and her partner and explored by the breast care nurse are set out in the Box.

BOX *Advantages and disadvantages of breast conservation and mastectomy*

Advantages

Breast conservation

- The operation is less disfiguring than a mastectomy; Caroline would be able to maintain her own body image
- It is also more cosmetically pleasing, with a smaller scar
- She would be able to wear clothing and underwear she likes

Mastectomy

- The operation is more extensive/radical, so she is less likely to need radiotherapy
- There is a shorter period of treatment when compared to breast conservation and radiotherapy, so she is likely to have a speedier recovery

Disadvantages

Breast conservation

- There is a risk that the tumour will be incompletely excised, so Caroline may need to undergo further surgery
- There is a slightly higher risk of local recurrence in the longer term than there would be if she chose a mastectomy
- She would need an additional course of radiotherapy to the breast and possibly the axilla
- There would be a longer period of treatment

Mastectomy

- Caroline's breast and nipple would be removed
- She would need to consider the options for recreating her own body image either by wearing an external breast prosthesis or opting to undergo breast reconstruction
- She would have a larger scar
- She may still require additional radiotherapy

Having received written information on both procedures, Caroline and her partner are given time to consider both options. The surgeon requests that Caroline make her decision prior to her hospital admission. She is given a contact number for the breast care nurse and is aware that they can meet again for further discussion, should she wish to.

Caroline and her partner choose for her to undergo a wide local excision and axillary sampling and radiotherapy. The procedure is performed within 10 days of her clinic attendance and proceeds without complications.

CASE STUDY 1 (*contd*)

Caroline and her partner return to clinic 1 week following surgery to discuss the histology results with both the consultant surgeon and the breast care nurse, and for the removal of her sutures. At clinic the following information is discussed:

- Grade of tumour
- Excision margins
- Lymph node status
- Oestrogen receptor result
- Presence of vascular or lymphatic invasion.

This information is particularly important when discussing whether further surgery, radiotherapy, chemotherapy or hormone treatment are recommended (see Ch. 4 about the staging of a breast cancer).

The results show the lump has been completely excised and her lymph glands were not involved. Her wound has healed well and she is delighted with the excellent cosmetic result.

Caroline is referred to the radiotherapist for consideration of additional, adjuvant treatments: chemotherapy, radiotherapy and hormone treatments (See Ch. 6 for detail on adjuvant medical treatments for breast cancer).

lymphatic system or the blood supply, surgical management of the axilla is extremely important, from both a staging and treatment management perspective. Some research has shown that the axillary lymph node status is the single best prognostic indicator (Dixon & Sainsbury 1993).

Surgery to remove some of the contents of the axilla includes:

- Axillary sampling
- Partial level 1 or 2 clearance
- Total axillary clearance/complete axillary dissection
- Sentinel node biopsy.

The British Association of Surgical Oncologists (BASO) Guidelines clearly state a minimum of four lymph nodes should be dissected to adequately stage the axillary contents (British Association of Surgical Oncologists 1998).

All women should be informed pre-operatively of the possibility of developing lymphoedema following any form of axillary surgery and given instructions on arm care and exercises (Fig. 5.1) (this is covered in more detail later).

Axillary sampling

An axillary sampling may be performed as a separate staging operation, following an excision biopsy, or in addition to either breast conservation or a mastectomy (see Fig. 1.2, Ch. 1, for the positioning of the loco-regional lymph nodes of the breast). During this procedure about 40% of the lymph nodes that are at the side border of the pectoralis minor muscle are removed. This means that usually only level 1 lymph nodes are sampled. However, palpable nodes from levels 2 or 3 may also be removed.

FIGURE 5.1

Shoulder exercises after breast and axillary surgery. Reproduced with kind permission of Oxford Medical Illustrations, the John Radcliffe Hospital, Oxford.

From first postoperative day

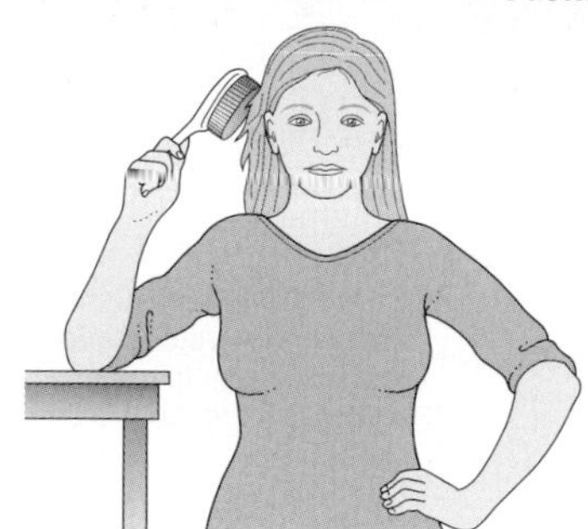

1. **Hair brushing:** Sitting down, rest your elbow on a table. Keep your head straight, start by brushing one side only and gradually increase to your whole head.

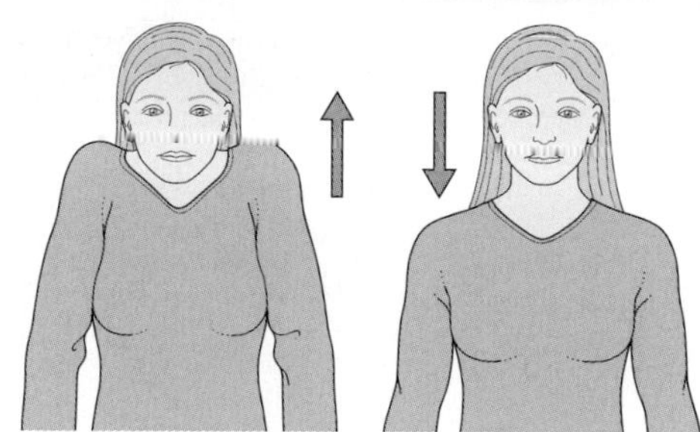

2. Shrug your shoulders upwards and downwards. Pull your shoulders forwards and backwards. Circle your shoulders. Repeat the process.

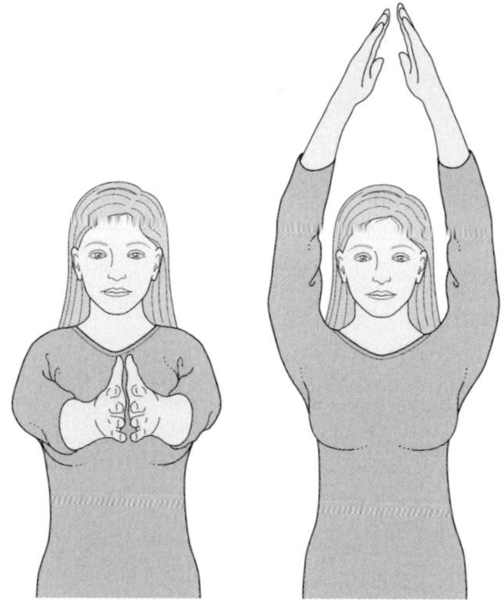

3. Hold your hands together. Keep your elbows straight. Lift both arms up, aim a little higher each time until full elevation can be reached.

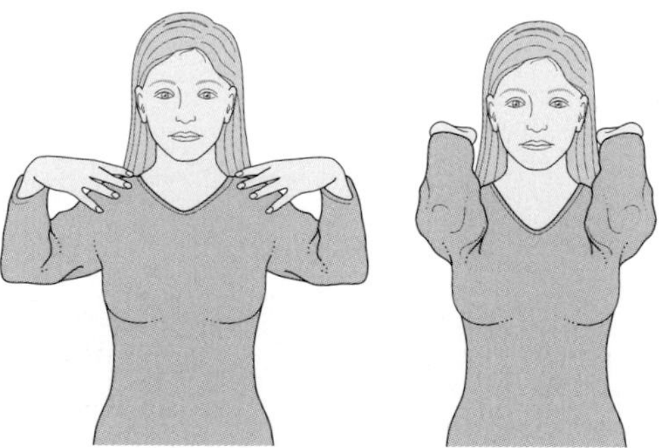

4. Place your fingertips on your shoulders. Concentrate on the direction of movement of your elbow. Lift your elbows forwards and backwards as far as possible. Lift your elbows away from your side.

FIGURE 5.1

Cont'd.

Following removal of your drain

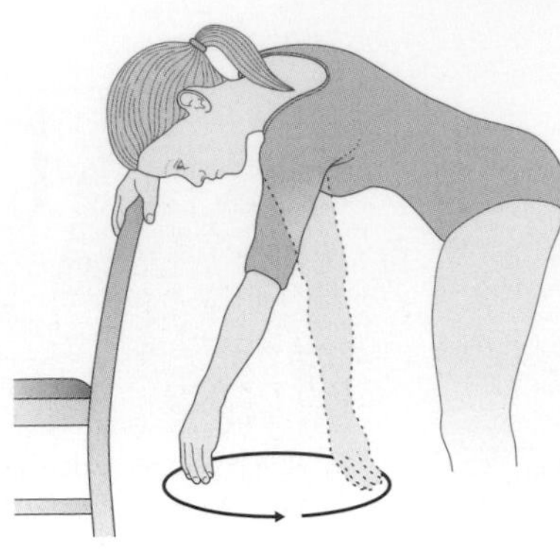

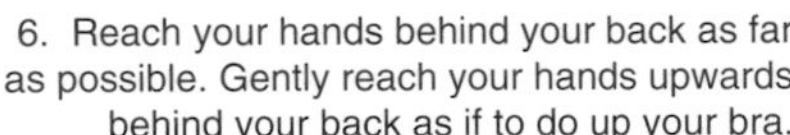

5. **Arm swinging:** Standing upright, lean forwards with support from your unaffected arm resting on a chair, allow your other arm to hang loosely. As your arm relaxes, gradually increase the size of each circle.

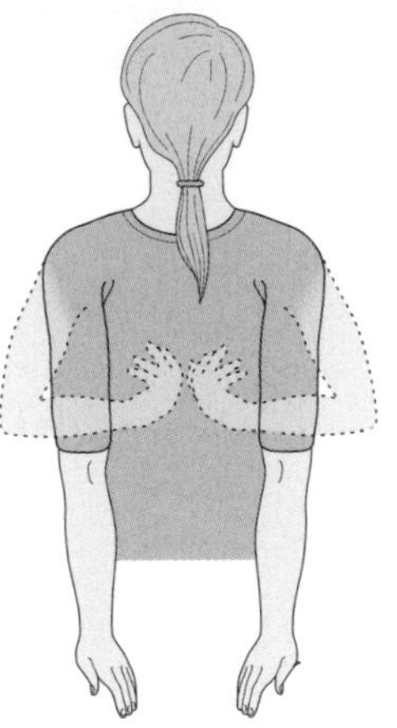

6. Reach your hands behind your back as far as possible. Gently reach your hands upwards behind your back as if to do up your bra.

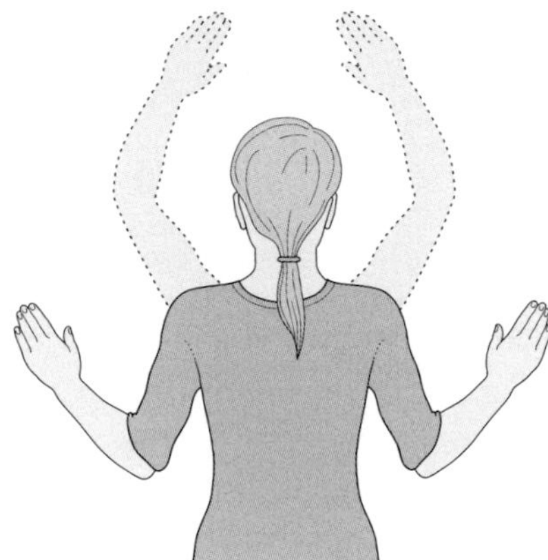

7. **Wall reaching:** Stand at arm's length facing a wall with hands at shoulder level. Place both hands up against the wall and slide back down to shoulder level. Aim a little higher each day.

At home

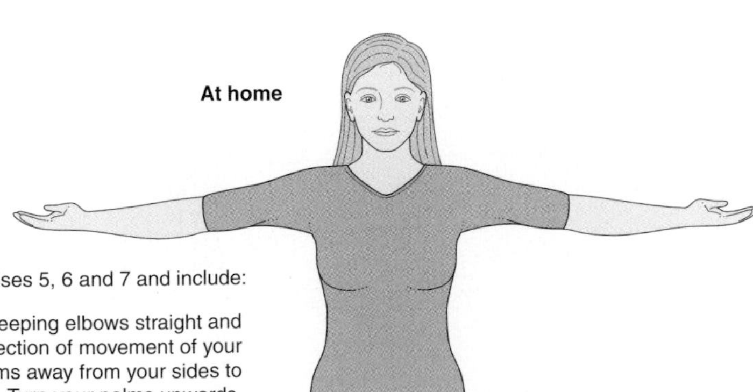

Continue exercises 5, 6 and 7 and include:

8. Whilst standing, keeping elbows straight and concentrating on the direction of movement of your hands – lift your arms away from your sides to shoulder level. Turn your palms upwards.

FIGURE 5.1

Cont'd.

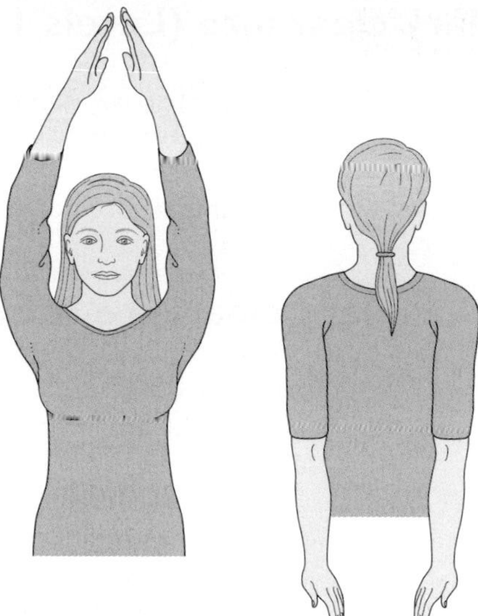

Continue to lift your hands above your head. Lower your arms and reach behind your back as far as possible.

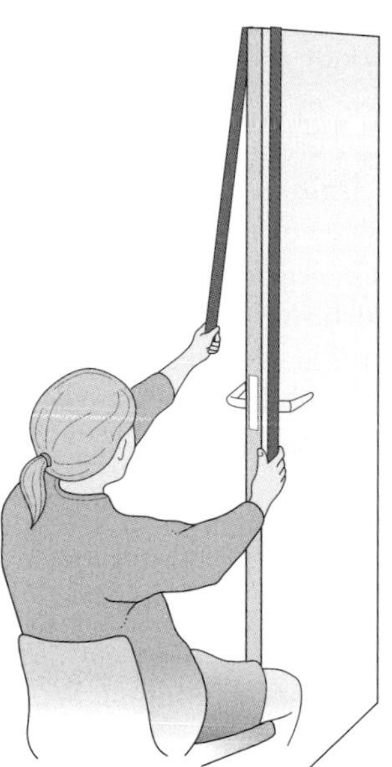

9. **Rope pulley:** Hang a rope or dressing-gown cord over an open door. Sit with the door between your legs. Hold lower end in your affected hand and gently pull down on the other end. Raise your arm as high as possible until full elevation is achieved.

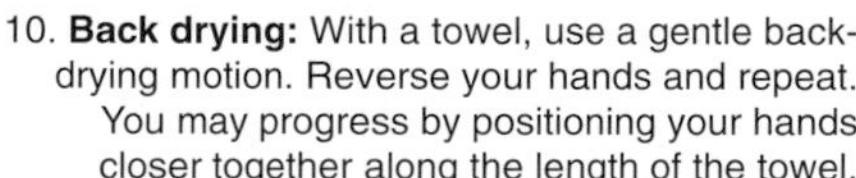

10. **Back drying:** With a towel, use a gentle back-drying motion. Reverse your hands and repeat. You may progress by positioning your hands closer together along the length of the towel.

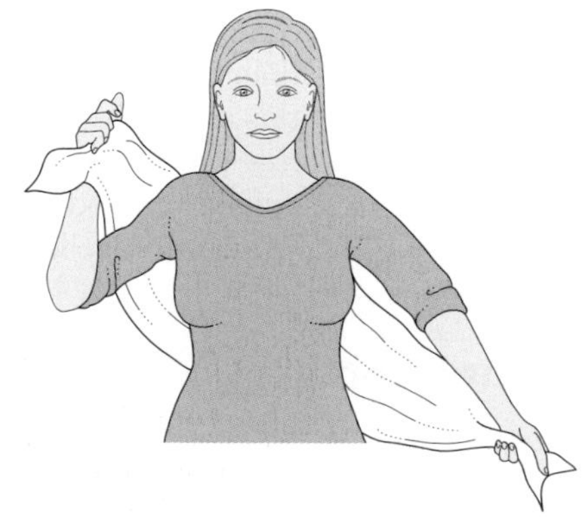

Axillary clearance (Levels 1 & 2)

During a partial axillary clearance, 70–80% of the contents of the axilla are removed. Adipose tissue that contains level 1 & 2 lymph nodes, around the pectoralis minor muscle is also dissected. The apex of the axilla and the pectoralis minor muscle are not removed.

Total axillary clearance (Level 3)

During a total axillary clearance, all the axillary contents from the three levels of the axilla are removed, including those medial to the pectoralis minor muscle.

The BASO Guidelines, 1998, recommend that all patients, irrespective of age, diagnosed with breast cancer, should have some form of axillary staging, as it has implications for future treatment and management of their disease.

As a result of axillary surgery, all patients are at risk of lymphoedema, reduced range of shoulder movement, loss of muscle power, and nerve damage (Baum et al 1995). Also, the risk of long-term physical morbidity increases the more the axillary contents are disturbed.

The immediate postoperative care of a patient following axillary surgery should be the same regardless of the extent of surgery. In a number of centres following an axillary sampling, a drain is not placed in the axillary cavity. Following a partial or complete axillary clearance, the majority of patients will have an axillary drain in situ, which normally stays in place until the serous drainage is less than 30 ml over a 24-hour period.

The surgical management of the axilla remains controversial; some surgeons promote axillary dissection/clearance, whilst others prefer to use axillary sampling with additional radiotherapy where necessary.

Sentinel node biopsy

A recent technique set to revolutionise the management of the axilla has been the introduction of the sentinel node biopsy technique. Whilst still in its infancy, this procedure sets out to identify the main lymphatic drainage system by injecting a radioactive dye around the tumour bed and then X-raying at regular intervals. Once identified, the main drainage node is removed and if it contains tumour cells, formal axillary staging is undertaken. If no cancer cells are present then no further axillary surgery is required and the morbidity associated with this surgery can be avoided. An accuracy rate of over 90% has been quoted for this procedure but research will continue until it is proved that this is a guaranteed method of assessing whether the axillary nodes have been infiltrated with cancer cells or not (Zurrida et al 1997).

Lymphoedema

'Lymphoedema is a chronic swelling due to primary failure of lymph drainage. It arises from a congenitally determined lymphatic abnormality or from damage to

> lymphatic structures by inflammation including infection, tumour, surgery or radiation. It is essentially incurable but the major manifestations namely swelling and infection (cellulitis) can be improved and controlled.'
>
> (British Lymphology Society 1998)

The incidence of lymphoedema after axillary surgery for breast cancer is difficult to estimate. A number of studies have been published and a range of 6–63% has been quoted by various authors (Mortimer & Regnard 1986 in Kirshbaum 1994).

Simple precautions recommended after axillary surgery that may reduce the risk of developing upper arm lymphoedema include:

- Using the arm normally as muscle activity helps prevent swelling
- Gently washing the skin daily, and avoid using perfumed soaps
- Drying the skin thoroughly, especially in-between fingers
- Moisturising daily with a bland cream (e.g. Aqueous Cream)
- Taking care in cutting nails, preferably using clippers
- Using gloves for washing up and gardening
- Avoid lifting or pushing heavy objects
- Removal of underarm hair – if possible using a depilatory cream or electric razor rather than an ordinary wet-shave razor
- Always treating cuts to that arm promptly by washing under running water. Applying an antiseptic cream as a precautionary measure and covering with a dressing or plaster. If any sign of infection develops (e.g. redness, heat, swelling or discharge) the woman may need a course of antibiotics.

Any trauma or damage to the affected arm may increase the patient's risk of developing lymphoedema. For more detail about care of chronic lymphoedema caused by breast cancer, see Chapter 8.

Trauma can be avoided by refraining from the following:

- Having blood pressure checked on that arm
- Having injections and blood taken from that arm
- Getting that arm sunburnt
- Insect bites
- Very hot baths.

Pain

As breast tissue is highly sensitive to touch and temperature change, it would be natural to assume that any surgery involving the breast tissue would be extremely painful. This is not necessarily so. In the majority of cases women who undergo local breast surgery are surprised at the minimal amount of pain they suffer. This is, in part, due to the fact that the majority of breast surgeons inject a local anaesthetic into the operation site at the time of surgery, which continues to numb the area for 6 hours postoperatively.

Other pain-relieving measures that may be useful and which may decrease postoperative discomfort include the application of a tight pressure dressing over the wound to decrease breast movement, or encouraging the patient to wear a soft, comfortable bra both day and night for 2 weeks after the operation.

Once the local anaesthetic has worn off, the ward nurse should offer other prescribed analgesics when required to obtain good pain relief. For those women that do not have a local anaesthetic injected into the wound at the time of surgery, an intramuscular injection or rectal non-steroidal anti-inflammatory medication should be offered until the woman can tolerate oral medication. Women who have undergone more extensive breast surgery, such as a mastectomy or some form of axillary dissection, are likely to have significantly more pain and discomfort than women who have undergone local breast surgery.

In a number of centres a patient-controlled analgesic (PCA) system is set up at the time of surgery to make the woman more comfortable during the first 24 hours postoperatively. This provides her with an element of control over her pain as she is able to self-administer analgesia at the press of a button. Overdose is prevented by restricting the maximum injectable dose in any one hour. Side-effects of the PCA system include nausea and dizziness. Once the immediate pain and discomfort has settled and the woman is tolerating food and fluids, the PCA system can be discontinued. Oral analgesia can be offered 4–6 hourly in the form of paracetamol or co-proxamol, depending on the patient's level of discomfort.

For those women unable to have a PCA system, intramuscular injections should be offered until they are able to tolerate oral medication.

Postoperative pain caused by bruising at the mastectomy site usually improves over a matter of days or weeks. However, intercostal nerve damage that is not noticeable during the immediate postoperative period due to numbness, can become quite troublesome. This is sometimes more problematic than the initial discomfort and may be in the form of axillary soreness, burning or pricking sensations that can be debilitating. It may interfere with arm and shoulder movement but women should be encouraged to continue their exercises. The nurse should reassure her patient that this is quite normal, and that it should eventually settle, whilst offering her oral analgesia to relieve it.

Wound care

According to Dixon & Sainsbury (1993), wound infections are reported to occur in approximately 4% of patients following excision biopsy. Postoperative observations are made for symptoms of pyrexia, inflammation, redness and swelling of the breast, formation of pus/offensive discharge and pain. Antibiotics may be commenced should any or all of these symptoms occur.

As breast tissue is highly vascular, the ward nurse should also observe the breast for haematoma formation. This accounts for approximately 2% of post-operative complications following any form of breast surgery (Dixon & Sainsbury 1993). Haematomas can present suddenly with swelling, bruising, pain and discomfort. Should this occur, the patient may be required to return to theatre for re-opening of the wound to evacuate the haematoma and to establish adequate haemostasis by cautery and suturing.

A similar complication is seroma formation. This is a collection of fluid that accumulates underneath the surgical wound usually following the removal of wound drainage tubes. If this persists it can sometimes be aspirated using a needle and syringe as an outpatient procedure. Aspirations can continue until the fluid stops collecting.

Women are encouraged to shower within days of their surgery. In the longer term some surgeons recommend the application of vitamin E cream to the scar, which can assist in the process of wound healing. Arnica is a herbal remedy prescribed or bought over the counter, to reduce bruising. Whilst frequently used, arnica is not always recommended by the surgeon and permission should be sought from the surgical team before it is taken.

Bras and prostheses

The pre-admission information sent to all women undergoing breast surgery should request that they bring a comfortable bra into hospital with them.

All women who are about to undergo a mastectomy should be given advice pre-operatively regarding the suitability of their bra, and offered an opportunity to see a picture of a mastectomy scar as well as temporary and permanent breast prostheses (Fig. 5.2). Many women wear ill-fitting bras that are the wrong size. Commonly, women report they have always worn the same bra size and have never been correctly measured and fitted (see Ch. 1 for how to be measured properly for a bra).

Pre-operatively the breast care nurse can provide the woman with an opportunity to be measured for her bra, and to discuss types of bras that are suitable following surgery. Generally, the bra should be full cupped, with adjustable straps, and have ample support under the arm, with at least two hooks to fasten at the back. If the bra is thought to be too tight, bra extenders can provide a temporary solution. Half cupped and underwired bras should be discouraged. Half cupped bras generally do not support a permanent breast form adequately. Underwired bras are thought to damage and reduce the life of the prosthesis by

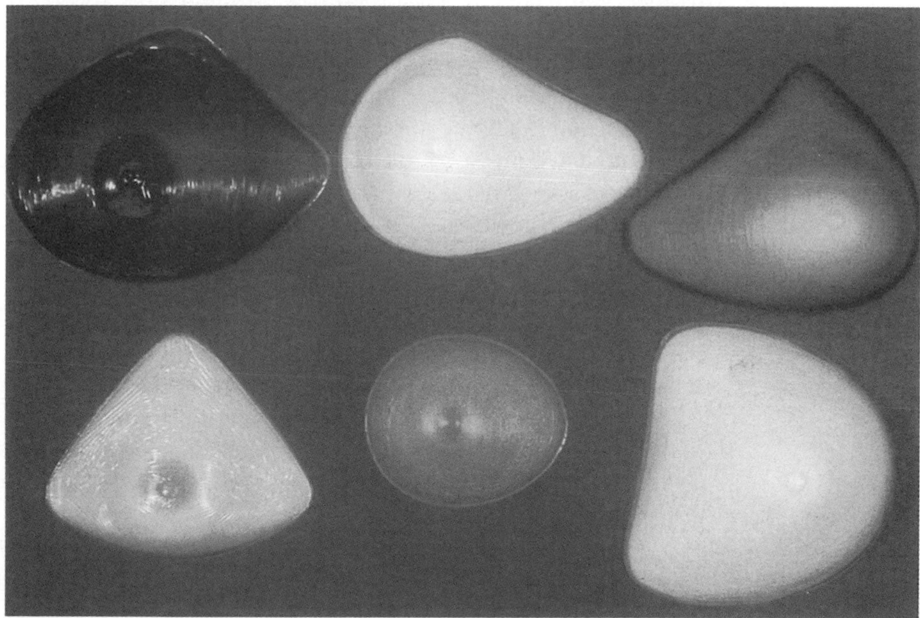

FIGURE 5.2

Breast prostheses. Reproduced with kind permission from Baum & Schipper, 1999, Fast Facts – Breast Cancer, Health Press, Oxford.

pressure and distortion. Women are advised to wear an older bra or crop top immediately postoperatively for comfort.

Following a mastectomy, and prior to discharge home every woman should be offered the opportunity to be fitted with a temporary breast prosthesis (sometimes known as a 'cumfie'). Temporary breast forms come in various sizes: small, medium or large, or 1–14 depending on make and shape. Individual sizes are adjustable allowing for the stuffing to be added and removed as the initial postoperative swelling settles. Some women find the cumfie moves upwards in the bra and can be advised to weigh the prosthesis down by securing it in place with safety pins. This should be fitted in a quiet, private area by the breast care nurse or a ward nurse who has been trained to fit temporary prostheses. This can be quite an emotional time for the woman, as she may see it as a major step forward in her recovery by recreating her external body shape. The nurse should approach the fitting with sensitivity and tact. Making the woman appear whole again may help to boost her confidence as to what she can safely and comfortably wear. The woman should be given the opportunity for her partner to be present throughout the fittings. For those women unable to wear a bra due to postoperative discomfort they can be advised to attach a cumfie inside a nightie or clothing using safety pins.

In centres where the permanent prosthetic fitting is carried out by the appliance officer, the ward nurse should ensure the patient has been referred to this person prior to her discharge home.

Once the initial postoperative swelling has settled and the wound has healed, a permanent breast form can be fitted. This usually takes place 4–6 weeks post-surgery. However, if radiotherapy is required the permanent fitting is delayed until 4–6 weeks after completion of radiation treatment, to allow skin soreness and the chest wall contour to settle.

All women who have undergone breast-conservation surgery, and who are conscious of a noticeable deficit between their treated and untreated breasts are eligible to be fitted with a permanent breast form. As the majority of these women will have had radiotherapy treatment, this should be fitted 4–6 weeks following the completion of radiation treatment as radiotherapy may reduce the size of the treated breast by about 10%.

The first permanent prosthetic fitting normally takes between 30 min and 1 hour. When making the appointment for the fitting, the nurse should encourage the woman to bring a couple of favourite tops. This fitting should be performed by the breast care nurse or an experienced female surgical appliance officer. The breast forms come in a variety of shapes, sizes, makes and also skin colours for ethnic minorities. Every attempt is made to match the remaining breast as closely as possible. There is also the opportunity to be fitted with a prosthetic nipple. To achieve a good cosmetic result it is essential the woman is wearing the correct-sized bra. For women who have larger breasts or do not fit the shapes available, there is a made-to-measure prosthetic fitting service.

During the consultation the woman should be informed of the care instructions, the expected life of the breast form, its length of guarantee and the procedure to follow when it needs to be replaced. She should also receive information and advice about evening wear and swim wear.

It is acknowledged that whilst the majority of women welcome being fitted with temporary or permanent breast forms, a small number prefer to wear nothing.

BREAST RECONSTRUCTION

Introduction

The female breast is viewed symbolically as a source of love, nourishment, comfort and sexuality (Parker & Scullion 1996) so the threat of breast loss can deeply effect these areas of a woman's life.

Tagliacozzi (1597 in Walsh Spencer 1996) draws together the impact of these issues beautifully in the context of breast reconstruction:

> 'We restore, repair and make whole those parts which nature has given but which fortune has taken away, not so much that they may delight the eye but that they may buoy up the spirit and help the mind of the afflicted.'

Breast reconstruction

Breast reconstruction following surgery refers to the replacement of breast tissue to restore breast symmetry, matching as nearly as possible the remaining normal breast. This can be done as an immediate procedure (at the time of the mastectomy) or as a delayed procedure, some months after the mastectomy. The aim of breast reconstruction is to replace breast tissue, to restore breast volume and cleavage, to help the patient regain their sense of 'wholeness' and to adjust to their breast loss.

For the majority of people having surgery for breast cancer, reconstructive surgery is a realistic option. However, in some instances the overall disease status precludes reconstructive surgery, such as a patient with locally advanced or metastatic disease at the time of presentation (Hart 1996). It is advisable to carefully consider this type of operation in relation to the following factors:

- A large invasive tumour because of the associated risk of local recurrence and secondary disease
- Tumour fixation to the chest wall
- Distant disease spread involving other major organs.

Emotional issues

Hart (1996) describes the difficult process women face when making choices about breast reconstruction, and outlines the factors that influence these decisions. Five specific factors are highlighted, which the nurse must bear in mind when assessing someone who is considering reconstructive surgery:

1. Self-knowledge – Understanding the reasons for preferring to have a breast reconstruction including how each woman sees herself, particularly her breasts
2. Economics – The impact of a lengthy period of recuperation upon work, finance, and quality of life, especially given the longer recovery time compared to other forms of breast surgery
3. Medical choices and safety – Ensuring women have free access to information about the full risks and benefits of surgery

4. Self-determined needs – Being able to make choices and act freely. This may involve making a decision without fear of upsetting a partner
5. Interpersonal relationships – The impact of breast surgery upon close relationships, including those at work and social life.

Hart (1996) goes on to highlight other issues that motivate and guide a woman's decisions about breast reconstruction. These are:

- To be able to wear more styles of clothing
- To prevent the need for an external prosthesis
- To feel less preoccupied with her body
- To feel more balanced
- To feel 'whole' again
- To feel more feminine
- To lessen preoccupation with cancer
- To improve marital or sexual relations.

When diagnosed with breast cancer, women experience many strong emotions. Usual ways of coping are disrupted, which makes thinking about information and considering complex treatment options quickly problematic. The breast care nurse and consultant are involved in providing each woman with an opportunity to talk about their expectations of surgery. Approaching this in an open, honest way helps each woman to fully understand what is realistic and achievable; many women find it helpful to know that our aim is for them to look normal in a bra. Realistically breast reconstruction produces a breast mound. The reconstruction may not have the same ptosis (droop) as the natural breast and there may be loss of nipple and skin sensation. The reconstructed breast may look smaller, higher and firmer than the natural breast, depending upon the type of reconstruction. These are important points to discuss when helping someone to prepare for this surgery and decide whether or not they want to go ahead.

Having talked about the range of options, showing photographs of different types of breast reconstruction can help a woman to have both a realistic expectation and outlook. However, this may not suit everyone and needs to be approached sensitively. Meeting a former patient can be helpful to see how someone else has coped with and recovered from surgery. Written information is available to support discussion and reinforce information. The British Association of Cancer United Patients (BACUP) booklet (1998) is particularly useful (see Ch. 7 for useful addresses).

Whilst these issues may seem obvious, the importance of involving each woman in the decision-making process should not be underestimated. The nurse should assess how the woman sees herself, including her femininity, her long-term emotional well-being, and her level of self-confidence. These issues if not explored fully can affect a woman's satisfaction with the final cosmetic result.

Surgical approaches to breast reconstruction

There are various approaches to breast reconstruction, used either at the time of operation (immediate reconstruction) or many months or years later (delayed reconstruction).

Immediate or delayed reconstruction?

It is suggested that women have positive psychological outcomes from undergoing immediate breast reconstruction that include feeling less embarrassed by breast loss. There may also be a reduction in emotional distress.

Delayed reconstruction arguably allows the patient time to adjust to breast loss and the shock of diagnosis. At the time of diagnosis, it is not unusual for a woman to be primarily concerned with having the cancer safely removed and some women decide to delay breast reconstruction in order to wait until they feel free of disease.

In spite of these advantages, breast reconstruction remains uncommon and partial or complete breast loss remains the norm. Patients may decide against breast reconstruction because of the following fears:

- A reconstruction may conceal cancer recurrence
- Reconstructed breasts may not live up to their expectations of how breasts normally look
- Uncertainty about surgery, fear of pain and discomfort (Schain et al 1985)
- Silicone-related problems, including leakage and rupture of the implant.

The techniques used for breast reconstruction (see diagram of breast and chest wall in Figure 1.2 in Ch. 1) are as follows:

- Insertion of a tissue expander placed subpectorally or subcutaneously
- Transfer of skin and muscle to form a breast mound using either latissimus dorsi or transverse rectus abdominus myocutaneous (TRAM) flaps.

Insertion of tissue expander

The insertion of a rough textured silicone tissue expander with a saline filled chamber, done either at the same time as the mastectomy or as a delayed procedure many months later assuming radiotherapy has not been given, is by far the simplest procedure.

This technique involves lifting the pectoralis major and fascia away from the chest wall and creating a pocket for an implant. The implant is placed inside this pocket. Suturing stabilizes the implant, preventing upward or sideways movement of the implant in future (Hinojosa & Layman 1996). A device called a ‘filling port’ attaches to the implant and is placed subcutaneously. A volume of saline is instilled via the port at the time of operation to begin stretching out the overlying skin. A useful way of describing the procedure is ‘blowing up a balloon-like device to stretch and grow new skin’ (Hart 1996). Further inflations begin approximately 2 weeks postoperatively, when the wound is well healed and any bruising and postoperative oedema has settled. This may continue over several weeks to achieve the breast mound. In order to achieve a degree of ptosis, some surgeons advise overinflation of the implant for 2–3 months followed by deflation to achieve symmetry. Patients can choose whether to have the subcutaneous port removed at a later date. This can be done as a simple day case procedure removing the port under a local anaesthetic. Figure 5.3 shows a reconstructed left breast using an inflatable tissue expander and Box 5.1 lists the advantages and disadvantages.

The more recent use and introduction of anatomically shaped implants has provided an alternative means of improving cosmetic results. Their use aims to reduce the problem of upper pole fullness as the reconstructed breast using

FIGURE 5.3

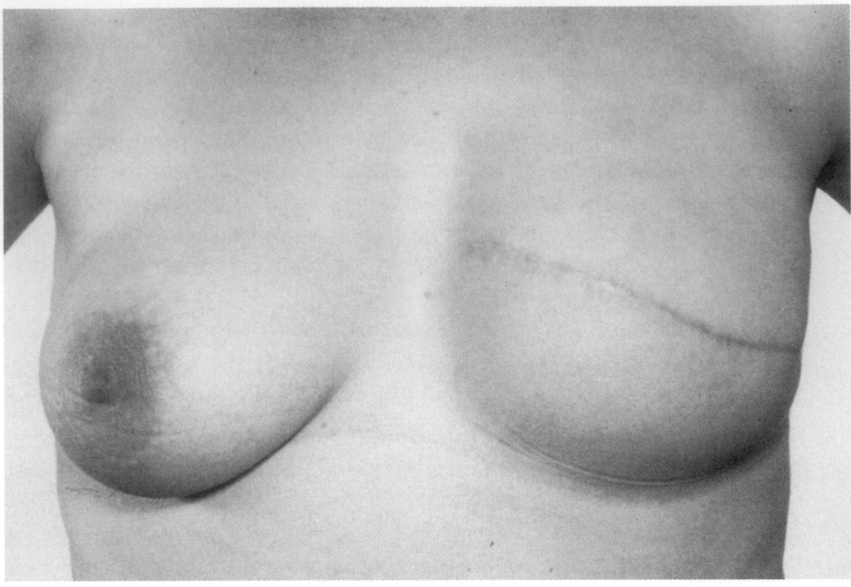

A left breast reconstruction using an inflatable tissue expander. Reproduced with kind permission from Oxford Medical Illustrations, the John Radcliffe Hospital Photography Department and Mr Humzah, Consultant Breast Surgeon.

BOX 5.1 ***Advantages and disadvantages of tissue expansion***

Advantages

- Simple procedure.
- Can be done as an immediate or delayed procedure.
- With small, firm-breasted women, may achieve good symmetry.

Disadvantages

- Expansion can be painful.
- Capsule formation – distortion and pain/discomfort.
- Intrinsic life of implant – approximately 10 years.
- Risk of rupture especially if not fully inflated and the implant wrinkles.
- Risk of infection.
- Cannot be done after radiotherapy.
- During over-inflation women need to wear an external prosthesis and adjust their bra size.
- Breast can look 'pert' because of upper pole fullness.
- Shape and size do not change with weight gain or loss.

hemispherical tissue expanders can look rather pert, although the result should be acceptable in a bra. In women who would like to have more evenly matched breasts, surgery to the other breast, such as a mastopexy or breast reduction, can be offered at a later date. The advantages and disadvantages of this procedure are noted in Box 5.1.

Is silicone safe?

Much concern and controversy has surrounded the use of silicone implants and there has been a great deal of scientific interest looking into these concerns. There is no evidence to support either an increased risk of breast cancer or autoimmune disorders thought originally to be caused by rupture or leakage of silicone into the body (Independent Review Group 1998). Until recently the limited use of soya-based implants provided an alternative to other commonly used implants. However, the Government has recently banned these due to reports of local complications in a small number of women.

Clearly, the need for fully informed consent in relation to any form of breast reconstruction remains important in light of these concerns.

Skin and muscle flaps

The use of skin and muscle flaps provide alternative approaches. Typically this type of surgery is used to move tissue from a distant site to correct a defect. This is useful surgery for someone with larger, ptotic breasts, who has undergone radiotherapy to the chest wall, leaving the skin less elastic and where tissue expansion would be unsatisfactory. Also, some women may not wish to consider the use of a tissue expander containing silicone or may wish to have a more natural looking breast.

Latissimus dorsi flap

The latissimus dorsi muscle is a flat, triangular muscle originating broadly from the spines of the lumbar and sacral vertebrae and the posterior iliac crest. It is supplied by the thoracodorsal artery. Overlying skin takes its blood supply from the muscle so that it can move with it. Figure 5.4 A, B and C shows the stages of a woman undergoing breast reconstruction with a Becker tissue expander and a latissimus dorsi flap.

During this procedure the latissimus dorsi flap consisting of overlying skin, fat and muscle is moved from the upper back. This is tunnelled through the axilla and placed onto the chest wall. If the muscle is too small, as is usually the case, an implant can be placed behind to match the size of the other breast. Advantages and disadvantages of this surgery should be explained fully to the patient (Box 5.2).

Reconstruction following breast conservation provides another way of improving cosmesis. This involves using a mini latissimus dorsi flap, where loss of breast tissue would leave too big a deficit if done alone (Fig. 5.5 shows a mini flap right breast reconstruction).

BOX 5.2 ***Advantages and disadvantages of latissimus dorsi flaps***

Advantages

- Gives good muscle cover for correct sized implant.
- Offers generous amount of skin. Good blood supply.
- Can be used following radiotherapy to the chest wall.

Disadvantages

- Scarring to the back.
- Differences in skin colour and texture.
- Muscle weakness is not usually a problem but should be discussed with women who are keen on sports.

TRAM flap

The TRAM flap reconstructive technique has been a well-established technique since the early 1980s. Surgery involves movement of lower abdominal fat and

FIGURE 5.4

Full LD flap breast reconstruction (A) before (B) the shoulder scar and (C) after. Reproduced with kind permission from Oxford Medical Illustrations, the John Radcliffe Hospital Photography Department and Mr Humzah, Consultant Breast Surgeon.

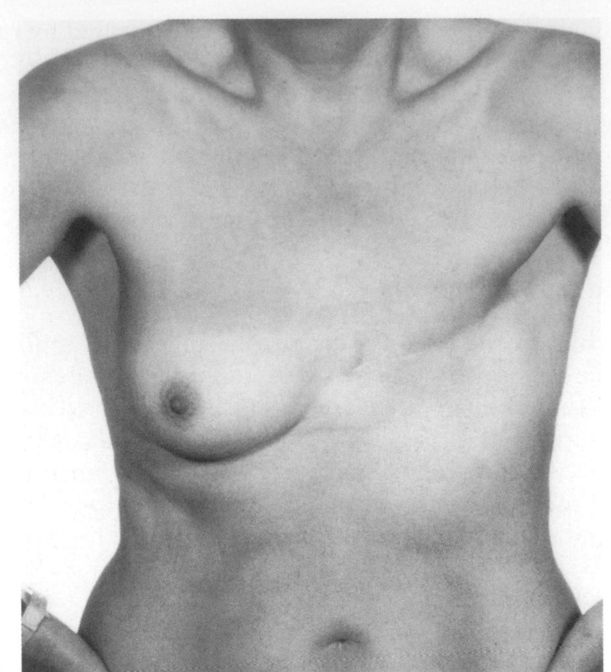

A

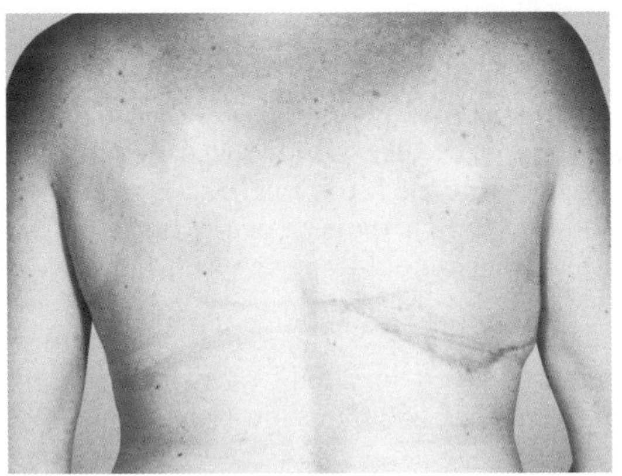

B

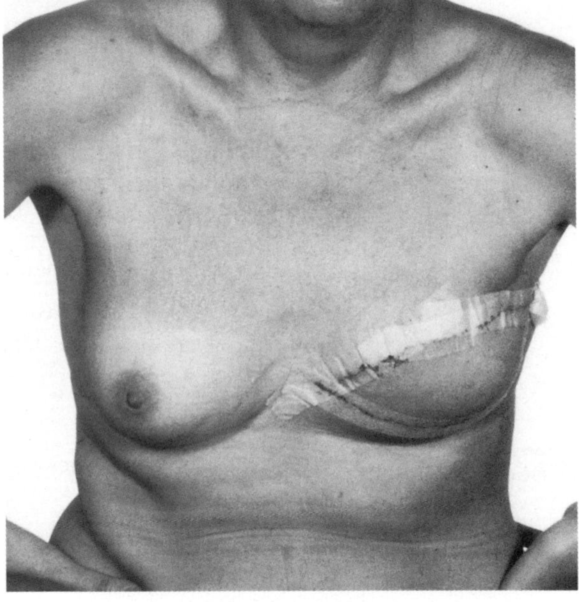

C

skin based on the rectus abdominis muscle (TRAM) flap. This muscle runs from the pubic bone to the breast bone. TRAM flaps are performed as either a pedicled flap based on the superior epigastric artery or a free flap using a microvascular anastomosis. This is acknowledged as giving the most attractive and natural cosmetic result and is the procedure of choice for someone with larger ptotic breasts, where a tissue expander would be unsuitable. This might also suit

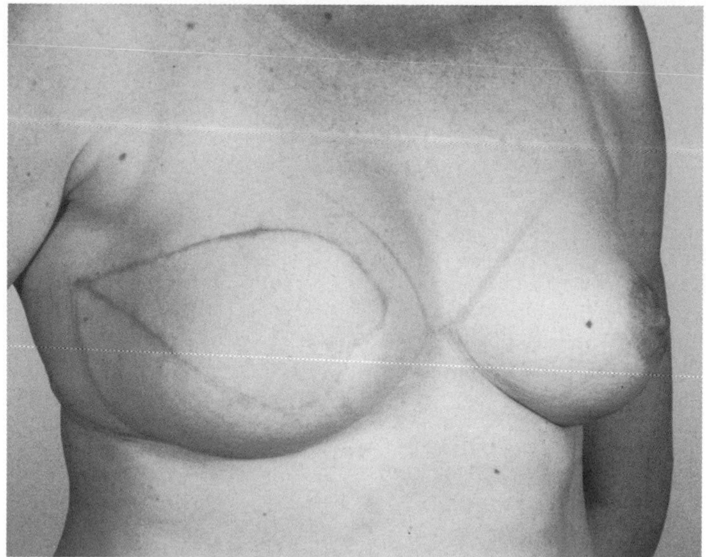

FIGURE 5.5

Mini flap right breast reconstruction. Reproduced with kind permission from Oxford Medical Illustrations, the John Radcliffe Hospital Photography Department and Mr Humzah, Consultant Breast Surgeon.

someone with a failed implant. See Figure 5.6 of a TRAM-flap-reconstructed left breast and abdominal scar.

Caderna et al (1995) reported increased satisfaction amongst women who have chosen to undergo breast reconstruction using their own skin and muscle. In contrast, patients have reported increased levels of anxiety about the length of operation, anaesthesia, hospital stay and prolonged period of recovery.

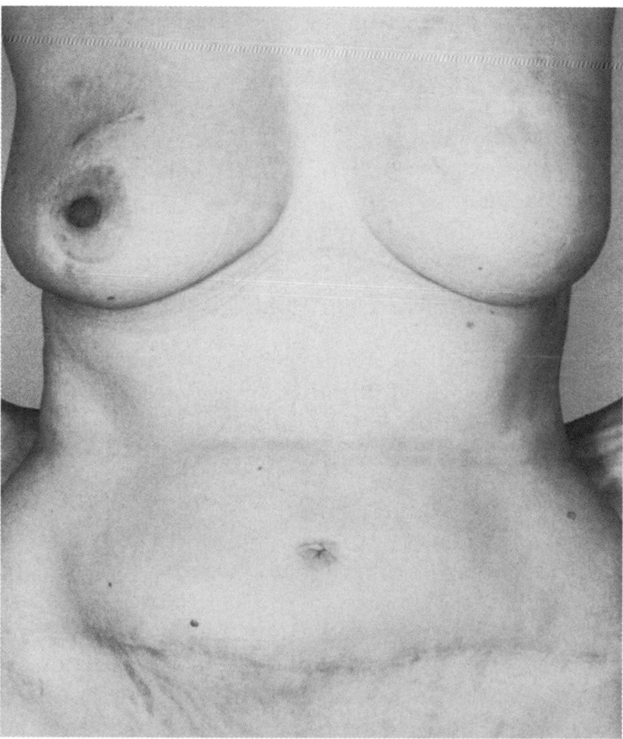

FIGURE 5.6

TRAM flap reconstructed left breast and abdominal scar. Reproduced with kind permission from Oxford Medical Illustrations, the John Radcliffe Hospital Photography Department and Mr Humzah, Consultant Breast Surgeon.

BOX 5.3 *Advantages and disadvantages of TRAM flaps*

Advantages

- Uses all patient's own tissue. Provides a 'tummy tuck'.
- Give a natural ptosis to the breast mound that can be adjusted to the correct size and shape.
- No need for an implant.
- Can be done for people who have previously had radiotherapy to the chest wall or who have had surgery leaving an extensive chest wall deficit.

Disadvantages

- Lengthy period of recuperation – up to 3 months.
- Lengthy anaesthesia – up to 7 hours' duration.
- Size of abdominal scar.
- Abdominal weakness, 'bulge' or hernia. This risk is less with a free flap.
- Discomfort and delayed healing creating difficulties with managing activities of daily living.
- Tissue death if blood supply to flap is obstructed.

Before embarking on this type of operation, a woman would need to be in a good state of physical and mental health. A lengthy surgical procedure and prolonged period of recovery pose immediate physical problems. The surgery requires adequate abdominal tissue and a previous abdominal scar may limit the availability of skin for reconstruction. The donor site scar should be discussed with the patient and should be an acceptable part of the operation. Enquiries need to be made about cigarette smoking as heavy smoking may compromise the blood supply to the flap.

The advantages and disadvantages of this operation are well documented (Box 5.3).

TRAM flap surgery is contraindicated in those:

- With previous scars to the abdomen
- People aged 65 years and over
- With other medical problems such as diabetes mellitus, pulmonary or cardiac disease or obesity
- Heavy smokers
- Patients with little in the way of redundant abdominal tissue.

Complications of breast reconstruction

Understanding the range of complications following breast reconstruction helps both the patient to be well informed when choosing whether or not to go ahead with breast reconstruction and the nurse to identify potential risks when caring for patients. These complications are outlined as follows.

Complications of tissue expanders

1. *Capsular contracture*: Placing any foreign substance under the skin causes the body to react by forming scar tissue around it. In time this capsule can become thickened and contracted. Being the commonest complication, these so-called 'fibrous capsules' shrink causing a noticeable hardness around the implant called a 'capsular contracture'. With the introduction of textured implants during the early 1980s, the reported incidence fell from 40–60% to approx-

imately 10% 1 year following surgery. Some people need a surgical procedure to release the fibrous capsule, known as a 'capsulotomy'. However, if the problems of pain, discomfort, and/or an unusually hard feel to the implant persist, removal of the implant may be considered. A new implant can be replaced at the time of operation, but recurrence of the capsule is not uncommon.

Teaching patients how to perform gentle massage around the implant has been advocated to reduce the risk of contracture (Hart 1996). One study compared two groups of patients 6 months following surgery. The experimental group was taught massage techniques beginning 3 days following surgery; the control group was not taught these exercises. Interestingly, there was a lower rate of capsular contracture in the experimental group compared to the control group (Riddle 1986). There is a need for more research to confirm these limited findings.

2. *Infection*: Chronic low-grade infection due to the presence of an implant is well documented. Associated symptoms may include fatigue and intermittent pyrexia. In the event of obvious infection with signs of pain, swelling, heat and discharge from the suture line the implant would be removed. To minimize the risk of infection, prophylactic antibiotics are commenced intra-operatively and then for 7 days following surgery.

3. *Rupture of implants* is reported to occur in 1% of all cases and is said to be a major concern to patients due to the potential leakage of silicone. Common causes of rupture include deterioration of the outer shell over time, undetected damage at the time of operation, a flaw in the original manufacture of the implant or trauma to the breast, e.g. a seat belt injury. Following rupture of an implant the gel or saline is contained within the fibrous capsule created by the body. Changes in the shape and feel of the breast gradually become more obvious. Deflation of a saline filled implant can usually occur within 24–48 hours. The saline is absorbed and eliminated naturally by the body, leaving the silicone outer shell in place.

This initial stage may be followed by spread of gel or saline beyond the fibrous capsule (known as extracapsular spread). Presence of gel outside the fibrous capsule may cause an inflammatory reaction and it can be possible to feel small lumps. At this stage distortion of the shape and size of the implant becomes obvious. In these instances both the implant and gel are removed surgically.

4. *Movement of the implant*: Creating a pocket too large to hold the implant can lead to its rotation. This is usually remedied with minor surgery.

Complications of myocutaneous flaps

1. *Flap necrosis due to vein and arterial thrombosis*: This is reported to occur in approximately 10% of patients undergoing pedicled TRAM flaps and less than 5% of free TRAM flaps, but is very rare in patients with latissimus dorsi flaps. In certain cases areas of necrotic tissue may need to be excised surgically and skin grafts applied to the defect.

2. *Abdominal weakness*: Abdominal herniation is reported in approximately 10% of patients undergoing TRAM flap reconstruction. Usually this is remedied with surgery.

3. *Muscle weakness* may be noticed following latissimus dorsi flap reconstruction in keen sportspeople such as climbers, rowers and swimmers.

4. *Breast asymmetry*: It may not be possible to match the degree of ptosis of the natural breast and so it is important to discuss further options for enhancing the overall symmetry. This involves either breast augmentation, mastopexy or reduction mammoplasty.

Lavine (1993) reports that implants often start out feeling firm and look high compared to the natural breast. Approximately 2–3 months later they usually soften and the position settles over several months. Where asymmetry is related to position of the implant a second operation may be needed to reposition the implant.

Nipple/areola reconstruction

Without doubt, the nipple and surrounding areola give the breast its identity. When faced with a life-threatening illness the absence of a nipple may not be a woman's main concern. It can be helpful to mention options from the outset but most people prefer to wait until they are fully recovered from surgery and any adjuvant treatment is completed. Nonetheless, it is now possible to recreate a nipple–areola complex using a variety of techniques with some excellent and pleasing cosmetic results for the patient. This can be offered within a range of options for breast reconstruction.

The simplest and most common method involves making prosthetic nipples. Initially, an impression is made of the remaining nipple and a colour-matched silicone nipple is prepared. The process usually involves between two and three outpatient visits with nipples usually being supplied within 1 month from the time of their first visit. The false nipple is held in position with a mild water-based adhesive. This can be worn whenever the patient wishes but will stay in place for between 4–6 weeks providing a shape for use under tight fitting clothing and swimwear. Many women say this improves their appearance, making their reconstruction look and feel complete. Alternatively, prosthetics companies produce prosthetic nipples that can be supplied through an appliance fitter or breast care nurse. However, these nipples are less realistic and may not be as pleasing to the patient.

Alternatively, a nipple may be reconstructed using a plastic surgical technique. It is generally advisable to wait 3–6 months before embarking upon nipple reconstruction to allow postoperative oedema to settle, the reconstructed breast to soften, and ideally, for any other treatment to be completed. In the case of radiotherapy, it would be advisable to reconstruct a nipple before treatment starts because treatment causes changes in the microcirculation that may affect nipple viability.

In order to create skin that looks similar to the areola, dark skin can be removed from the upper inner thigh or from the contralateral areola. Excellent results can be achieved by tattooing (micropigmentation). Although the colour may fade with time, it is possible to repeat this process and is recommended for its ease of use and low complication rate.

The tattooing procedure is normally done by a plastic surgeon or by a nurse certified in intradermal micropigmentation, ideally no sooner than 1 month following nipple reconstruction as an outpatient. It is possible to use a combination of different pigments to closely match the colour of the other nipple–areola complex. The tattoo gun, or pen, applies the tattoos using a small cluster of six needles, which pierce the skin using permanent colour. It may be advisable to use local anaesthetic for this procedure depending upon the degree of sensation that the person has in the area to be tattooed. Rare complications include infection and allergic reactions to the dye used. Bleeding is usually minimal but patients are advised of this prior to the procedure so as not to alarm them.

CONCLUSION

Whilst there have been many advances in the management of breast disease, surgery remains the primary treatment of choice. This chapter highlights the key role played by the breast care nurse in providing information and support for women undergoing breast surgery – from simple lump excision to reconstructive surgery, including their potential complications.

The decision-making process is complex and poses a tremendous challenge to women newly diagnosed with breast cancer and their health care team. As we enter the 21st century, the demands on the team are likely to increase in order to meet the diversity of patient needs.

REFERENCES

BACUP 1998 Understanding Breast Reconstruction. Lithoflow Limited, London

British Association of Surgical Oncologists (BASO) Guidelines for Surgeons in the Management of Symptomatic Breast Disease in the United Kingdom (1998 Revision). The BASO Breast Speciality Group

Baum M, Saunders C, Meredith S 1995 Breast Cancer – A guide for every woman. Oxford University Press, Oxford

Baum M, Schipper H 1999 Fast Facts – Breast Cancer. Health Press Ltd, Oxford

British Lymphology Society 1998 Strategy for Lymphoedema Care, Caterham, Surrey

Caderna P S, Yates W R, Chang P, Cram A E, Ricciardelli E J 1995 Post mastectomy reconstruction: Comparative analysis of the psychosocial, functional and cosmetic effects of transverse abdominis musculocutaneous flap vs. breast implant reconstruction. Annals of Plastic Surgery 35(5): 458–468

Dixon M, Sainsbury R 1993 Handbook of Diseases of the Breast. Churchill Livingstone, London

Hart D 1996 The Psychological Outcome of Breast Reconstruction. Plastic Surgical Nursing, Fall 16(3): 167–171

Hinojosa R J, Layman A S 1996 Breast Reconstruction Through Tissue Expansion. Plastic Surgical Nursing, Fall 16(3): 139–145

Independent Review Group 1998 Silicone Gel Breast Implants: The Report of the Independent Review Group. Rogers Associates, Cambridge

Kirshbaum M 1994 The management of lymphoedema after treatment for breast cancer – Clinical Practice Guidelines – Department of Health

Lavine D M 1993 Saline Inflatable Prostheses: 14 years' experience. Aesthetic Plastic Surgery 17: 325–330

Oberle K, Allen M 1994 Breast augmentation surgery: A women's health issue. Journal of Advanced Nursing 20: 844–852

Parker J, Scullion P 1996 Susan's breast reconstruction: a case study and reflective analysis. British Journal of Nursing 5(12): 718–723

Riddle L B 1986 Expansion exercises: modifying contracture of the augmented breast. Research in Nursing and Health 9: 341–345

Sainsbury J R C, Anderson T J, Morgan D A L 1995 Breast Cancer. In: Dixon J M (ed) ABC of Breast Diseases. BMJ Publishing Group, London

Schain S, Wellisch D K, Pasnau R O, Landsverk J 1985 The sooner the better: A study of psychological factors in women undergoing immediate versus delayed breast reconstruction. American Journal of Psychiatry 142(1): 40–46

Tagliacozzi F, De Curtorum (1597 in Walsh Spencer K 1996) Significance of the Breast to the Individual and Society. Plastic Surgical Nursing, Fall 16(3): 131–132
Zurrida S, Galimberti V, Veronesi P et al 1997 Can sentinel lymph node biopsy avoid axillary dissection in node negative breast cancer patients? The Breast – Churchill Livingstone, Edinburgh

FURTHER READING

BACUP 1998 Understanding Breast Reconstruction. Lithoflow Limited, London
BASO Guidelines for Surgeons in the Management of Symptomatic Breast Disease in the United Kingdom (1998 Revision). The BASO Breast Speciality Group
Baum M, Saunders C, Meredith S 1995 Breast Cancer – A guide for every woman. Oxford Medical Publications, Oxford University Press, Oxford

ACKNOWLEDGEMENT

The authors would like to acknowledge the advice and support of Miss P J Clarke, Consultant Surgeon, the John Radcliffe Hospital, Oxford.

6 Medical Treatments for Breast Cancer

Karen Burnet and Catherine Oakley

At the end of this chapter the reader should be able to understand:

- The need for additional medical treatment after primary surgery for breast cancer
- The different types of medical therapy and when they are used to treat breast cancer
- The effect of these medical treatments on the patient and the nursing care of any side-effects caused by these treatments
- The safety issues involved when dealing with radioactive sources and with chemotherapy
- The use of complementary therapies to help with the symptoms of the treatment for breast cancer.

INTRODUCTION

Complete treatment for breast cancer often involves several therapeutic modalities. Once the primary surgery has been performed the nature of the tumour should be known. Its size, grade, position in the breast and whether there are clear margins of normal tissue around the tumour and the axillary node status of the woman will help the clinician to make a decision about further adjuvant treatment. Adjuvant treatment means any treatment that is given alongside, or just after, the primary surgery.

It is well recognised that good breast care is provided by a multidisciplinary team with close liaison between surgeons and oncologists (Breast Surgeons Group of the British Association of Surgical Oncology 1995). Treatment decisions are usually made once the grade of the tumour is known, using the tumour node metastases (TNM) classification system, and the Nottingham Prognostic index (see Ch. 4). There may be some question as to whether the tumour has been completely removed from the breast and the surgeon may feel that re-excision of the tumour bed is required. The prospect of another operation for a woman who will know that she has cancer can be very distressing. The nurse should explain with tact and understanding clearly why a further anaesthetic and more surgery is necessary.

Radiotherapy will be offered as a local treatment to the breast for women who have their breast cancer removed by wide local excision, or after mastectomy, if the margins between the cancer and the normal tissue are close. Most women will undergo radiotherapy if: (1) they have positive node status, (2) they have received primary chemotherapy to shrink the breast tumour, or (3) the tumour cannot be completely surgically excised. Adjuvant chemotherapy will usually be offered to pre- and some postmenopausal women with positive node status (Sledge 1996) and there is gathering evidence to support all young pre-menopausal women with breast cancer receiving adjuvant chemotherapy (Early Breast Cancer Trialists' Collaborative Group 1998a and b, Kroman et al 2000, Dixon & Hortobagyi 2000). Between 50% and 60% of patients have breast cancers that need some level of oestrogen to continue to grow and are oestrogen receptor positive (Powles 1983, Fenlon 1996). For these patients some form of hormone manipulation is another useful adjuvant treatment.

Adjuvant medical treatment is given so that the woman receives the optimal local and systemic treatment to prevent the cancer from returning (i.e. cure) or to prolong the time before it recurs (i.e. time to disease relapse).

This chapter will consider radiotherapy, hormone therapy, and finally chemotherapy. New advances in medical treatments are also discussed. In addition to being used adjuvantly, all these treatments can be utilised in the treatment of recurrent loco-regional breast cancer or metastatic breast cancer, which is covered in greater detail in Chapter 8.

RADIOTHERAPY

Why is radiotherapy used?

Radiotherapy as part treatment for early breast cancer

Surgical treatments for breast cancer have become less radical with the introduction of wide local excision of the tumour plus radiotherapy, and the use of primary chemotherapy to reduce the size of the tumour. The surgeon will have tried to remove all of the tumour cells but there is always the small risk that some cancer cells will have been left behind or that a separate focus of cancer has been missed. To complete the treatment of the breast, and as added insurance against local recurrence, radiotherapy is given. It has been demonstrated that mastectomy can safely be replaced by wide local excision and radiotherapy (Fisher et al 1995). In addition, there is now evidence that radiotherapy may contribute to the systemic control of the disease, improving overall survival of the patient as well as preventing local relapse in the treated breast (Overgaard et al 1997).

Radiotherapy as local treatment for advanced breast cancer

Women who have a large and inoperable tumour may receive radiotherapy as a primary treatment to shrink the tumour and perhaps make future surgery possible. The plan of treatment may change as the treatment continues.

What is radiotherapy?

Radiotherapy is the use of ionising radiation to damage tumour cells. The radiation interacts with the DNA molecules of the tumour cells, producing biological effects that are harmful to the tumour. From the end of the 19th century to the present day, clinical and laboratory research has facilitated the use of radiation to treat and cure many cancers.

X-rays were discovered by Röntgen in 1895. He produced them by heating an electrode in a sealed vacuum tube, and applying a voltage across it, which accelerated the electrons towards a target plate. Striking the target, the electrons change their kinetic energy into energy in the form of X-rays. The term 'X' was coined because at the time the nature of the rays was not known. The potential for medical diagnosis was immediately recognised; an early photograph exists of Röntgen's wife's hand, demonstrating how well bones could be seen even with the earliest of equipment.

The idea of using X-rays as a therapy followed shortly after; the first radiotherapy treatment was given in 1896. In the same year Becquerel described radioactivity, and his name is given to the modern unit of its measurement (Bq). Shortly after, the Curies discovered radium, a radioactive substance, contributing further to the understanding of radiation. Their name was given to the first unit of radioactivity (Ci). X-rays (produced by electrons hitting a target) and gamma (γ) rays (produced by the decay of the nucleus of a radioactive atom), are identical forms of electromagnetic radiation. Of all the electromagnetic wave spectrum, which includes lightwaves, infrared and radiowaves, only X-rays and gamma rays have the right amount of energy to produce ionisation of atoms, which takes place when radiation passes through living tissue. These are the main sources of therapeutic radiation that are used today.

In the recent past women with breast cancer were treated with ^{60}Cobalt machines, which were found in nearly all cancer treatment centres across the UK. ^{60}Cobalt decays at a steady rate, with a half-life of 5 years, emitting gamma rays with high energy. The output of gamma rays does not change with any external factor, such as temperature or pressure, and together with its steady and predictable rate of decay, this physical fact makes it a very reliable source of radiation.

The ^{60}Cobalt machine exposes the radioactive source every time the patient is treated but keeps the source shielded at all other times. Today these machines have mostly been replaced by the superior linear accelerators, or 'Linacs', which produce X-rays. Such machines accelerate electrons along a radiofrequency electromagnetic wave, to almost the speed of light, before they hit a target to produce X-rays. Some Linacs are equipped to allow use of the electron beam (beta particle radiation) itself to treat the patient. Linacs produce a sharper beam than ^{60}Cobalt machines and are able to achieve greater depth doses through tissue (Souhami & Tobias 1986, Cotton 1996).

The very first unit of radiation dose, actually a measure of the amount of ionisation produced in a chamber containing air, was called the Röntgen. Nowadays, radiation dose is measured as the amount of energy that is absorbed by tissue. The unit of dose used to be the 'rad' or the radiation absorbed dose. Today, this unit of measurement has been replaced by the SI (Système International) unit termed the 'gray', abbreviated Gy. One gray is equal to one joule of energy absorbed per kilogram of tissue treated. Sometimes doses are expressed in centigray (cGy) or 100th of a gray, which is the equivalent of the older rad (Cotton 1996).

The high penetrating power of high energy X-rays and gamma rays means that some normal tissues will be irradiated as well as the tumour. However, it is important to include normal tissue around the site of the tumour itself, since this can be a site of microscopic spread. With electrons, the radiation dose decreases rapidly in normal tissue, the depth of penetration depending on the energy of the beam. This is useful for giving a 'boost' to the site of the tumour, since dose to the deeper structures of the chest wall is minimised.

How does radiotherapy kill cancer cells?

Radiation kills cancer cells by:

- A direct hit, when the radiation damages DNA directly
- By an indirect hit, when the radiation produces free radicals in the water adjacent to the DNA, which then react with it.

This DNA damage leads to breaks in chromosomes. If a cell is unable to repair these breaks it will die when it tries to multiply. In some haematological malignancies, radiation can induce programmed cell death or apoptosis, but this does not occur in solid tumours such as breast cancer.

Sensitivity to radiation occurs mostly when the cells are in M and G phases of cell division (Hall & Cox 1994). The damaging effects of radiation are less marked in cells that are hypoxic (have a limited oxygen supply) and as some areas of tumour are not well vascularised these cells are usually radiation resistant. In early breast cancer, the tumour mass to which this might apply, has been removed surgically.

Cell death is proportional to the amount of radiation given – the more radiation given the greater the cell kill. Unfortunately, the surrounding normal tissues will also receive a high dose of radiation and would become permanently damaged if very high doses of radiation were used (Souhami & Tobias 1986). Some sparing of normal tissue is achieved by dividing the course up into a number of treatments, called 'fractions'. The challenge for the radiotherapist is to deliver the prescribed radiation to those parts of the patient that need it, and a low dose to those areas that do not.

How is radiotherapy given to the woman with breast cancer?

Radiotherapy for the treatment of breast cancer can be given in two ways: as an external beam from a Linac or ^{60}Cobalt unit, or in certain circumstances as an implant, called brachytherapy. Most women in the UK receive external beam radiotherapy. Brachytherapy has its place, particularly for local recurrence of breast cancer, where external beam radiotherapy has already been given. This is discussed later in this section (Sainsbury et al 1995, Cotton 1996).

External beam radiotherapy

External beam radiotherapy is given in divided doses, known as fractions, on a daily or every other day basis. It usually begins about 1 month after chemotherapy has finished or 1 month to 6 weeks after the surgery, if no chemotherapy is given. Most radiotherapy services do not treat breast cancer patients at the weekend except in clinical emergencies of spinal cord compression or superior vena caval obstruction, sites of potential breast cancer recurrence. In the UK there is some disparity nationwide in the dose and number of fractions of radiotherapy given, with little consensus agreement between radiotherapists (Yarnold et al 1995). Generally, treatment fractions are given at a 2.0 Gy/day in 25 fractions, over 5 weeks, or as 2.67 Gy/day in 15 fractions over 3 weeks. A national trial has been implemented to discover which treatment regimen is the optimal. Called Standardisation of Breast Radiotherapy (START), the trial randomises women requiring radiotherapy between regimens of differing dose and fractions (Standardisation of Breast Radiotherapy Protocol 1998).

Planning radiotherapy

An individual treatment plan is worked out for each patient receiving radiotherapy. The woman's first visit to the radiotherapy department will include her being simulated, that is, an accurate plan is made of where her radiotherapy will be given (Cotton 1996). The radiotherapy plan is based on pictures taken from an X-ray machine linked to an image intensifier called a 'simulator', and an outline of the shape of the chest. The simulator reproduces the movement of the actual treatment machines so that angles and distances between the woman and Linac radiotherapy machine can be calculated. Marks are made on the woman's skin that will later be used to ensure that the treatment beam is accurately directed at the precise area required, avoiding the delicate structures of the lung and heart. These marks are made with a semi permanent pen with an additional permanent, tiny 'tattoo' from a small drop of indian ink introduced under the skin with a small bore needle. This procedure is quick and painless but the need for this mark introduces yet another assault on the woman's body image, which she can find very difficult and it needs to be explained carefully and with sensitivity.

During the planning, which for complex treatments may take up to 1 hour, the woman will be asked to keep quite still, and, if the radiotherapy is being given to the breast after a wide local excision, she will be asked to keep her hands behind her head. She will remain supine during her treatment (Cotton 1996). Figure 6.1 is a photograph of a Linac radiotherapy machine.

If the woman has undergone a wide local excision of her tumour, the whole breast will be treated, plus a 'boost' given to the tumour bed. The position of the boost is worked out by using the surgical scar as a guide. For women who need radiotherapy to the chest wall following a mastectomy, the chest wall is the target, and a boost is not usually required. Some primary breast tumours which have not been removed are visible to the naked eye or their dimensions can be defined with mammogram and ultrasound. Depending on the surgical clearance of the axilla and the lymph node positivity, and the radiotherapist's preference, the axillary lymph nodes and supraclavicular nodes may also be treated. There has been some discussion about the treatment of the axilla with radiotherapy because of the rare but serious complication of brachial nerve damage or plexopathy (Royal College of Radiologists 1995, Bates & Evans 1995) and an increased risk of lymphoedema. At present there is no consensus of opinion as to whether the axilla should be routinely treated or not, although standardisation of what areas of the breast and loco-regional nodes are to be irradiated is under consideration (Rodger 1998).

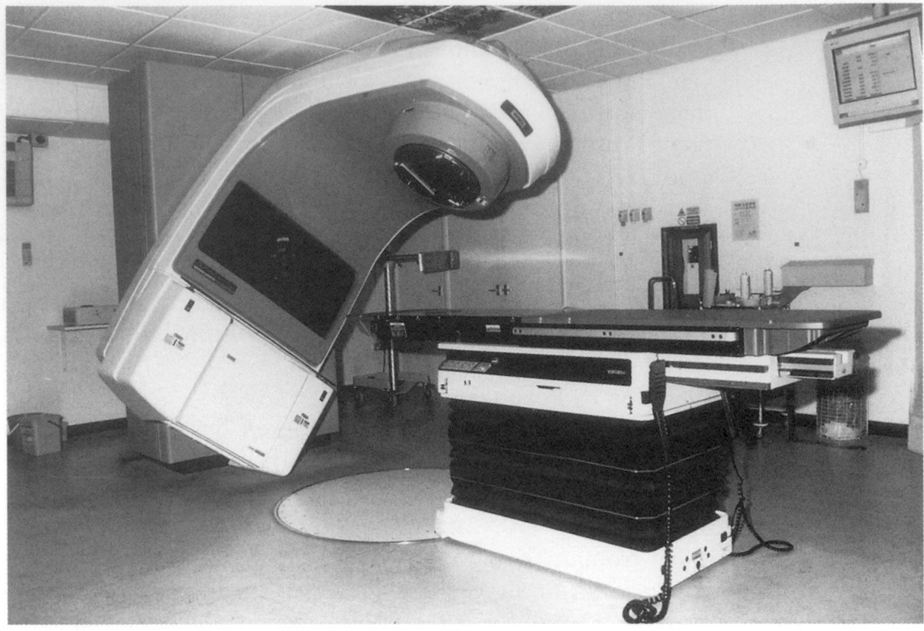

FIGURE 6.1

A Linac radiotherapy machine. Reproduced with kind permission of the Addenbrooke's NHS Trust Photographic Department.

The volume of tissue to be irradiated and the number of fields to be used is assessed by the radiotherapist and the therapy radiographer. Sometimes, for more difficult plans, the radiation physics department will be involved. For treatment to the breast it is usual to use two directions of radiation beam so that the beams intersect within the breast. This gives the most radiation to the tumour or the tumour bed whilst sparing the skin and normal tissues as much as possible. Since the chest wall is curved and radiation travels in straight lines, it is inevitable that the ribs and a small amount of the lung are treated. When treating the left side, where the heart lies just below the chest wall, it is especially important to minimise doses to the heart.

Once simulated to the satisfaction of the radiotherapist, the woman is expected to adopt the exact position each time she is treated. Laser beams projected onto the patient are used to ensure that accuracy of positioning is maintained throughout the weeks of treatment.

Each time the patient is treated she is left alone in the treatment room whilst the radiographers work the Linac. This can be quite frightening for some women who have been diagnosed with a serious condition and then find themselves isolated whilst they receive the radiotherapy, yet another unknown experience. Sometimes a radio or tape cassette is left on in the treatment room making the solitude easier and the radiographers who operate the machinery have an audio link with the woman. Clear explanation of the procedure and the approximate time for which the woman is left alone can help to relieve her anxiety. For a two-field treatment to the breast alone, the whole treatment lasts only about 10 min, and the woman is alone in the room for much less than this. If the woman has undergone a wide local excision, a boost of radiotherapy may be given to the site of the tumour or the tumour bed after the whole breast has been treated. Treating the tumour bed will be by a single small electron beam that can be produced from many Linacs.

Brachytherapy

This is the use of sealed sources of radioactive material placed within, or near to, the area of the tumour. The radioactive source used to treat breast cancer is usually iridium wire. Inert, empty catheters will be placed into the breast by a radiotherapist when the patient is anaesthetised. Two alternative systems are used to deliver the radiation. One option is to insert the radioactive wires into the catheters manually. The degree of radioactivity is usually fairly low, and the implant takes several days to deliver the required dose of radiation. For the safety of staff and other patients, the woman is nursed in a lead-lined room and behind lead shields to minimise exposure to others. The radioactive implants will remain in until the calculated dose of radiation has been given (usually a few days) and will be removed along with the inert tubes.

The second option is to use iridium wire that is very much more radioactive, after-loaded into the inert catheters by a remote controlled machine. These treatments take a matter of minutes, but have to be repeated in a daily, fractionated way. Using this remote after-loading machine, the radioactive sources are withdrawn if the nurse or doctor wishes to enter the room, so there is no exposure to staff.

Safety concerns

For any staff caring for an inpatient with radioactive implants, there are three watch words to bear in mind: time, distance and shielding (Langmack 1998). The nursing care of the patient should be carefully planned before going into the patient's room and the nurse should spend as little time as possible near the patient while providing her needs. The nurse should keep a good distance between herself and the patient when she is in the same room. The energy of radiotherapy reduces in strength as the distance from the radiation point source increases, according to the inverse square law. This means that if a nurse doubles her distance from the patient she will reduce her radiation exposure to one-quarter. The room in which the patient is cared for is usually lead lined and movable lead shields are also available for added staff protection. The area where someone is being treated with radiotherapy should be marked very carefully with internationally recognised symbols and any visitors should also be made aware. The area should be avoided by pregnant woman and young children.

Levels of radiation for individuals can be measured if they wear badges containing radiation-sensitive film. When this film is developed the photographic film provides a record of how much radiation that individual has been exposed to. Each badge is assigned to a specific individual and assessed for a set time period.

Nursing care

The woman is isolated when the radioactive implants are in situ and will only be able to have limited visitors and this should be explained to her before she embarks on her treatment. The woman should be prepared for the isolation by bringing in books and other distractions to help pass the time. A television is usually available in the treatment room. Limited emotional support is essential as the woman is not only coping with breast cancer but the loneliness of being nursed in virtual isolation. This time away from others may provide her with time to reflect on her situation and to ponder her future. When with the woman, the nurse should make a little time to listen to her concerns whilst being mindful of her own exposure to the radiation.

Any sign of a wound infection should be reported to the clinician in charge of the woman's care so that antibiotics may be prescribed. Any pain or discomfort should be assessed and treated with appropriate analgesia.

Safe practice with radiotherapy

There are significant and known hazards associated with the insertion and removal of radioactive sources and working around radioactive substances, but radiation protection is not within the remit of this book. The Ionising Radiations Regulations (HMSO 1999) provide guidance on which local radiation protection policies are written. All staff working in areas where radiation treatment is given have a responsibility to themselves, their colleagues and their patients to be aware of these and any other local policies that their hospital Trust follows, and should practise strictly according to them.

Early effects of radiotherapy to the breast

The normal tissue effects of radiotherapy can be complicated. For further details of both early (acute) and late radiotherapy reactions see Perez & Brady 1998.

Skin reactions

The skin is composed of several layers of cells; normal mature cells are constantly shed from the skin surface and replaced by new cells from the basal layer. This continual state of reproductivity accounts for the relative radiosensitivity of the skin. Although the skin is not the primary target, the radiotherapy beams must pass through the skin to treat the underlying breast or chest wall.

Erythema, or a reddening of the skin may be the only manifestation of mild radiation sensitivity for some women, and may develop 2–3 weeks after radiotherapy treatment has started. In some women, if their skin is particularly sensitive, the erythema may progress to dry desquamation where there is scaly loss of some of the epidermal layer, or moist desquamation, where there is loss of all of the dermal layer producing a small ulcer. This is more common where skin folds meet, such as the inframammary fold. Dry desquamation can be itchy and uncomfortable, but responds well to hydrocortisone cream 1%, although it may mask fungal infections and should be used with caution (Cotton 1996). Radiotherapy may be interrupted to allow healing if the woman develops moist desquamation, though this is not usually necessary. After the radiotherapy has been given, healing may be slow but is usually complete and leaves minimal evidence of the acute damage except for pigmentation. The same amount of radiation given in the same way can cause completely different skin reactions in different women. Skin sensitivity to radiation differs across the population and cannot be routinely tested for at the moment (Burnet et al 1998).

Nursing care

All women who receive radiotherapy to their breast will be given advice about skin care during their treatment. If erythema develops advice should be sought at the review appointment with the radiotherapist who will see the patient throughout their treatment. Moisturising the breast with simple Aqueous Cream or E45 lotion will be encouraged and should ease the effects of dry desquamation. If severe moist desquamation develops, this is an indication for a break in treatment.

The treated breast can be washed carefully with tepid water but the skin should be patted, not rubbed, dry. If there are marks that need to be preserved, this should be explained and the woman will be encouraged not to wash the skin roughly. Perfumed products such as deodorant and perfume should not be used in the treatment area.

Hair follicles and sweat glands are also radiosensitive due to their high rate of growth. For this reason women who receive axillary radiotherapy will lose underarm hair on the treated side and may temporarily stop sweating from that axilla, although the sweat glands usually recover after the treatment. Axillary hair does not normally grow back.

Clothing covering the treatment field should be loose fitting and made of natural fibres. Tight fitting bras should be avoided and, as treatment continues, it may be appropriate to stop wearing a bra and to use a crop top or a loose cotton T shirt.

When receiving radiotherapy the treatment area should not be exposed to full sunlight. After treatment the woman should be advised to not expose the treatment area to sunlight until it has completely healed. If, after several months the woman wishes to sunbathe she must use a high factor sun cream on the treated area and should not continue to sunbathe if the area becomes red or sore. The skin will stay sensitive to sun for at least 1 year after treatment and caution in future years may need to be taken.

Fatigue

Fatigue is very common among patients who have cancer and this tiredness may be compounded by receiving a course of radiotherapy. There may be many practical reasons why radiotherapy makes the patient tired:

- Recovering from surgery
- Receiving concurrent chemotherapy
- Pain
- Frequency of visits to the hospital.

In her research Faithfull (1998) found that patients attending for radiotherapy became very tired. She suggests that this fatigue may be related to the accumulation of metabolites and cell destruction from tissue damage caused by the radiation. Encouraging the patient to take naps during her treatment can help and pre-treatment explanation will help to prepare the woman for this side-effect.

Late changes

Radiation pneumonitis may have two components. Acute inflammation, with cough, can occur during or just after a course of radiotherapy but is uncommon with radiotherapy for breast cancer. It is the result of inflammation of the alveolar wall plus the accumulation of exudate in the alveolar air space, similar to pneumonia. Later changes can lead to fibrosis of the lung tissue and thickening of the pleura. Such changes reduce respiratory function in the area treated, but the degree of disability is related to the amount and condition of the remaining lung tissue. It is rarely noticeable by the patient after breast radiotherapy.

Damage to the myocardium and the coronary arteries has been recognised as a serious late change to the left side of the chest wall or the left breast caused by radiotherapy (Cuzick et al 1994). With the increased use of adjuvant anthracycline chemotherapy, which also damages the myocardium, cardiac tolerance can be further compromised. Clinicians are aware of this problem and now make every effort to individualise treatment planning to reduce the amount of heart tissue that is irradiated in order to reduce cardiac toxicity.

The ribs are often treated by adjuvant radiotherapy as they fall within the treatment field. There can be immediate rib tenderness and, over time, the ribs can become more brittle and susceptible to pathological fracture. This is a rare complication.

Lymphoedema

Swelling of the arm can be caused by surgery due to interruption of the lymphatic channels and postoperative scarring, and by radiotherapy, due to fibrosis. For more detail on care of lymphoedema see Chapter 7.

Conclusion

These side-effects of radiotherapy for the the treatment of breast cancer are rare and with better treatment planning systems are becoming more a problem of the past.

Specific nursing care of a woman undergoing radiotherapy

For many women the thought of undergoing radiotherapy is a daunting prospect. They may have preconceptions about their treatment, of being burnt badly or of being very unwell. Some may believe that they will lose their hair and be nauseated despite being treated on the chest wall or the breast.

Most people never see a radiotherapy machine until they are being treated so some of their nursing care is about helping them to understand the unknown and to support them through their treatment. For many women who have had adjuvant chemotherapy, radiotherapy is not as hard work but they find that they are still recovering from the physical side-effects of their chemotherapy. In reality, radiotherapy is painless and quick once the planning has taken place and for most women the only side-effects they experience are fatigue and some skin sensitivity. Other side-effects do occur but these are rare and the severity of such effects depends on the dose of radiation, the individual's sensitivity and the treatment site. If the woman knows what sort of side-effects to expect, and that there are measures to alleviate them, she is usually able to cope much better. Having to attend daily or every other day for radiotherapy may cause some problems for a mother or for someone who has a particularly demanding job.

Although most radiotherapy centres are working to full capacity, it is often possible for a woman's treatment to be scheduled for early in the morning or later in the day to help her organize her life better. Each woman needs to be assessed and cared for as an individual. Women are seen regularly throughout their treatment by the clinician and the radiographers, so this can be an opportunity to see how things are going as well as assessing the physical effects of the radiotherapy. Most patients find that radiotherapy is not as bad as they were expecting and meeting other women that are going through the same treatment can help the individual cope with her fears and anxieties better.

HYPERTHERMIA

Some radiotherapy centres have offered the use of hyperthermia as an additional treatment, particularly when treating a local recurrence of breast cancer. The theoretical basis for this treatment is that the tissue to be treated is heated sufficiently to kill any cells that are in S phase, when they are the least radiosensitive. Radiotherapy is used concurrently to kill the cancer cells that are in the other phases of the cell cycle and the treatments are thought to work synergistically. Hyperthermia is also thought to work on hypoxic cells when radiotherapy has a limited chance of cell kill. Heating the tissue to be treated can be achieved in several ways, but in this context is usually done with microwaves. Side-effects include discomfort or pain during the procedure, and local skin reaction, pain, fever, and rarely, cardiac arrhythmias.

Nursing care

This treatment needs to be clearly explained to the patient. Comfort throughout the procedure and afterwards is an important nursing consideration. The integrity of the skin following treatment should be assessed carefully. Only a few centres in the UK offer this treatment and it remains a partly experimental treatment.

ENDOCRINE THERAPIES

The normal growth of breast tissue is stimulated by several steroid hormones, particularly oestrogen. In pre-menopausal women, oestrogen is mostly produced by the ovaries and in postmenopausal women, a small amount of oestrogen is produced by the adrenal glands. Breast cells contain receptor sites for oestrogen within their cytoplasm and are stimulated to grow when oestrogen binds to these receptor sites. Some breast cancer cells have this cytoplasmic receptor. Pre-menopausal women have a lower incidence of oestrogen-receptor-positive tumours (30%) than postmenopausal women (60%), and peri-menopausal women have the lowest rate at only 10% (Fenlon 1996). Surprisingly, a small number of women who have receptor-negative tumours will respond to anti-oestrogen therapy.

Oestrogen receptors (ERs) are measured in femtomoles per milligram of cytoplasmic protein, ranging from 0 to more than 1000. The breast cancer tissue will be examined after surgical removal for the grade and type of cancer cells, and the concentration of ER. If the ER is more than 10 Fmol/mg, then the breast cancer is said to be ER positive (Fenlon 1996). The percentage of ER receptors present can also be given; the higher the percentage, the more ER receptors.

In general, endocrine therapies act by interfering with the synthesis of oestrogen or by preventing oestrogen from exerting an effect on the cancer cells. Endocrine therapies can be used in four ways to treat breast cancer:

1. To prevent 'at risk' women, e.g. those with certain types of benign breast disease, or a family history of breast cancer, from getting breast cancer in the first place. Studies in the USA using the oestrogen-blocking agent tamoxifen as a protective agent for women at risk have reported positive results after an interim analysis of their data. Similar trials run in the UK have not demonstrated such positive effects, but the long-term results of these trials will not be be available for several years (Powles et al 1998).
2. As an adjuvant therapy started at the time of the primary surgery for breast cancer. It is known that tamoxifen improves survival and reduces the incidence of a second primary breast cancer if it is given to women when they are first diagnosed and treated for breast cancer (EBCTCG 1992).
3. The endocrine therapy tamoxifen can be given as a primary breast cancer treatment for older women with inoperable breast cancer. Such treatment has been shown to produce a partial response in 75% in women who are ER positive (Richards & Smith 1995).
4. To treat metastatic disease. Hormone therapies can present a relatively non-toxic but effective treatment for women with metastatic breast cancer (Fenlon 1996).

Types of endocrine therapy

Tamoxifen

Tamoxifen is a synthetic non-steroidal anti-oestrogen and, at the moment, is the most widely used endocrine therapy. Tamoxifen competes with oestrogen receptors in the cytoplasm of the cell and blocks endogenous oestrogen from stimulating breast cancer cell growth. Tamoxifen has a long half-life (7 days) and takes 4 weeks to reach a steady state drug concentration in the blood. It has been found to be effective in many women with breast cancer and is thought to reduce the death rates from breast cancer by 20–30% (Baum & Schipper 1999), but generally is more effective in women who are postmenopausal and have high levels of oestrogen receptors. This drug is very widely given in view of its relatively few side-effects and its proven efficacy (ECTGB 1998b).

Pre-menopausal women who take this drug usually experience menopausal symptoms and postmenopausal women may experience a resurgence of their menopausal symptoms, especially if they have recently stopped taking hormone replacement therapy (HRT). Other reported side-effects of tamoxifen include vaginal discharge, mild fluid retention and transient nausea. Although originally developed as an anti-oestrogen, tamoxifen is also an oestrogen agonist. This agonist action can have the positive side-effects of preventing post menopausal osteoporosis as well as reducing cholesterol but can also cause problematic side-effects such as thrombosis, an increased risk of endometrial cancer and cataracts (EBCTCG 1992, Pritchard et al 1996, Dhingra 1999). Very occasionally thrombocytopenia is a problem and the individual taking tamoxifen should be advised to report increased bruising or bleeding from her gums. Any abnormal vaginal bleeding, shortness of breath or rapid deterioration in eyesight should also be investigated (Bruzzi 1998). At present tamoxifen is usually prescribed as a 20 mg tablet per day and is being taken by most women for 5 years, although current research aims to find out if it should be taken for 10 years (Rea et al 1998).

Selective oestrogen receptor modulators

To overcome the potential side-effects of the oestrogen agonist effects of tamoxifen, a new range of drugs are being developed that have more appropriate, tissue selective, oestrogen antagonist or agonist effects. Selective oestrogen receptor modulators (SERMS) are being compared with tamoxifen for their anti-tumour effect and some women in the UK are being asked to enter such trials. A new selective oestrogen inhibitor, raloxifene, is thought to have the right mix of antagonistic and agonist effects with oestrogen and does not cause endometrial stimulation. This is the most popular SERM at present, although research is ongoing into better alternatives (Osborne 1999, Dhingra 1999, Lien & Lonning 2000).

Aromatase inhibitors

Despite their ovaries no longer working, postmenopausal women still have a small level of circulating oestrogen. Androstenedione, secreted from the adrenal glands, is synthesised to oestrogen by the action of the enzyme aromatase. This process occurs mostly in extraglandular tissue and the synthesised oestrogen is released into the bloodstream (Fenlon 1996, Harvey 1998). Historically, adrenalectomy was a treatment used to reduce the levels of circulating oestrogen in postmenopausal women. Aminoglutethimide was the drug designed to supersede the adrenalectomy.

Aminoglutethimide blocks or inhibits all adrenal hormone production including that of hydrocortisone. Because of this consequence the side-effects of aminoglutethimide can be quite severe and include lethargy, skin rash, hypotension, dizziness and depression. Hydrocortisone was given with aminoglutethimide to prevent some of these side-effects and also to prevent the pituitary overriding the suppression of the adrenal glands.

Because of these significant side-effects and the need for more effective treatments for breast cancer, a new generation of aromatase inhibitors has been developed. Anastrazole (Arimidex), letrozole (Femara), exemustane (Aromasin) and vorozole (Rizivor) are presently being trialed and are set to replace aminoglutethimide.

Anastrazole (Arimidex), an oral tablet taken daily, is probably the most widely used aromatase inhibitor in the UK and is being used as the optimal second-line agent after tamoxifen for the treatment of advanced breast cancer. As a selective aromatase inhibitor, Arimidex prevents the synthesis of oestrogen and so reduces the levels of circulating oestrogen (Harvey 1998). Arimidex has fewer side-effects than aminoglutethamide, although it can cause slight headaches, hot flushes, tiredness and fatigue (Chapman & Goodman 1997). The role of aromatase inhibitors in other clinical settings and as potential breast cancer chemopreventatives is yet to be determined (Njar & Brodie 1999).

Ovarian ablation

Ovarian ablation has a long history in the treatment of breast cancer. At the end of the 19th century several medical reports appeared about the beneficial effects of the surgical removal of the ovaries in pre-menopausal women with advanced breast cancer. For women who are still menstruating and who are taking tamoxifen, the levels of circulating oestrogen can be significantly reduced by preventing the ovaries from releasing oestrogen. Today this can be achieved in the following ways:

- By surgical oophorectomy
- By radiation ablation of the ovaries
- By inducing a temporary menopause by using luteinising hormone-releasing hormone (LHRH) inhibitors such as goserelin (Zoladex), or buserelin (Suprecure).

The hypothalamus controls the ovaries by releasing LHRH, which stimulates the pituitary to release both luteinising hormone (LH) and follicle-stimulating hormone (FSH) which, in turn, stimulate the ovaries to release oestrogen. If an LHRH analogue is given it blocks the action of the pituitary gland and inhibits the release of LH and FSH which, in turn, effectively switches off the ovaries. This chemically induced menopause dramatically reduces the levels of circulating oestrogen. Such drugs include goserelin (Zoladex) and buserelin (Suprecure).

Zoladex is a widely used LHRH inhibitor and is given as a monthly or 3-monthly subcutaneous depot injection. The practice nurse can give this injection subcutaneously so saving the woman an unnecessary trip to hospital. Unlike surgical oophorectomy or radiation ablation, once the injection is stopped the menopausal effect is reversed. In the younger woman this may be a more acceptable way of stopping the ovaries from producing oestrogen, especially if the woman wants to have a family after her treatment for the breast cancer has finished.

The side-effects of ovarian ablation will include menopausal symptoms such as hot flushes, weight gain and may cause transient nausea.

Progestin therapy

The action of progestins is unclear but they appear to inhibit the stimulatory effect of oestrogen on tumour growth. Megestrol acetate is a progestin that is often used as a third-line hormone therapy in the treatment of recurrent breast cancer. It can have a response rate of up to 30% (Honig 1996). Given as a daily oral dose this drug is well tolerated but does have the side-effects of weight gain and an increase in appetite and vaginal bleeding. For some patients it can promote a feeling of wellbeing (Fenlon 1996, Chapman & Goodman 1997).

Endocrine treatments in metastatic disease

Endocrine therapy is the first-line treatment for most women who present with metastatic disease and are oestrogen receptor positive. Endocrine therapy has the added advantage of causing a few manageable side-effects whilst offering an effective treatment for metastatic disease, which is an important consideration when cure of the breast cancer is no longer possible.

Responses to endocrine treatments in metastatic breast disease are seen in about 30% of all patients and are more likely in oestrogen-receptor-positive patients. Response rates of 25% are seen in second-line endocrine treatments and only 10–15% respond to third-line treatment (Leonard et al 1995). Endocrine therapy is used in women who have a non-aggressive relapse in the bones or lymph nodes, have a long disease-free interval and an oestrogen-positive tumour. Widespread bone disease often responds to hormonal treatment such as tamoxifen, Arimidex (anastrasole) or Zoladex. The older aromatase inhibitors such as aminoglutethimide, have been superseded by Arimidex, although are still available for use for women who are unable to take Arimidex (Coleman 1999). In rare instances the hormone therapy, particularly oestrogens, can make the metastatic breast disease worsen before responding to the treatment. This 'flare' of disease can result in hypercalcaemia, an increase in bone pain or growth of skin nodules (Fenlon 1996). The symptoms of hypercalcaemia should be reported immediately as this could be a life-threatening situation. See Chapter 8 for more detail on the use of hormones for recurrent breast cancer and hypercalcaemia.

Nursing care of the woman receiving endocrine therapies

Assessment of a woman's symptoms is crucial when trying to identify her particular problems with hormone therapy. As can be seen, symptoms will differ slightly according to the therapy being taken, but the most frequently reported side-effects are menopausal symptoms. Explaining to the woman how the endocrine therapy works may help her understand why it is being used to treat her breast cancer. This information should also help her to understand why she is experiencing menopausal symptoms such as hot flushes and sweating. Knowing about a particular treatment and the associated side-effects can help the woman take control of her situation, which may help her cope better with her symptoms. The nurse should take into account the woman's social role as a wife or a mother and how much her symptoms are affecting her work and home life. Hormone therapies are sometimes considered an easier treatment, but for a few women, severe menopausal symptoms can significantly affect their lives.

Menopausal symptoms

Hot flushes are a frequently reported symptom of endocrine therapies. The frequency and intensity of these flushes differs between individuals but most women find them a nuisance. Hot flushes are often associated with night or day sweats. These episodes of flushing and sweating can cause sleepless nights and leave a woman feeling tired and drained. Home life and work can be affected if the woman is not getting enough rest. Hot flushes and sweats can be worsened by:

- Alcohol intake
- Caffeine intake
- Cigarette smoking
- Hot and spicy foods
- Hot weather

(Abernethy 1997).

The first treatment to be considered for hot flushes would probably be oestrogen replacement therapy, although this is contraindicated in women who have been treated for breast cancer (Fenlon 1996). The drug clonidine, which was used to treat migraine, has been found useful although it has side-effects of dry mouth, dizziness and headaches. Avoiding hot drinks, hot food and alcohol, and cutting down on smoking and caffeine may help, although it is recognised that most women do not want to live a very restricted lifestyle.

Comfort can be maintained by wearing cotton next to the skin and several layers of clothing so that the layers can be removed when the woman feels a hot flush coming on. Several layers of bedding can be used following the same principle for when the woman is asleep (Fenlon 1996).

Menopausal symptoms can be reduced by behavioural relaxation methods (Freedman & Woodward 1992). Learning to relax during a hot flush may not be easy but it could reduce the intensity of the flush (Abernethy 1997). Fenlon (1996) writes of women being taught to face hot flushes with a positive attitude, which may help make the experience less distressing. Generally reducing stress in a woman's life may also be of value. Some ways to reduce stress include:

- Relaxation and visualisation
- Gentle exercise (providing permission has been sought from the woman's clinician)
- Meditation
- Acupuncture (providing permission has been sought from the woman's clinician).

Feeling embarrassed by a hot flush can be a distressing experience for a woman as she may feel that others are noticing her. Reassurance can be given that most people do not notice.

Muscle and joint pains

As oestrogen levels reduce in the body the bones start to get brittle due to calcium loss. There is no known way of preventing calcium loss but bone strength can be maintained through gentle exercise. Any woman that comments on an increase in bone pain should tell her clinician of these symptoms.

Dry skin and hair

A lack of oestrogen can cause the skin and hair to become dry and some women have reported increased hair loss. Advice can include eating a well-balanced diet with a reduction in the total fat, sugar and salt intake and an increased intake of starches, cereals and fibre, fruit and vegetables to maintain general health (Abernethy 1997). The skin can be kept in good condition by using rich moisturisers and by washing the skin with mild non-drying soap. Hair should be washed less frequently and liberal use of a conditioner may help (Fenlon 1996). If hair loss is severe advice about getting a wig may be helpful, although the subject should be approached with tact and understanding.

Dietary supplements

Vitamin and mineral supplements such as vitamin E and oil of evening primrose zinc and magnesium have been reported to help some women with thei menopausal symptoms but there is no definitive research to support these claims. Women wishing to take these supplements would be advised to check with their clinician.

There has been some interest in the use of plant-derived phyto-oestrogens for the treatment and relief of menopausal symptoms (Nestel et al 1999). Phyto-oestrogens can be found in soya, red clover and most legumes (Zava 1998). Research is being conducted that is studying the effect of these phyto-oestrogens on women who have had breast cancer but are experiencing menopausal symptoms and it may be that these are a safe and effective solution to hot flushes and sweats.

Bladder symptoms

A drop in oestrogen levels can have a significant effect on bladder function (Abernethy 1997). Typical bladder symptoms include stress incontinence and frequency of micturition. Referral for urodynamic studies should be considered for women whose lives are severely affected by their bladder symptoms.

Sexual function

A decline in oestrogen levels can result in changes to the vagina and vulval area, causing the vagina to shorten, become less elastic and to have less vascularity and be easily irritated. This can result in vaginal dryness and dyspareunia (painful lovemaking) making sexual intercourse difficult. Intercourse should continue but be made easier with the use of vaginal lubrication such as KY jelly or 'Senselle'. Another hormonal vaginal moisturising gel called Replens is also available. The vulval area should be washed with non-drying soap, perhaps one of the pH-adjusted soaps and moisturised if necessary. The vagina is more susceptible to candida infection (thrush) and any sign of this should be treated with antifungal medication. For pre-menopausal women advice should be given about contraceptives as some of the endocrine therapies do not automatically stop ovulation.

Sexuality

Endocrine therapies can reduce or increase a patient's libido. These side-effects should be explained at the beginning of the woman's treatment. It is thought that oestrogens decrease the libido whilst progestins increase the libido. During her treatment the woman should be given the opportunity to discuss her experiences with the treatment and be offered emotional support if required.

Weight gain

The progestins can cause an increase in appetite and weight gain and many women who take tamoxifen complain about an increase in weight soon after starting the tablets. Warning the woman that this may occur can help her prepare for this problem. Referral to a dietician may be appropriate for someone who has gained weight.

Gastric disturbances

Gastric upsets, nausea and diarrhoea are uncommon with tamoxifen. The progestins may cause nausea and occasionally vomiting, which can be treated with anti-emetics.

Menstrual disturbances

For pre-menopausal women who are taking tamoxifen, it may be that their periods stop or become much lighter. When an endocrine therapy is stopped, it may be that the woman experiences a withdrawal bleed and she should be prepared for this. Any unexpected bleeding should be reported to the clinician in charge of the woman's care.

Emotional support

The physical effects of endocrine therapies are well documented. The loss of or increase of libido, the potential weight gain, and the dryness of the skin can have a profound and longlasting effect on how the woman perceives herself and her body image. She may have a loss of self-esteem, which in itself may cause her to function less well at work and at home. This loss of self-esteem may also cause difficulties in her interpersonal relationships, particularly if she has sexual problems. When the woman comes to clinic for assessment it is important that she is seen in an environment where she can discuss openly her feelings about her endocrine therapy and the effects it is having on her life. Sometimes just to be heard can make the physical and emotional effects easier to deal with. If the nurse explains why the woman is experiencing such effects and that these effects are not unusual, this can be reassuring. By understanding the woman's problems, it may be that the nurse can help to identify practical methods of dealing with the symptoms of endocrine therapy and identify goals for future management.

CHEMOTHERAPY

At the end of this section the reader should have an understanding of chemotherapy with regard to:

- Its use in breast cancer
- Clinical trials
- Physical effects of treatment
- Psychological and social effects
- Complementary therapies that may be used to alleviate symptoms
- Home chemotherapy.

The side-effects and care for a woman undergoing chemotherapy will be described in this section. The treatment of breast cancer with an increasing focus on chemotherapeutic treatments (EBCTCG Overview of ASCO 1999) will be discussed.

How chemotherapy works

This section will explore the way in which chemotherapy works against cancer cells. Cytotoxic drugs are defined as 'cell killing drugs' and they act against cancer cells in two main ways: (1) to kill dividing cancer cells and (2) to interfere with cell division. In this way such drugs eradicate or control cancer cell growth. However, cytotoxic drugs do not specifically attack cancer cells but can affect all cells that are in a state of division. Because of this non-specific effect, women who are undergoing a course of chemotherapy will experience some side-effects from their treatment. To understand the action of specific cytotoxic drugs, the mechanism of cell division will now be outlined. This is represented below and consists of the following stages:

G0: Cells are inactive having travelled out of the cell cycle. They remain so until stimulated to re-enter the cell cycle and divide

G1: The initial resting phase. This is the point of decision to replicate or differentiate

S: The synthetic phase, leading to replication of the DNA

G2: The second resting or pre-mitotic phase. RNA and the protein necessary for mitosis is synthesised

M: Mitosis or cell division occurs.

The body is made up of three basic types of cells:

1. *Dividing cells*. In adults these cells are continuously replicating and include blood cells, hair, the lining of the gastrointestinal tract and the mouth.
2. *Non-dividing cells*. These cells divide and differentiate, and are unable to divide again, for example nerve and brain cells.
3. *Resting cells*. Cells that leave the cell cycle and don't divide unless stimulated to reactivate and re-enter the cycle, e.g. liver cells.

Cells are not all cycling or in the same phase of cycle at the same time. The overall circulating time varies depending on the type of cell.

How chemotherapy interferes with cell division

Affecting DNA

Cytotoxic drugs attack DNA in three ways: (1) by interfering directly with DNA or (2) the enzyme required for DNA or RNA synthesis, and (3) by killing cellular proteins required for the manufacture of DNA.

Action on the cell cycle

Cytotoxic drugs are either cell cycle specific or cell cycle non-specific. Cell cycle specific drugs attack a particular stage of cell division and are most effective against dividing tumours. Cell cycle non-specific drugs are active in all phases of cell division and are most effective against large tumours.

Combination chemotherapy

In most of the chemotherapy regimens given for breast cancer, the drugs are given in combination. When more than one cytotoxic drug is used, the drugs are usually from different groups and have different mechanisms of action, targeting different stages of cell division. When given in combination they enhance the effect of each other. All of these factors promote maximum cell kill. The individual drugs have different toxicities and timing of toxicities, which reduces the side-effects for the patient (Table 6.1).

TABLE 6.1 ***Cytotoxic drugs used for breast cancer***

Drug and mode of action	Potential side-effects
Alkylating agents Cell cycle non-specific Acts on previously formed nucleic acid causing DNA strand to be misread, the DNA molecule to fracture and the DNA strand to cross link	Risk of infertility. Risk of second malignancy (leukemia).
Cyclophosphamide	Hot flush/dizziness/metallic taste, during intravenous administration. Nausea and vomiting. Bone marrow depression. Haemorrhagic cystitis. Alopecia in high doses. Cardiotoxicity.
Cisplatin Non-classic alkylating agent Heavy metal compound	Nausea and persistent vomiting. Diarrhoea at high doses. Nephrotoxic. Bone marrow depression. Peripheral neuropathy. Tinnitus, high frequency hearing loss. Hyperuricaemia.
Vinca alkaloid Spindle poison. Blocks G2/S Phase *Navelbine (vinorelbine)*	Bone marrow depression. Alopecia (mild). Nausea and vomiting. Peripheral neuropathy. Autonomic neuropathy: constipation which rarely leads to paralytic ileus.
Antimetabolites S phase specific Folic acid antagonist Block essential enzymes necessary for DNA synthesis or become incorporated into the DNA and RNA so that false message is transmitted	
Methotrexate	Sore ulcerated mouth and gums. CNS effects (dizziness, malaise, blurred vision). Nausea rare. Bone marrow depression. Rashes. Pruritus. Photosensitivity. Hepatotoxicity. Renal failure (high dose). Cystitis. Pulmonary changes.
5-Fluorouracil	Diarrhoea. Occasional nausea. Darkening/ discoloration of veins with prolonged infusions. Bone marrow depression. Stomatitis. Hyperpigmentation.

TABLE 6.1 *contd.*

Antibiotics **Anthracyclines** Cell cycle non-specific active in all phases of cell cycle (maximum in S phase) Disrupts DNA transcription and RNA synthesis by altering cell membranes and inhibiting certain enzymes produced by bacteria and fungal organisms	
Doxorubicin *Epirubicin* (Synthetic analogue of doxorubicin)	During infusion, red flush/aching local reaction in higher doses/sensitive veins. Red urine. Stomatitis. Nausea and vomiting. Bone marrow depression. Alopecia. Thrombophlebitis. Cardiotoxic. Nail pigmentation. Vesicant drug (risk of venous pain and damage to local tissues if tissuing occurs).
Mitozantrone	Green urine. Nausea and vomiting mild. Bone marrow depression. Minimal alopecia.
Mitomycin C Antibiotic miscellaneous	Nausea and vomiting in high doses. Lethargy. Fatigue. Nephrotoxic. Stomatitis. Bone marrow depression. Delayed recovery. Pruritus. Vesicant drug (risk of venous pain and damage to local tissues if tissuing occurs).
Taxanes New group of drugs developed from the Yew tree. Inhibits mitosis	Alopecia. Bone marrow depression. Short-lived arthralgia/myalgia following administration. Peripheral neuropathy. Allergic reaction. Nausea and vomiting. Diarrhoea. Stomatitis.

(Eli Lilley 1998)

History of chemotherapy

Chemotherapy was first identified by Paul Ehrlich's research into antibiotics in the 1800s. During the First World War the potential for nitrogen mustard as a treatment for cancer was highlighted. An explosion of nitrogen mustard gases in Naples, Italy caused damage to the lymph glands and bone marrow of soldiers exposed to the gases, resulting in their deaths. Following this, nitrogen mustard was used to treat lymphomas. In 1947 methotrexate was discovered as a treatment for leukaemia. By the 1970s, after much research, chemotherapy had become an established treatment for cancer.

Clinical trials

Progression in the efficacy of chemotherapy has come about as a result of clinical trials. The aims of these trials are to improve knowledge and treatments for breast cancer. The three main types of trials are phases 1, 2 and 3. Phase 1 studies are designed to establish the effective dose, i.e. how much can be given safely, how often, the method of administration and any side-effects. Phase 2 studies are designed to establish how effective the drug is. If the drug is effective, it is moved onto a phase 3 study. Phase 3 studies are randomised, controlled trials that compare new treatments with established effective treatments or a placebo where none exist. Such studies are based on protocols, approved by regional and local ethics committees. Informed consent is an essential aspect of clinical trials. The oncologist and research nurse have an important role to play in obtaining informed consent. The patient is given an information sheet about the study, which is also explained to them. The patient is then given time to think about the study before deciding whether to participate. If the patient decides to take part, they sign a consent form. It is explained to the patient that they have the right to decline entry into the study, which will not compromise their care in any way.

Chemotherapy in breast cancer

It is rare for breast cancer patients to have detectable metastatic disease at presentation. However, it is thought that the presence of micrometastases at diagnosis are responsible for the large number of patients who develop metastatic disease. Prognosis is directly correlated to the presence and number of lymph node metastases. Women who do not have cancerous spread to their lymph nodes at presentation have the best prognosis, with up to 70% being cured. However those with spread to the lymph nodes have a poorer outlook. Prognosis is directly correlated to the presence and number of lymph node metastases (Miller et al 1995). Between 60% and 80% of women who present with cancer in four or more lymph nodes will go on to develop metastatic disease (Anglo Celtic Cooperative Oncology Group 1996).

Chemotherapy has an important part to play in the treatment of breast cancer. The treatment aims to cure some women, but for others who are not going to be cured from their breast cancer, to prolong life and affect or palliate symptoms. There is a constant striving to improve the effectiveness of these drugs through research. This next section will outline the chemotherapy drugs used to treat breast cancer and include the ongoing clinical trial work. The role of chemotherapy in breast cancer will now be discussed. Approaches include adjuvant, neoadjuvant, high-dose and palliative treatments.

Adjuvant chemotherapy

This approach involves the administration of chemotherapy following local treatment to the tumour with surgery or radiotherapy. The aim of adjuvant treatment is to reduce the risk of metastatic disease and it is normally used for women who have poor prognostic factors such as lymph node metastases. Cyclophosphamide, methotrexate and 5-fluorouracil (CMF) is the standard adjuvant treatment for breast cancer. It was developed by Bonadonna et al (1995) and modified in Milan. However, there is an increasing body of evidence to suggest that the addition of an anthracycline chemotherapeutic drug to the

CMF regimen has a place in the adjuvant setting (Buzzoni et al 1991, Bonadonna et al 1995). Research in this area is ongoing.

Neoadjuvant chemotherapy

Chemotherapy may be used as a first-line treatment for large breast tumours. The aim of this approach is to shrink the tumour prior to surgery, thus avoiding a mastectomy or rendering inoperable breast tumours operable (Mansi et al 1989). This method of treatment has been shown to prevent 90% of women from undergoing a mastectomy. The most effective chemotherapeutic drugs in women with large breast tumours are the anthracyclines (doxorubicin and epirubicin), which are normally given with cyclophosphamide. Current research is investigating the role of taxanes in combination with anthracyclines.

High-dose chemotherapy

This approach involves the administration of high doses of chemotherapy in an attempt to permanently eradicate the cancer. High-dose chemotherapy for breast cancer was first trialed on women whose cancer had progressed following conventional treatment (Eder et al 1986). None of these women were cured despite 50% responding to the chemotherapy and approximately 25% achieving complete remission. At the time of this research, high-grade toxicities were associated with this way of giving chemotherapy and the associated mortality rate was approximately 25%.

Today, this treatment still has many side-effects, including a profoundly low white cell count, but is over relatively quickly and provides women with a poor prognosis another treatment choice (Ayash et al 1994). High-dose treatment has become a much safer option than previously thought. Drugs are now available that stimulate blood cell production thus negating the need for bone marrow transplants; the medical teams caring for such patients have become more skilled in coping with the treatment-associated toxicities.

So far, the research trials on high-dose chemotherapy have not been encouraging. Several international trials looking at high-dose chemotherapy for the treatment of metastatic breast cancer, or as an adjuvant treatment for women at high risk of a cancer relapse have shown that there was no significant survival advantage for women treated in this way (Berger 1999). Further randomised studies will be necessary to demonstrate whether this treatment provides a real advantage to such women (Rodenhuis et al 1998).

Palliative chemotherapy

The aim of palliative treatment is:

> 'The active total care of patients whose disease is not responsive to curative treatment. Control of pain, of other symptoms, and of psychological, social and spiritual problems, is paramount. The goal of palliative care is achievement of the best quality of life for patients and their families. Many aspects of palliative care are also applicable earlier in the course of the illness in conjunction with anticancer treatments.'
> (World Health Organization 1990)

Chemotherapy is no exception to this and should be used to treat symptoms associated with metastatic disease (such as liver pain). Because it is not possible to cure this group of patients, or prolong life, optimal quality of life is a priority of treatment. It is important to closely monitor the patient's progress to ensure that their quality of life outweighs the toxicity of treatment. The most common regimen used to treat metastatic breast cancer is cyclophosphamide, methotrexate and 5-fluorouracil (this is also discussed in Ch. 8).

Chemotherapy administration and handling

In this section the management of breast cancer patients requiring chemotherapy will be outlined, including strategies in self-care. Areas to be covered include provision, handling chemotherapy, information, and physical and psychological side-effects of chemotherapy.

Handling chemotherapy

Chemotherapy may be administered in several different ways. The most common routes of administration for breast cancer patients are intravenous and oral routes. Specially trained nurses working as part of a multidisciplinary oncology team should administer chemotherapy (Calman & Hine 1995). Such nurses have a high level of knowledge surrounding the holistic care of the patient requiring chemotherapy. They provide the patient and significant others with information, assess and manage toxicities associated with treatment and provide ongoing support. There are certain hazards for staff and patients, associated with chemotherapy drugs, which are minimised by skilled handling and knowledge. The Control of Substances Hazardous to Health (COSHH) Report (1994) provides guidelines for the safe handling of hazardous substances. However, the available research does not show a connection between the handling of chemotherapeutic drugs and long-term health risks to staff (Goodman 1999). The most important point to remember for non-cancer nurses who may be involved in handling oral preparations is that gloves must be worn and that tablets should not be crushed.

Preparing the patient

Before a patient begins chemotherapy the nurse provides them with written and verbal information regarding their treatment. Information has been shown, in a review of the literature by Ream & Richardson (1996), to reduce distress and aid adaptation to living with cancer and its treatments. Preparing the patient for the sensory experience of treatment, i.e. touch, smells, sounds and the sight of chemotherapy is highlighted by Ream et al (1997) as being particularly important.

Effects of chemotherapy and implications for nursing care

Patients experience side-effects from chemotherapy because the drugs used cannot distinguish between normal and cancerous dividing cells. The side-effects experienced depend upon the drugs or combination of drugs used and are usually transient due to the ability of normal cell division to recover. It could be assumed that i.v. drugs cause more side-effects than oral medication. However, side-effects are dependent on individual chemotherapy drugs and not the method of administration. The experience of women receiving chemotherapy for breast cancer and strategies to manage toxicities will now be outlined.

Physical Side-effects of chemotherapy

Veins

A woman undergoing chemotherapy treatment faces multiple needle sticks for blood testing and i.v. cannulation. Needle phobia is common in patients who are having chemotherapy and may be more distressing than having the chemotherapy for some. This may be a pre-established phobia or may develop if venous access becomes difficult and results in multiple needle stick attempts. Venous access is often limited to one arm in this group of patients due to lymph node damage caused by surgery or metastasis in the axillary nodes. Use of the affected arm for venous access could increase the risk of lymphoedema and potential skin damage.

Chemotherapy nurses are usually experts in venous access device care. The nurse assesses the condition of the patient's veins and any needle phobia at the start of each treatment. The nurse also takes into account the drugs that are to be administered and the length of the treatment schedule. If a peripheral cannula is deemed suitable, the nurse will insert this and can be very expert in accessing difficult veins with minimal discomfort to the patient. Small paediatric-sized cannulae are used, which minimises pain and damage to the veins. When administering i.v. chemotherapy, particular care is taken with vesicant drugs such as Doxorubicin, Epirubicin and Mitomycin C, which can cause venous pain. These drugs are also dangerous if they leak into the surrounding tissue, which can result in tissue necrosis.

Long-term central venous catheters may be used to prevent damage to veins, relieve needle phobia and allow easy venous access for patients with difficult veins. Blood samples may be taken from these lines and chemotherapy administered. Two types of central venous lines are commonly used in chemotherapy units and may be seen in Figures 6.2 and 6.3. Skin-tunnelled lines of the Hickman type are catheters that are inserted through the chest into a large vein leading to the heart. The visible part of the line is skin tunnelled along the chest wall. These lines may be left in place for several weeks or months. More recently peripherally inserted central catheter (PICC) lines have become popular in cancer treatment. Insertion involves a minor surgical procedure and venous access is obtained through a vein in the antecubital fossa. These lines may be inserted by a specially trained nurse on the ward or in the outpatient department. Research has shown that PICC lines have a low rate of complication, such as thrombosis (Merrell et al 1994) and infection (Goodwin & Carlson 1993). Recent research by Oakley et al (1998) found that a holistic nurse-led PICC line service was well received by patients, community and hospital-based nurses. Ongoing education and support was especially important for patients and

FIGURE 6.2

PICC line. Reproduced with kind permission from the Journal of Cancer Nursing, Peripherally inserted central venous catheters: the experience of a specialist oncology department. 1(1): 50–53.

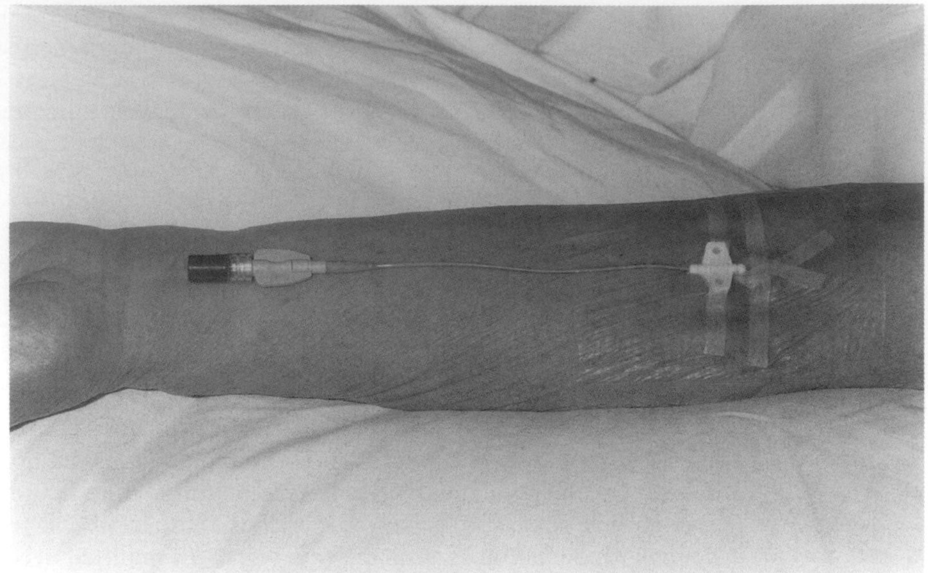

FIGURE 6.3

Hickman line. Reproduced with kind permission from Andrews G (ed) 2001, Women's Sexual Health, 2nd edn, Baillière Tindall, Edinburgh.

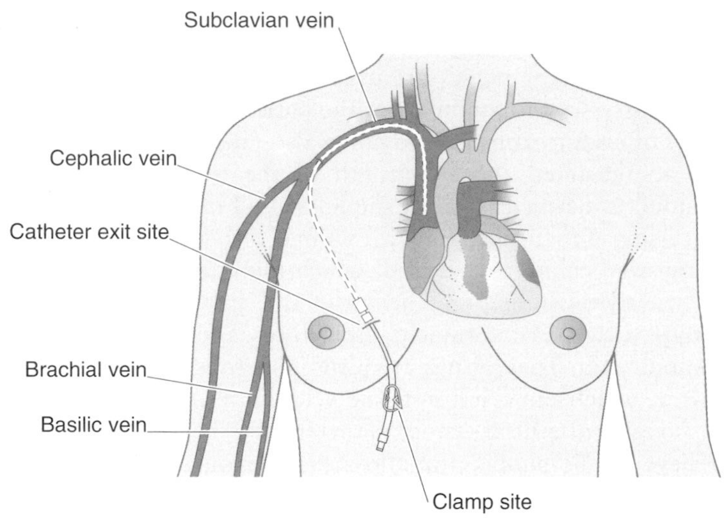

community nurses. The study also appeared to demonstrate less alteration in body image with PICC lines than Hickman lines (Figs 6.2 & 6.3). Complications associated with PICC and Hickman lines, strategies to reduce these and management of complications are highlighted in Tables 6.2 and 6.3.

Hair loss or alopecia

Hair loss or alopecia is one of the most distressing side-effects of chemotherapy (Dougherty 1996) and is associated with an alteration in body image (Gallagher 1992, Freedman 1994). This is particularly difficult for women with breast cancer who are at high risk of body image changes as a result of their disease or other

TABLE 6.2 *PICC lines – common complications*

Complication	Symptoms	Action
Mechanical phlebitis (vein inflammation) Most common problem, usually occurring during first week post insertion. Caused by catheter irritating the vein/use of powdered gloves to insert line.	Tenderness/pain. Redness/warmth. Venous cord. Induration/Swelling.	Inform oncology team. Apply heat to the upper arm three times a day for 24 h. If no improvement after 48 h consider line removal.
Infection Caused by: Poor insertion technique/after care. Immunosuppression.	Pyrexia/rigors – may occur after line flush. Redness, drainage or swelling at site. Pain or tenderness at the site or along the vein.	Inform oncology team. Antibiotics. Line blood cultures. Possible line removal and tip culture.
Thrombosis Problem for cancer patients. Increased risk with foreign body in the vein. Patients to take 1–2 mg of warfarin daily to reduce the risk.	Swelling of the neck/arm on the side of the line. Dilated veins across wall of the chest. Pain in the chest or arm.	Inform oncology team. Venogram. Line removal. Anticoagulation
Occlusion **1.** Unable to take blood but able to flush – may be caused by fibrin sheath on tip of catheter or tip pressing against vein wall. **2.** Blood clot in catheter lumen due to blood reflux. Caused by improper flushing (especially after blood removal) or patient vomiting, coughing, heavy lifting.	Inability to flush line/withdraw blood.	Inform oncology team. Urokinase 5000 iu/ml may relieve blockage.
Mechanical failure **1.** Fragile lines which easily puncture or break. Fracture most commonly occurs due to excessive pressure when flushing a blocked line.	Torn line. Line leaks when flushed.	Inform oncology team. Line may be repaired.
2. Valve failure.	Blood flow down the line when not in use.	Line may require removal.
Accidental removal		Apply pressure. Contact oncology team.

TABLE 6.3 *Skin tunnelled lines – common complications*

Complication	Symptoms	Action
Exit site infection Usually due to organisms on the skin.	Redness. Pain. Discharge. Heat.	Inform oncology team. Take a swab. Patient may require oral or intravenous antibiotics.
Infection in the catheter lumen Caused by poor insertion technique/aftercare. Increased risk with neutropenia.	Fever. Rigor after line has been accessed. Redness/tenderness/pain. Discharge. Heat.	Inform oncology team. Take blood cultures from the line and peripherally. Start intravenous antibiotics. Possibly remove line if infection does not resolve.
Thrombosis Problem for cancer patients. Increased risk with foreign body in the vein. Patients to take 1–2 mg of warfarin daily to reduce the risk.	**Related to impaired blood flow** Shoulder tip pain. Swollen arm. Distended veins in the neck. Swollen face. Changes in skin colour/temperature. Shortness of breath.	Venogram to confirm thrombosis. Remove line. Anticoagulation.
Occlusion **1.** Unable to take blood but able to flush – may be caused by fibrin sheath on tip of catheter or tip pressing against vein wall. **2.** Blood clot in catheter lumen due to blood reflux. Caused by improper flushing (especially after blood removal) or patient vomiting, coughing, heavy lifting.	Inability to flush line/withdraw blood.	Inform oncology team. Urokinase 5000 iu/ml may relieve blockage.
Split line – internal Risk of chemotherapy leaking into subcutaneous tissue and tissue necrosis if vesicant drug being administered.	Pain when line flushed. Redness swelling across chest wall.	Do not use the line and stop any infusion. Inform oncology team. Seek radiologist's opinion. Remove the line if split.
Split line – external Avoid using scissors to remove dressings.	Line leaks when flushed.	Inform oncology team. Line may be repaired.

treatments such as surgery or radiotherapy. Doxorubicin, epirubicin and Taxol cause complete hair loss including loss of scalp hair, eyebrows, eyelashes and pubic hair (Gallagher 1992). Cyclophosphamide causes hair thinning but in high doses will cause total alopecia. Hair loss may start within a few days or weeks of treatment depending on the drugs used. The hair usually starts to grow 4–6 weeks following the final treatment, with most patients having a good head of hair at 6 months.

Scalp cooling may be used to reduce hair loss associated with chemotherapy treatment. The aim of scalp cooling is to cool the circulating blood flow to the scalp, consequently preventing the chemotherapy from reaching the hair follicles. Scalp cooling involves placing a cold cap on the patient's head 15 min before the i.v. chemotherapy is administered. The hats are then changed every 45 min. The number of hats used depends on the plasma half-life of the chemotherapy drug. Taxol requires seven hats whereas epirubicin requires three or four hats, depending on the dose. Despite scalp cooling, some hair loss will occur and total hair loss cannot always be prevented.

Scalp cooling is most ineffective in patients who have liver disease. These patients do not excrete the drugs as quickly as those with normal liver function. The effectiveness of scalp cooling is unclear and needs to be further researched (Tierney 1987; Gallagher 1992).

Scalp cooling can be uncomfortable, upsetting and lengthy for the patient (Dougherty 1996). However, a pilot study by Dougherty (1996) found that patients felt that scalp cooling was beneficial, even if some hair loss occurred. These patients also felt that it should be made available in all chemotherapy units.

The chemotherapy nurse plays a vital role in supporting women through the threat of hair loss. Information is vital so that the woman is aware that she may lose her hair (Dougherty 1996). Information should include a description of the actual hair loss process, including the dramatic nature of this (Gallagher 1992) and the scalp-cooling procedure. A wig would be offered and the best time to consult a wig specialist is before hair loss starts. Gallagher (1992) states that careful consideration should be given to the meaning of hair loss for each individual patient and ways of coping with this explored. Advice on scarves and hats has also been found to help women cope with this distressing side-effect. One service that is available across the UK, is Look Good Feel Better. This registered charity offers free consultations on make up and skin care for women with cancer. The aim of the service is to improve self-esteem for women with cancer.

Sore mouth

Chemotherapy attacks the cells that form the lining of the mouth. This can result in an inflamed mouth, or stomatitis, and an opportunistic thrush infection. These patients may also develop mouth ulcers and a herpes simplex virus. Damage to the mouth can result in pain, distress and difficulty in eating and drinking (Jones 1998). Methotrexate, doxorubicin and epirubicin are the drugs most likely to cause stomatitis. A patient can reduce the risk of a sore mouth when receiving methotrexate by taking folinic acid rescue tablets 24 hours following chemotherapy administration.

A healthy diet is important to promote healing, and careful mouth care to prevent infection and soothe the mouth. The patient should be advised to use a soft toothbrush, which should be rinsed well after use. Jones (1998) suggests that crusting on the lips is removed with warm water, and petroleum jelly applied. If stomatitis is present in the mouth, it is advisable to gently clean with swab sticks soaked in warm water, or a thin layer of chlorhexidine gel or chlorhexidine mouth wash (0.2%) (Jones 1998). Herpes simplex (cold sores) may be treated with Zovirax cream and ulcers with sucralfate mouthwash. Saliva substitutes are available for the relief of a dry mouth.

Mouthwashes containing local anaesthetic and anti-inflammatory properties, such as Difflam are available from most pharmacies. Chlorhexidine gluconate is an effective mouthwash because it reduces plaque (Turner 1996) and has antibacterial and fungicidal properties (Jones 1998). The patient should also rinse the mouth with nystatin to prevent oral thrush. If thrush develops, then an additional antifungal drug such as fluconazole should be prescribed.

Cystitis

Cyclophosphamide can cause cystitis, which can be treated through a good fluid intake.

Bone marrow suppression

The most worrying side-effect of chemotherapy is the destruction of blood cells, particularly white cells. Patients typically experience a drop in their white cell count between 10 and 14 days following treatment. Occasionally the white count can drop to a level where the patient cannot fight infection normally. If a patient has any sign of infection the chemotherapy unit should be contacted. The patient would require an immediate blood test to assess the white cell count. If the count were low the patient would require i.v. antibiotic treatment as an inpatient. Sometimes the blood count does not recover in time for the next chemotherapy treatment and this would be delayed, usually by 1 week.

If patients persistently have problems with low blood counts the dose of the chemotherapy may be reduced or granulocyte colony stimulating factors (GCSFs) used to stimulate white cell production.

Gastrointestinal symptoms

Nausea and vomiting

Nausea and vomiting are some of the commonest complications associated with chemotherapy. Vomiting is coordinated via the vomiting centre in the brain. There are four stages associated with chemotherapy-induced nausea and vomiting:

1. The anticipatory stage before chemotherapy is administered
2. The acute stage occurs within minutes of chemotherapy being given
3. The subacute stage within 6–12 h of treatment
4. The delayed stage at least 24 h after chemotherapy.

Anticipatory nausea and vomiting is difficult to control and is associated with worsening acute nausea and vomiting (Goodman 1997). Triggers for anticipatory nausea and vomiting include association with chemotherapy such as the chemotherapy nurse, hospital, smells and auditory stimulation.

Predisposing factors associated with nausea and vomiting will now be addressed and include: chemotherapy regimens, prior experience of chemotherapy, gender, alcohol, disease status, fear of needles, previous experience with non-chemotherapy-induced nausea, and excretion of drugs.

Some chemotherapeutic drugs, for example cisplatin, epirubicin and doxorubicin are more emetogenic than others. The emetogenic potential of drugs is also dependent on the frequency and method of administration, and duration of treatment. Patients who have not had previous experience with chemotherapy are less likely to encounter nausea and vomiting (Morrow 1992). Also, patients who have experienced uncontrolled chemotherapy-induced nausea tend to have similar problems throughout treatment, despite changing anti-emetic cover or chemotherapy regimens (Italian Group for Anti-emetic Research 1995). Anticipatory nausea and vomiting is more common in women than men and has been identified in women receiving CMF chemotherapy for breast cancer (Jacobsen et al 1993). Previous alcohol abuse reduces nausea and vomiting in patients receiving chemotherapy (Goodman 1997). Disease status can also have an impact on the incidence of nausea and vomiting, for example, a woman with metastatic breast cancer may have symptoms associated with high calcium, brain metastases, renal status, ascites, dehydration, abnormal urea and electrolyte blood levels. Distress caused by a fear of needles is associated with nausea. Some women may have a predisposed tendency to nausea, having experienced motion sickness or sickness during pregnancy. Finally, delayed excretion of drugs caused by liver impairment can result in protracted nausea and vomiting.

Anti-emetics interrupt the stimulation of the vomiting centre. These drugs are chosen to match the emetic potential of the chemotherapy drugs. Anti-emetic protocols direct the health care professional to prescribe the most effective anti-nausea drugs. These protocols guide the health care professional to prescribe a stronger anti-emetic if the current treatment is ineffectual. New anti-emetics are now available, which have drastically reduced the instance of nausea and vomiting associated with chemotherapy. These 5HT3 antagonists (e.g. ondansetron and granisetron) are most effective for the first 48 h of chemotherapy and are generally reserved for the most emetogenic drugs such as cisplatin, epirubicin and doxorubicin. Their effect is enhanced when used in combination with dexamethasone. Other common anti-emetics include metoclopramide, domperidone and cyclizine. Generally, the patient is given anti-emetics prior to chemotherapy and for at least 5 days following treatment. The aim of anti-emetic therapy is to prevent nausea and vomiting.

The patient should be taught about the potential risks of nausea and vomiting and to report any symptoms so that anti-emetics may be changed. Also, it is worth remembering the side-effects of anti-emetics as these may outweigh the benefits. Steroids for example can cause hyperactivity, sleeplessness and weight gain.

Anorexia

Anorexia may occur in women with breast cancer and is associated with loss of taste, smell and nausea and vomiting. In metastatic disease it may be confounded by physical symptoms. However, it should not be assumed that weight loss will be a problem in women receiving adjuvant treatment. These women may experience weight gain, which can be due to the steroids used to control nausea, decreased activity, and the feeling of nausea in the stomach that is alleviated by eating. If anorexia is a problem this should be explored with the patient and a referral made to an oncology dietician.

Diarrhoea

Diarrhoea may occur due to the destructive effect of cytotoxics, such as 5-fluorouracil, on the lining of the gastrointestinal tract. Patients may experience abdominal cramps and varying degrees of diarrhoea. Normally diarrhoea may be controlled with loperamide and dietary measures such as a low-residue, high-calorie and protein diet. A stool specimen should be taken to ensure that the cause is not infection. However, occasionally the patient experiences a severe episode of diarrhoea, which may require hospital admission and rehydration.

Fatigue

Fatigue, which has been identified as the worst symptom of chemotherapy treatment, has become an increasing focus in recent years. The reason that fatigue has become more evident has been attributed to the improved control of physical symptoms such as nausea and vomiting (Coates et al 1983, Griffin et al 1996). Richardson & Ream (1998) in a review of the literature, stated that the impact of fatigue for patients is often underestimated by health care professionals and rated more highly by primary care givers. Fatigue is a subjective experience, influenced by multiple factors including cancer treatments, the physical effects of cancer and psycho-social influences (Richardson & Ream 1998). Patients find it difficult to express and describe the effect of fatigue associated with chemotherapy. The effects are usually most profound during the few days following treatment and when the white blood cell count is at its lowest. The symptoms of fatigue may continue after treatment has stopped (Pearce & Richardson 1998, Ream & Richardson 1997).

Self-care strategies for managing fatigue identified through research suggest that exercise is most effective in combating fatigue (Macvickar et al 1989, Mock et al 1997). Berger (1998), in a study looking at women with breast cancer, also found that patients should monitor fatigue and balance exercise with rest. Diversional therapies (Cimprich 1993) and psycho-social interventions (Forester et al 1985) are also beneficial in reducing fatigue.

Infertility/menopausal symptoms

Cytotoxic drugs can damage the ovaries, causing infertility and amenorrhoea. Drugs used in breast cancer, which are known to cause such damage, include cyclophosphamide and cisplatin. The effects of cyclophosphamide, methotrexate and 5-fluorouracil (CMF) have been studied in women with breast cancer and have demonstrated that an early menopause is common in women over 30 years. The average risk of amenorrhoea for women receiving CMF is 40% for those under the age of 40 and 75–80% for those over 40 years of age. Amenorrhoea is usually irreversible in older women, but in younger women, menstruation may return within 2–3 years. Larger doses of cyclophosphamide or prolonged courses of CMF increase the risk of amenorrhoea. Effects on sexual function may occur during treatment, but normally recover after it has stopped. If the menopause is induced the patient will experience normal symptoms including mood swings, hot flushes and vaginal dryness. Hormone replacement therapy (HRT) would normally be prescribed for women experiencing menopausal symptoms. However, medical opinion is divided on the risk of HRT prescription for women who have experienced breast cancer and it is not considered suitable for women under 45 years old.

The chemotherapy nurse would explore the risks of infertility and a premature menopause with the woman prior to the start of her chemotherapy. Chemotherapy cannot be considered as a method of contraception and protection against pregnancy should be used during treatment and for 1 year after. Theoretically, in the first trimester chemotherapy can have a mutagenic effect on the fetus. However, a higher rate of birth defects compared to the general population has not been identified in children conceived following treatment. Fertility treatment can be offered to women who have damaged ovaries as a result of chemotherapeutic treatment. Egg storage prior to the commencement of chemotherapy is in the early stages of development and may offer benefits to women in the future.

Psycho-social impact of chemotherapy

Breast cancer is often associated with mutilating surgery and frightening chemotherapy treatment (Fallowfield et al 1990, Fredette 1995). Hughes (1986) suggests that the psychological and physical impact of disease and treatment may be the precipitating causes of anxiety and depression. Adjuvant chemotherapy has been shown to increase the risk of psychological morbidity (Hughson et al 1987) with Maguire et al (1980) finding the risk to increase the more toxic the treatment. There is some evidence that chemotherapy affects cognitive state. However, this is difficult to distinguish from psychological distress (Silberfarb et al 1980). Perceived loss of control is a common concern amongst cancer patients (Northouse 1981), with uncontrollable life events, such as cancer, being shown by Brown & Harris (1978), to increase the probability of breakdown of mental health. Cancer patients may feel a lack of internal control with the cancer and health care professional appearing to take control.

Woodcock (1997) states that chemotherapy regimens may result in a lifestyle change, change of role and subsequent lowering of self-esteem and ability to interact with individuals. This may be the result of the disruption caused through attending the hospital for chemotherapy, and also, through the effects of chemotherapy, such as alopecia, diarrhoea or nausea and vomiting. Breast cancer itself and chemotherapy treatment may also affect the patient's sexuality and body image. This includes the intrusion of i.v. lines (Price 1990). The Royal College of Nursing (RCN 1995) noted that skin-tunnelled lines can act as a constant reminder of cancer.

The adaptation to difficult and changing physical and emotional circumstances is considered by Fallowfield to be a good outcome of coping for breast cancer patients. In order to reduce anxiety related to treatment, an aim of care could be to identify the patient's perceived threat of treatment, loss of control and the benefit of previous coping strategies. Suitable strategies could then be promoted and adjusted according to changing needs, in order to enhance quality of survivorship.

Home chemotherapy

Home or domicilary chemotherapy for cancer patients in the UK is becoming increasingly available. Oncology units have been instrumental in establishing home chemotherapy services (Richardson 1988, Daniels 1995, Oakley 1997) and several home care companies are now available to provide chemotherapy at home (Watters 1997). This shift of care from the hospital to the home environment is largely driven by the Calman–Hine report (1995). This report looked at the reconfiguration of cancer services in the UK and stated that the focus of cancer care should be in the community. This move is also driven from the overcrowding experienced in chemotherapy day units. However, it is important to identify the treatment setting most appropriate to patients and their families. This may be the patient's home or the hospital. Correct allocation should facilitate optimal patient quality of life and allocation of resources.

COMPLEMENTARY THERAPIES

Women who are being treated for breast cancer undergo a whole range of physical and psychological challenges. More women are turning to complementary therapies to help them cope with the effects of their cancer and complementary therapies are an increasingly acceptable facet of cancer treatment in the UK. Such therapies appear to assist patients and their carers to regain a degree of control over their cancer and more traditional cancer treatments such as chemotherapy (Gates 1998). At a recent conference Dr R Daniel, the Medical Director of the Bristol Cancer Help Centre, stressed the benefits of complementary therapies. She stated that they help improve health and energy, give a new meaning and value to life and empower patients and their carers to help themselves, thus reducing feelings of helplessness.

Studies have shown that chronic stress has a negative impact on survival in cancer patients (Reighlin 1993). This has been strongly linked to the depressing effect of emotions on the immune system (Felton et al 1985, McEwen & Stellar 1993). It is thought that complementary therapies help patients to deal with their emotions, therefore increasing their immunity and ability to fight cancer and deal with the physical effects of cancer and its treatments.

Research into the effectiveness of complementary therapies has shown that psychotherapy improves survival of patients with metastatic breast cancer (Spiegel et al 1989). Fawzy et al (1993) have demonstrated similar findings in psychiatry for patients with metastatic melanoma. Massage has also been shown to benefit cancer patients in research. Corner (1995) randomised cancer patients to receive essential oil or plain oil massage; these patients reported significantly reduced anxiety levels and improvements in physical and emotional symptoms. The benefits of the oils themselves was not proven in this study. However, Wilkinson (1995), in a similar study demonstrated a statistically significant improvement in the aromatherapy group for quality of life, physical symptoms and anxiety. Aromatherapy, the use of essential oils, can be used very successfully with therapeutic massage. If a patient wishes to undergo therapeutic massage, it is advisable to check with their oncology consultant and to choose a masseuse who has an International Therapy Examination Council (ITEC) qualification (Hildebrand 1994).

Few studies have explored the impact of complementary therapies in controlling symptoms associated with chemotherapy. Research has shown that visualisation and relaxation reduce nausea (Redd et al 1993, Troesh et al 1993). Anecdotal reports of the use of complementary therapies suggest that patients receiving chemotherapy experience fewer side-effects. For example, Stevenson (1996) has found acupuncture effective for the control of nausea. A service offered at the Hammersmith Hospital found complementary therapies helped patients to feel calm and more able to cope with their treatments (Bell 1998). More specifically, Bell found aromatherapy burners in the chemotherapy room effective against nausea and that reflexology helped combat nausea, especially anticipatory nausea, which can be extremely difficult to treat.

Other therapies may have a place in helping the woman take some control over her situation by helping her physical symptoms and making them easier to cope with such as:

- Macrobiotic diet
- Homoeopathy
- Use of therapeutic touch
- Relaxation
- Visualisation.

Any complementary therapy should be discussed with the medical team caring for her in case there are particular contraindications. For more detail on such supportive therapies the reader is referred to *Well's Supportive Therapies in Health Care* (Wells & Tschudin 1994).

NEW THERAPIES

New cytotoxic therapies are being researched all the time and immunotherapy may be an area that offers another choice of treatment to the woman with breast cancer. One of these therapies is Herceptin, a genetically engineered antibody, that has been developed to block the HER-2/*neu* growth factor receptor found on the surface of the breast cancer cell. This receptor is overexpressed in about 25–30% of breast cancers, specifically in young women. Herceptin is administered by i.v. infusion, usually over 1 h and may be given in conjunction with other chemotherapy. The main side-effects of this treatment are fever and chills, mild pain, headache and nausea. Herceptin has also been associated with cardiotoxicity. This drug is currently offered in a few centres in the UK and is being tested in women with metastatic disease (Hadden 1999). Theratope and other experimental vaccines are also being developed. By provoking the immune system to recognise abnormal cancer cells the body produces antibodies to fight the breast cancer (Hadden 1999).

Although experimental, immune therapies usually have few side-effects and offer another choice of treatment to women who have metastatic disease.

CONCLUSION

There are many permutations of medical treatments that a woman who has breast cancer may undergo. Although there are guidelines for treatment, each treatment plan should be, within reason, tailored to the individual patient. Despite many of these treatments being medically directed and prescribed, there is a great deal of scope for nurses to be creative with their practice to enhance the patient's treatment experience. The next chapter will deal with the issues concerning the patient if their breast cancer returns.

REFERENCES

Abernethy K 1997 The Menopause and HRT. Baillière Tindall, London

Andrews G 2001 Women's Sexual Health, 2nd edn. Baillière Tindall, Edinburgh

Anglo Celtic Oncology Group 1996 Intensive chemotherapy for high risk breast cancer. (BR9505)

Ayash L, Elias A, Wheeler C et al 1994 Double dose intensive chemotherapy with autologous marrow and peripheral blood progenitor cell support for metastatic breast cancer: a feasibility study. Journal of Clinical Oncology 12(1): 37–44

Bates T, Evans R G 1995 Report of the independent review commissioned by the Royal College of Radiologists into brachial plexus neuropathy following radiotherapy for breast cancer. Royal College of Radiologists, London

Baum M and Schipper H 1999 Fast Facts – Breast Cancer. Health Press Ltd, Oxford

Bell L 1998 Integrating complementary therapies into cancer care. Reflexions, March: 4–5

Berger A 1998 Patterns of fatigue and activity and rest during adjuvant breast cancer chemotherapy. Oncology Nursing Forum 25(1): 51–62

Berger A 1999 High dose chemotherapy offers little benefit in breast cancer, new article BMJ 318: 1440

Bonadonna G, Valagussa P, Moliterni A, Zambetti M, Brambilla C 1995 Adjuvant cyclophosphamide, methotrexate and 5-fluorouracil in node-positive breast cancer: the results of 20 years of follow-up. New England Journal of Medicine 332(14): 901–906

British Surgeons Group of the British Association of Surgical Oncology 1995 Guidelines for surgeons in the management of symptomatic breast disease in the United Kingdom. European Journal of Surgical Oncology 21(Suppl. A): 1–13

Brown G W, Harris T 1978 Social origins of depression: a reply. Psychol Med 8(4): 577–588

Bruzzi P 1998 Tamoxifen for the prevention of breast cancer. Important questions remain unanswered, and existing trials should continue. BMJ 316(7139): 1181–1182

Burnet N G, Johansen J, Turesson I, Nyman J, Peacock J H 1998 Describing patients' normal tissue reactions: Concerning the possibility of individualising radiotherapy dose prescriptions based on potential predictive assays of normal tissue radiosensitivity. Steering Committee of the BioMed2 European Union Concerted Action Programme on the Development of Predictive Tests of Normal Tissue Response to Radiation Therapy. International Journal of Cancer 79: 606–613

Buzzoni R, Bonadonna G, Valagussa P, Zambetti M 1991 Adjuvant chemotherapy with doxorubicin plus cyclophosphamide, methotrexate and 5-fluorouracil in the treatment of resectable breast cancer with more than three positive axillary lymph nodes. JCO 9: 2134–2140

Calman K, Hine D 1995 A Policy for Commissioning Cancer Services. A Report by the Expert Advisory Group on Cancer to the Chief Medical Officers of England and Wales. Department of Health, London

COSHH (Control of Substances Hazardous to Health) Regulations 1994 HSE IND(G) 136L (revised) 10/96 C2000

Chapman D, Goodman M 1997 Breast Cancer. In: Groenwald S L, Goodman M, Frogge M H, Yarbro C H. Cancer Nursing: Principles and Practice, 4th edn. Jones and Bartlett, MA, USA Ch 34, p 916–979

Cimprich B 1993 Developments of an intervention to restore attention in cancer patients. Cancer Nursing 16(2): 83–92

Coates A, Abraham S, Kaye S, Sowerbutts T, Frewin C, Fox R, Tattersall M 1983 On the receiving end; patient perception of the side effects of cancer chemotherapy. European Journal of Cancer Clinical Oncology 19(2): 302–308

Coleman R E 1999 Medical management of bone metastases. Continuing Medical Education Bulletin 1(3) 70–75
Corner J 1995 Innovative approaches in symptom management. Eur J Cancer Care (Engl) 4(4): 145–146
Cotton T 1996 Radiotherapy for Breast Cancer. In: Denton S (ed) Breast Cancer Nursing. Chapman and Hall, London
Cuzick J, Stewart H, Rutqvist J et al 1994 Cause-specific mortality in long term survivors of breast cancer who participated in trials of radiotherapy. Journal of Clinical Oncology 12(3): 447–453
Daniels E L 1995 Developing a home chemotherapy service. International Journal of Cancer Nursing 1(2): 81–85
Dhingra K 1999 Antiestrogens–tamoxifen, SERMs and beyond. Invest New Drugs 17(3): 285–311
Dixon J M, Hortobagyi G 2000 Treating young patients with breast cancer. The evidence suggests that all should be treated with adjuvant therapy. British Medical Journal 320: 457–458
Dougherty L 1996 Scalp cooling to prevent hair loss in chemotherapy. Professional Nurse 11(8): 507–509
Early Breast Cancer Trialists' Collaborative Group (EBCTCG) 1992 Systemic treatment of early breast cancer by hormonal, cytotoxic or immune therapy. 133 randomised trials involving 31,000 recurrences and 24,000 deaths among 75,000 women. Lancet 330: 1–15, 71–85
Early Breast Cancer Trialists' Collaborative Group (EBCTCG) 1998a Polychemotherapy for early breast cancer: an overview of the randomised trials. Lancet 352: 930–942
Early Breast Cancer Trialists' Collaborative Group 1998b Tamoxifen for early breast cancer: an overview of the randomised trials. The Lancet 351: 1451–1467
Eder J P, Antman K, Peters W P et al 1986 High dose combination alkylating agents chemotherapy with autologous bone marrow support for metastatic breast cancer. Journal of Clinical Oncology 4: 1592–1597
Eli Lilly 1998 The Royal Marsden Cytotoxic Handbook. Eli Lilly, London
Faithful S 1998 Fatigue in patients receiving radiotherapy. Professional Nurse 13(7): 459–461
Fallowfield L, Hall A, Maguire G P, Baum M 1990 Psychological outcomes of different treatment policies in women with early breast cancer outside of a clinical trial. British Medical Journal 302: 575–580
Fawzy I et al 1993 Malignant melanoma, effects of an early structured psychiatric intervention, coping and affective state on recurrence and survival six years later. Archives of General Psychiatry 50(a): 681
Felton D et al 1985 Noradrenergic sympathetic innervation of lymphoid tissue. Journal of Immunology 135
Fenlon D 1996 Endocrine therapies for breast cancer. In: Denton S (ed) Breast Cancer Nursing. Chapman and Hall London, ch 8, p 104–123
Fisher B, Anderson S, Redmond C K, Wolmark N, Wickerham D L, Cronin W M 1995 Reanalysis and results after 12 years of follow-up in a randomized clinical trial comparing total mastectomy with lumpectomy with or without irradiation in the treatment of breast cancer. New England Journal of Medicine 333(22): 1456–1461
Forester B, Kornfeld D, Fleiss J 1985 Psychotherapy during radiation: effects on emotional and physical distress. American Journal of Psychiatry 142: 22–27
Fredette S L 1995 Breast cancer survivors, concerns and coping. Cancer Nursing 18(1): 35–46
Freedman R R, Woodward S 1992 Behavioural treatment of menopausal hot flushes: evaluation by ambulatory monitoring. American Journal of Obstetrics and Gynaecology. 167: 436–439
Freedman T G 1994 Social and cultural dimensions of hair loss in women treated for breast cancer. Cancer Nursing 17(4): 334–341
Gallagher J 1992 Women's experience of hair loss associated with cancer chemotherapy. Unpublished dissertation. University of Massachusetts
Gates E 1998 A compliment to care. Nursing Times 94(9): 55–57
Goodman I 1999 The administration of cytotoxic chemotherapy (Recommendations). Royal College of Nursing, London
Goodman M 1997 Risk factors and antiemetic management of chemotherapy-induced nausea and vomiting. Oncology Nursing Forum 124(7): supplement 20–32
Goodwin M, Carlson I 1993 The peripherally inserted catheter; a retrospective look at three years of insertions. Journal of Intravenous Nursing 16(20): 92–103
Griffin A, Butow P, Coates A, Childs A, Ellis P, Dunn S 1996 On the receiving end: patient perceptions of the side effects of cancer chemotherapy in 1993. Ann Oncol 7: 189–95

Hadden J W 1999 The immunology and immunotherapy of breast cancer: an update. International Journal of Immunopharmocology. 21(2): 79–101

Hall E J, Cox J D 1994 Physical and biologic basis of radiation therapy. In: Cox J D (ed) Moss's Radiation Oncology: Rationale, Technique, Results 7th edn. St. Louis Mosby-Yearbook Inc., p 3–66

Harvey H A 1998 Emerging role of aromatase inhibitors in the treatment of breast cancer. Oncology-Huntington 12(3): 32–35

Hildebrand S 1994 Therapeutic massage and aromatherapy. In: Wells R, Tschudin V (eds) Wells' Supportive Therapies in Health Care. Baillière Tindall, London

HMSO 1999 The Ionising Radiations Regulations

Honig S F 1996 Hormonal therapy and chemotherapy. In: Harris J R, Lippman M E, Morrow M, Hellman S (eds) Diseases of the Breast. Lippincott Raven, Philadelphia, 669–718

Hughes J 1986 Depression in cancer patients. In: Stall B (ed) Coping With Cancer Stress, Martinus Nijhof, Chichester

Hughson A, Cooper A, McArdle C, Smith D 1987 Psychological impact of adjuvant chemotherapy in the first two years after mastectomy. British Medical Journal 293: 1265–1271

Italian Group for Antiemetic Research 1995 Persistence of efficacy of three antiemetic regimens and prognostic factors in patients undergoing moderately emetogenic chemotherapy. Journal of Clinical Oncology 13: 2417–2426

Jacobsen P, Bovbjerg D H, Redd W H 1993 Anticipatory anxiety in women receiving chemotherapy for breast cancer. Health Psychology 12: 469–475

Jones C V 1998 The importance of oral hygiene in nutritional support. British Journal of Nursing 17: 274–283

Kroman N, Jensen M, Wohlfhart J, Mouridson H T, Anderson P K, Melbye M 2000 Factors influencing the effect of age on prognosis in breast cancer: population based study. British Medical Journal 7233: 474–478

Langmack K A 1998 Factors influencing occupational radiation doses to brachytherapy nurses. Radiography 4: 141–146

Leonard R, Rodger A, Dixon J 1995 Metastatic Breast Cancer. In: Dixon J M (ed) ABC of Breast Diseases. BMJ Publishing Group, London p 45–49

Lien E A, Lonning P E 2000 Selective oestrogen receptor modifiers (SERMs) and breast cancer therapy. Cancer Treat Rev 26(3): 205–227

Macvickar M, Winningham M, Nickel J 1989 Effects of aerobic interval training on cancer patients' functional capacity. Journal of Nursing Research 38(6): 348–351

Maguire G P, Tait A, Brooke M et al 1980 Psychiatric morbidity and physical toxicity associated with adjuvant chemotherapy after mastectomy. British Medical Journal (ii): 1179–1180

Mansi J L, Smith I E, Walsh G et al 1989 Primary medical therapy for operable breast cancer. European Journal of Cancer and Clinical Oncology 25(11): 1623–1627

McEwen B S, Steller E 1993 Stress and the individual mechanisms leading to disease. Archives of Internal Medicine 153: 2093–2101

Merrell S W, Peatross R N, Grossman M D, Sullivan J J, Harker W G 1994 Peripherally inserted central venous catheters, low risk alternatives for ongoing venous access. Western Journal of Medicine 160(1): 25–30

Mock V, Hassey Dow K, Meares C, 1997 Effects of exercise on fatigue, physical functioning and emotional distress during radiation therapy for breast cancer. Oncology Nursing Forum 24(6): 991–1000

Miller W R 1995 Prognostic factors. In: Dixon J M (ed) ABC of Breast Diseases. BMJ Publishing Group, London

Morrow G R 1992 Behavioural factors influencing the development and expression of chemotherapy-induced side effects. British Journal of Cancer 19: S54–S61

Nestel P J, Pomeroy S, Kay S et al 1999 Isoflavones from red clover improve systemic arterial compliance but not plasma lipids in menopausal women. Journal of Clinical Endocrinology and Metabolism 84(3): 895–898

Njar V C, Brodie A M 1999 Comprehensive pharmacology and clinical efficacy of aromatase inhibitors. Drugs 58: 233–255

Northouse L L 1981 Mastectomy patients and the fear of recurrence. Cancer Nursing 4(3): 213–220

Oakley C 1997 Home or hospital intravenous therapy for cancer: A pilot instrument to aid professional decision making. Unpublished dissertation. University of Manchester

Oakley C, Wright E, and Ream E 1998 The experiences of patients and nurses with a nurse led peripherally inserted central venous catheter line service. Unpublished research

Osborne C K 1999 Aromatase inhibitors in relation to other forms of endocrine therapy for breast cancer. Endocr Relat Cancer 6(2): 271–276

Overgaard M, Hansen P, Overgaard J et al 1997 Postoperative radiotherapy in high risk premenopausal women with breast cancer who receive adjuvant chemotherapy. New England Journal of Medicine 337: 949–955

Pearce S, Richardson A 1998 Fatigue in cancer: a phenomenological perspective. European Journal of Cancer Care 5(2): 111–115

Perez C A, Brady L W 1998 Principles and Practice of Radiation Oncology. Lippincott-Raven, Philadelphia

Powles T J 1983 The role of aromatase inhibitors in breast cancer. Seminars in Oncology 10 (Suppl 4): 4

Powles T, Eeles R, Ashley S et al 1998 Interim analysis of breast cancer in the Royal Marsden Hospital tamoxifen randomised chemoprevention trial. Lancet 352: 98–101

Price B 1990 A model for body image care. Journal of Advanced Nursing (15): 585–593

Pritchard K I, Paterson A H G, Paul N A, Zee B, Fine S, Pater J 1996 Increased thromboembolic complications with concurrent tamoxifen and chemotherapy in a randomised trial of adjuvant therapy for women with breast cancer. For the National Cancer Institute of Canada Clinical Trials Group Breast Cancer Site Group. Journal of Clinical Oncology 14: 2731–2737

Rea D, Poole C, Gray R 1998 Adjuvant tamoxifen: how long before we know how long? British Medical Journal 316: 1518–1519

Ream E, Richardson A 1996 The role of inflammation in patients' adaption to chemotherapy and radiotherapy: a review of the literature. European Journal of Cancer Care 5: 131

Ream E, Richardson A 1997 Fatigue in patients with cancer and chronic obstructive airways disease: a phenomenological enquiry. International Journal of Nursing Studies 34(1): 44–53

Ream E, Richardson A, Alexander-Dann C 1997 Patients' sensory experiences before, during and immediately following the administration of intravenous chemotherapy. Journal of Cancer Nursing 1(1): 25–31

Redd W H et al 1993 Nausea induced by mental images on chemotherapy. Cancer 72(2): 629–636

Reighlin S 1993 Mechanisms of disease: neuroendocrine-immune interactions. New England Journal of Medicine 329: 1246–1253

Richards M, Smith I E 1995 Role of systemic treatment for primary operable breast cancer. In: Dixon J M (ed) ABC of Breast Diseases. BMJ Publishing Group, London

Richardson J 1988 The administration of chemotherapy in the patient's home – a new perspective. In: Pritchard P (ed) Cancer Nursing – A Revolution in Care. Proceedings of the Fifth International Conference on Cancer Nursing. 4–9 September. Macmillan Press, London

Richardson A, Ream E 1998 Recent progress in understanding cancer-related fatigue. International Journal of Palliative Nursing 4(4): 192–198

Rodenhuis S, Richel D, van der Wall E et al 1998 Randomised trial of high dose chemotherapy and haemopoietic progenitor cell support in operable breast cancer with extensive axillary lymph node involvement. Lancet 352: 515–521

Rodger A 1998 Fears over radiotherapy fractionation regimens in breast cancer. Proposed UK trial needs to define techniques as well as numbers of treatments. British Medical Journal 317: 155–156

Royal College of Nursing 1995 Skin tunnelled catheters guidelines for care. Royal College of Nursing, London

Royal College of Radiologists 1995 Management of adverse effects following breast radiotherapy. Royal College of Radiologists, London

Sainsbury J R, Anderson T J, Morgan D A L 1995 Breast cancer. In: Dixon J M (ed) ABC of Breast Diseases. BMJ Publishing Group, London

Silberfarb P M, Maurer L H, Crouthamel C S 1980 Psychosocial aspects of neoplastic disease: functional status of breast cancer patients of different treatment regimens. American Journal of Psychiatry 137(4): 450–455

Sledge G W 1996 Adjuvant therapy for early stage breast cancer. Seminars in Oncology 23 (Suppl 1–2): 51–54

Souhami R, Tobias J 1986 Cancer and its management. Blackwell Scientific, Oxford

Spiegel D, Bloom J R, Kraemer H, Gottheil E 1989 Psychological support for cancer patients. Lancet 2(8677): 1447

Spiegel D, Bloom J R, Kraemer H C, Gottheil E 1989 Effect of psychosocial treatment on survival of patients with metastatic breast cancer. Lancet 2(8668): 888–891

START Standardisation of Breast Radiotherapy Protocol 1998 A randomised comparison of fractionation. Regimes after local excision or mastectomy in women with early stage breast cancer. START Trials Office, Institute of Cancer Research

Stevenson C 1996 Complementary therapies in cancer care; an NHS approach. International Journal of Palliative Nursing 2(1)

Tierney A J 1987 Preventing chemotherapy-induced alopecia in cancer patients: is scalp cooling worthwhile? Journal of Advanced Nursing 12: 303–310

Troesh L M et al 1993 The influence of guided imagery on chemotherapy related nausea and vomiting. Oncology Nursing Forum 20(8): 1179–1185

Turner G 1996 Oral care. Nursing Standard 10(28): 51–54

Watters C 1997 The benefits of providing chemotherapy at home. Professional Nurse 12(5): 367–368, 370

Wells R, Tschudin V 1994 Wells' Supportive Therapies in Health Care. Baillière Tindall, London

Wilkinson S 1995 Aromatherapy and massage in palliative care. International Journal of Palliative Nursing 1(1): 21–30

Woodcock J 1997 An oncological perspective. In: Salter M (ed) Altered Body Image; The Nurse's Role. Baillière Tindall, London

World Health Organization (WHO) 1990 Cancer Pain Relief and Palliative Care. Technical Report Series 804. World Health Organization, Geneva

Yarnold J R, Price P, Steel G G 1995 Treatment of early breast cancer in the United Kingdom: radiotherapy fractionation practices. Clinical Oncology 5: 330–332

Zava D T, Dollbaum C M, Blen M 1998 Estrogen and progestin bioactivity of foods, herbs, and spices. Proc Soc Exp Biol Med 217(3): 369–378

FURTHER READING

Abernethy K 1992 The Menopause and HRT. Baillière Tindall, London

Denton S 1996 Breast Cancer Nursing. Chapman and Hall, London

Chapman D, Goodman M 1997 Breast cancer. In: Groenwald S L, Goodman M, Frogge M H, Yarbro C H. Cancer Nursing: Principles and Practice, 4th edn. Jones and Bartlett, MA Ch. 34, p 916–979

Wells R, Tschudin V 1994 Wells' Supportive Therapies in Health Care. Baillière Tindall, London

7 Informational and Psychological Aspects of Breast Care

Nicki De Zeeuw (Part 1) and Siobhan Carroll (Part 2)

This chapter is divided into two sections, the first is dedicated to information giving, and the second to the psychological care of a woman with a breast problem. All the chapters in this book stress the need for good communication and have emphasised the need for psychological as well as physical care. This chapter intends to give some guidance in both these areas.

PART 1

INFORMATIONAL SUPPORT

Nicki De Zeeuw

At the end of this section the reader should have a greater understanding of:

- The facts and influence of the media
- Information sources other than the media
- Benign breast disease
- Information and the patient with cancer
- How to facilitate effective information giving and communication.

INTRODUCTION

Giving information and answers to people with concerns about their health is often synonymous with emotional support. This section is dedicated to giving information to those with breast disease and how information is conveyed.

BREAST DISEASE: THE FACTS AND THE INFLUENCE OF THE MEDIA

Much of the information about breast disease is 'out there'. Thanks to media exposure, pressure groups and the Internet, women know the facts:

- Breast cancer is the commonest of all malignant diseases in women and the leading cause of death in women aged 35–54
- One out of every 12 women will develop breast cancer during their lifetime
- Some breast cancers are hereditary, so if a mother develops the disease, her daughters may be at risk (CRC 1996).

These powerful and increasingly accessible facts about cancer mean that breast disease is greatly feared, whether benign or malignant. As Maguire (1994) states,

> 'Most women who present with breast lumps are emotionally distressed. A substantial proportion of women whose lumps prove to be benign remain distressed and may become clinically depressed.'

It is probably true that more is commonly known about breast cancer than benign breast conditions. A woman finding a lump or irregularity in her breast is far more likely at first to fear cancer than to consider benign causes. The word 'cancer' represents to most people a threat to their lives and so the potential connection between a lump in the breast and cancer causes great anxiety. The increased awareness of the signs of breast cancer is largely due to a high media profile, sponsored by the Government and by women themselves, in light of the high death rates from the disease (14 000 deaths per annum in the UK (Hall 1998)). Increased awareness has certainly enabled women to assert their rights to be seen by breast specialists rather than merely their GPs. Governmental guidelines have been laid down advising GPs of their responsibilities (Clarke 1998); it should no longer be acceptable for a GP to tell a woman her breast lump is benign without referring her to a specialist, i.e. a surgeon or a rapid diagnosis clinic (Mead 1997).

Unfortunately the media, which has been a predominant tool for the Government in passing on information, is not particularly reliable. The media has an agenda of its own and in many cases news is sensationalised and incomplete. Often the frightening, negative statistics hit the headlines whilst more positive achievements receive less exposure. Some of these statistics are as follows:

- Successful screening and treatment means mortality rates are dropping – on average 64% of women with breast cancer are still alive 5 years later (CRC 1996)
- Only an estimated 5–10% of all breast cancers are hereditary (CRC 1996)
- The overwhelming majority of young women with breast lumps *do not* have cancer (Austoker 1994).

The haphazard, selective mode of information giving in the media can backfire by increasing the fear of cancer, whilst failing to dispel the cancer myth. This culminates in women delaying attendance to GPs with breast problems and being afraid to attend screening programmes because of a paralysing fear of the word 'cancer'. There must be more reliable sources than media coverage to help these women. Indeed, the challenge is to ensure that the public have access to accurate, unbiased information from credible sources. This should reduce anxiety about breast disease, improve compliance with screening programmes and so lead to early detection of those symptoms that do represent cancer.

CONTRIBUTION OF SOURCES OTHER THAN THE MEDIA

The fact that so much interest is generated by media coverage of health issues reflects a sea change in public opinion. There are more people now who are interested in their health and who are willing to be proactive to make a difference. As Healy (1997) observes:

> 'The consumers' growing role in medical care is here to stay – and in that context the informed consumer is medicine's greatest ally.'

Professional and governmental advice now reflects the fact that patients and families wish to have access to information about their health problems. This is illustrated in the *Patient's Charter*:

> '...your health authority must provide information about the specific services it has arranged. In addition, your health authority will set up more general information services to help people to find their way around the NHS and to understand what is available.' (DOH 1991)

and in the Calman–Hine report on cancer services:

> 'Patients, families and carers should be given clear information in a form they can understand about treatment options and outcomes available to them at all stages of treatment from diagnosis onwards.' (DOH 1994)

In the same vein, the Government White Paper / The new NHS (DOH 1997) proposes a helpline staffed by nurses and an information Website for patients. Though the Internet can be complicated and misleading for the medical amateur, it cannot be ignored as an increasingly accessed gateway to medical information. By providing a Website, the Government is acknowledging this and adding credibility to it. Nevertheless, it should be remembered that not all things found on the Internet are reliable, accurate or indeed available in this country (much information comes from the USA and mentions treatments not yet licensed in the UK). There is as yet no governing body regulating the Internet, so Websites on health issues should be validated or approved by health care professionals before being recommended to the public. Patients should also be advised of the above mentioned problems with the World Wide Web. Some useful Websites have been listed at the end of this chapter.

There is an increasing demand for public involvement in government papers on health; groups set up by patients for patients such as the National Cancer Alliance (NCA) have helped to influence the slant of these documents. Pressure groups and charities such as the Women's National Cancer Control Campaign (WNCC), Cancer Research Campaign (CRC) and Macmillan Cancer Relief also seek to raise women's awareness of the importance of screening for, and early detection of female cancers.

Facts presented by the above reports, patient groups and committed charities may serve to dispel some of the myths around cancer and reassure concerned women of the real risks, thus balancing the media bias.

In their local areas, health care professionals are looking to implement the recommendations of government health reports. The giving of information is a large factor in this and here the nurse's role is vital. From primary care through investigations, surgery and cancer treatment, nurses work closely with patients as part of the multidisciplinary team. This is particularly true in breast disease, where pressure groups and the frightening cancer statistics have led to hundreds of specially trained breast care nurses being appointed across the country. Nurses in general are ideal information givers because of their communication skills and advocacy roles. Indeed as Leino-Kilpi (1993) states:

> '...information is essential to the success of nursing. Patients who understand more about their condition will also show closer compliance to their treatment and work to advance the ultimate goals of nursing care.'

There is great interdependency between information giving and effective nursing, which can be capitalised on when dealing with the fear surrounding breast disease.

BENIGN BREAST DISEASE

Bearing in mind that the overwhelming majority of young women with breast lumps do *not* have cancer, the public needs to be more aware of benign breast disease and particularly the differences between this and cancer. As the media publicise the dangers of breast cancer, anxious women are turning to professionals for reassurance. The role of the nurse, particularly the practice nurse in this instance, is very important. Unless cancer is suspected, a woman will not be referred to a fast-track diagnosis clinic. She may not meet a breast care nurse specialist, as these nurses tend to be found in cancer care. Much benign breast disease is diagnosed and treated in the primary health care setting by GPs and practice nurses. Baum et al (1995) write:

> 'Often it is only when a woman develops breast symptoms that she realises she is unsure of their significance.'

At this stage a woman will be anxious and receptive to advice. It is the responsibility of GP practices to have the resources to inform and reassure. Current leaflets on breast awareness and information on benign breast problems such as mastalgia and fibroadenomas should be displayed. Similarly, practice nurses should work to stay up-to-date with current thinking: rather than strict teaching for all women on breast self-examination, it is now recommended that an individual knows her own breasts and what is normal for her, so that she can recognise changes. If women feel their local practice is approachable and helpful, they are less likely to delay in seeking advice or information about breast problems. Information from a reliable source will reduce anxiety and instill confidence, as opposed to impersonal media warnings. For current information/leaflets on breast problems, see the list at the end of this chapter. See Chapter 2 for more details on benign breast disease.

INFORMATION AND THE CLIENT WITH CANCER

Although information giving is important in all aspects of illness, the person with cancer has special informational needs and much of the literature relates to this group. Thus, whilst relevant to all women with breast disease, the following advice is based on the experiences of those with cancer and their families.

Benefits of information giving

Faced with a health scare or uncertainty about a diagnosis, the majority of people will use information seeking as a coping strategy (Denmark Friedman 1980). The giving of that information can serve as a therapeutic intervention in its own right (Slevin et al 1996). For nurses, therefore, information giving is an integral part of the emotional support they offer patients. This is particularly true in cancer care, where fear and anxiety are obstructive to normal coping mechanisms.

If the information to be given is not positive, for example a diagnosis or a recurrence of cancer, it can be difficult to impart. There is a temptation for health care professionals to withhold some details or disguise them, to avoid causing distress. However, research among those with cancer has proved that paternalistic behaviour does not facilitate coping. Fallowfield (1994) found that 96% of cancer patients wanted as much information as possible, good or bad; Bilodeau & Degner (1996) found that women with breast cancer ranked having information about the stage of disease, likelihood of cure and treatment options available as their three most important needs. Thus, at diagnosis, most women with breast cancer need not only empathy and psychological support, but an explanation of the disease and a realistic expectation of what is to follow.

Northouse & Northouse (1987) wrote:

> 'Information is generally beneficial because it gives patients a framework for interpreting and clarifying a life threatening event, and because it helps them feel that their responses to the uncertainties of that event are reasonable and normal.'

The informed patient and family feel more in control of the cancer experience and function in partnership with the health care team. Helping the cancer patient feel even a little in control of such a demoralising illness is empowering and generates hope. Books and articles written by patients with cancer illustrate this:

> 'A stage three ovarian adenocarcinoma had been discovered, which was inoperable and we both thought I was unlikely to be alive at Christmas. Having faced this hopeless situation I found that the visit by my medical oncologist brought hope beyond our wildest dreams. He told us that the chance of eradication was only 20% and despite the fact that the treatment offered would be difficult to endure and that chances of success were not very great, this offer gave us something to strive for. At this interview we established a relationship of communication and trust on which we could build.' (Clement Jones 1985)

Clement Jones was a doctor who established the cancer charity the British Association of Cancer United Patients (BACUP) as a result of her experiences. BACUP, along with other cancer organisations have published guides for professionals. These are based on consultations with patients about how important information, communication and support are to them, and include *The Right to Know Summary* (BACUP 1995) and *Patient-centred Cancer Services? – What Patients Say* (National Cancer Alliance 1996). By giving patients what they need, professionals will improve compliance with treatment programmes and earn the respect of patients and their families. Partnership between patients and professionals builds patients' self-esteem and is thus mutually beneficial.

Quite aside from the supportive aspects of information giving, there is the legal consideration of informed consent. Verbal and written consent is required for both surgical and oncological interventions for breast disease. It is based on the principle of the physician giving an adequate explanation of all likely sequelae (CRC 1996). There are those who argue that a signed consent form does not necessarily mean a patient has fully understood the implications or even had them properly explained. However, in the light of the evidence we have of what patients need, nurses could use the legal requirements of informed consent to their advantage, advocating for full explanations of disease and treatment options for their patients.

PITFALLS OF INFORMATION GIVING AND HOW TO AVOID THEM

Cancer diagnosis

In some areas of Europe, doctors still hide a diagnosis of cancer from their patients (Grahn 1996). As mentioned on page 141, this sort of paternalism has been found to be unhelpful to people in this country. In recognition of this, doctors in the UK generally strive to be truthful. Unfortunately, their methods often let them down. A major problem in giving information that is of great emotional significance to the recipient, is that if it is done badly, it can cause trauma. This adversely affects coping mechanisms and can even precipitate anxiety and depression (Fallowfield 1994). As Buckman (1996) writes:

> 'Centuries of systematic, insensitive deception cannot be instantly remedied by a new routine of systematic, insensitive truth telling.'

Similarly, in his book on psycho-oncology, Guex (1994) states:

> 'The way in which the cancer diagnosis is communicated will bring with it, in the patient and his family, reactions that will determine the whole course of the disease. Emotional adaptation begins on the day of diagnosis.'

Breaking bad news is a heavy responsibility and many doctors feel insufficiently trained to do it well (Watts 1995). However, research indicates that most patients prefer to hear their diagnosis from a hospital doctor, rather than a nurse or other member of the health care team (Meredith et al 1996). Whilst there is more emphasis now on communication skills in medical education, doctors will nevertheless need support in breaking bad news. There is much value in a multidisciplinary approach here. This is used successfully in the fast-track cancer diagnosis and screening clinics where specialist breast care nurses have a pivotal role in support around diagnosis.

Nurses working in other areas where cancer is diagnosed, such as outpatient clinics, wards or GP surgeries can be influential by creating standards for breaking bad news. These should be agreed by the multidisciplinary team, who then have no excuse not to adhere to them! Senior nurses should ensure that the agreed standards become fully integrated into routine practice. Standards should include: ensuring a suitable environment, providing nursing support during and after consultations and referring to a relevant nurse specialist (Maher et al 1996). Having a nurse present in the 'bad news consultation' not only supports patients but improves interdisciplinary communication around this crucial experience for the patient. Standards also need to be audited regularly to ensure their continued relevance.

Amount of information

Another common problem is that too much information is given to patients for them to take in. Many patients describe shock and numbness around the crisis of diagnosis, which reduces their cognitive abilities:

> 'I just couldn't do anything, I couldn't think, I couldn't read, I couldn't work, I couldn't concentrate and it went on for weeks. I didn't know what to make for supper. I kept wishing it would go away. I went through each day but I don't know how. I wasn't listening when people would talk to me.' (Hagopian 1993)

Unfortunately, the initial phase of diagnosis and treatment necessitates a lot of information being shared with the patient. There are often decisions to be made about treatment options or clinical trials, and the patient is thrown into a world of unfamiliar terminology. It is important to offer emotional and psychological support at this time (see the section on psychological care). However, many other things are vital to improve this experience for patient and family. These include:

- Repeating information as necessary
- Confirming whether information has been understood
- Backing verbal information up with written booklets or leaflets (see pp. 147–150)
- Providing a contact telephone number for questions arising after the consultation
- Allowing patients some time to consider the options before signing consent
- Encouraging patients to bring a relative or friend to the consultation, who can help them remember what was said.

Many of the above things can be coordinated and improved by nurses, who have a valuable role in ensuring information is understood.

However nurses should not feel that they must always know the answer. Information needs to come from a credible source, so it is perfectly acceptable to admit lack of knowledge, as long as the patient is then referred to someone who can answer their questions accurately, i.e. a doctor, senior nurse or specialist nurse. Patients and families are very vulnerable at this time and inaccurate or 'guessed at' information can damage the build up of trust that is so important between professional and patient. Patients and their families are also more likely to respect the professional who is honest.

Negative attitudes

Another pitfall for professionals giving information about cancer is the risk of passing on negative attitudes and beliefs. Dora Paraskevopoulou (1996) a breast cancer sufferer, wrote:

> 'How can a nurse reply with confidence, to questions patients ask, like, "Will I live and for how long?"; "Will my companion in life still like me?"; "How can I tell my children?" when the nurse herself may hold deeply negative attitudes about cancer. Women with cancer may have died in the arms of the nurse, while the thousands who have survived may just be statistics to her.'

Many cancer nurses will identify with this point. Patients relapsing or dying of their cancer is a regular occurrence for oncology professionals. The patients that do well or are in remission are seen less often. The emotional cost of caring for this group of patients can lead to professionals distancing themselves emotionally (Faulkner & Maguire 1994), or developing unnecessarily negative beliefs about prognosis and survival (Solodky et al 1986). Advice for dealing with supervision issues can be found in Part 2 of this chapter.

Doctors too are often guilty; those working on medical/surgical wards or clinics may not be fully aware of the wide range of treatments available for cancer, and convey negative messages, directly or indirectly, when giving the diagnosis. This should be guarded against. There are many treatments or interventions that can aid quality of life and give even the most unlikely cases some hope, yet many patients are left feeling hopeless or that they are about to die. Health care professionals need to be aware that their perspectives on a patient's outcome may not be shared by the person facing possible death, who needs some degree of hope to carry on. As Maggie Jencks (1995), another breast cancer patient wrote:

> 'Telling it as it is should never cut the patient off without leaving a chink of hope and some area of manoeuvre.'

However, this need not be hope of cure or even of remission. Doctors sometimes give unrealistically positive prognoses to patients, misguidedly thinking this is the only thing that will foster hope, but patients given a survival time of 10–15 years who develop metastatic disease 6 months later will be very angry that they were not prepared for a potential relapse. Indeed, disguising the truth in this way is more likely to destroy hope and paralyse coping mechanisms. Many less tangible things than cure or the promise of longer life foster hope for these patients, such as being with them, taking time to talk, indicating that you value them, answering questions honestly and sharing information (Koopmeiners et al 1997). Taking hope away unnecessarily by conveying beliefs about cancer that may not be true can have profoundly adverse effects on psychological adjustment (Maguire 1994).

POINTS TO CONSIDER WHEN PROVIDING INFORMATION

Differing needs

People's character, background and intellectual ability will affect how they process information and how much or little information they need. Degner &

Sloan (1992) looked at the role patients with serious illness wished to play in their treatment. They found that people fell into three categories:

1. An active role, which was more autonomous
2. A collaborative role, which shared responsibility with the doctor
3. A passive role, which relied totally on the doctor.

Astute judgements need to be made by health care professionals that are tailored to the individual. A balance needs to be drawn between the necessity and timing of information giving, respecting individual differences and working to make allowances for them within the system. Again, a multidisciplinary approach has the best chance of success, with specialist nurses often providing the personal touch that is so valued by the individual.

Family

A diagnosis of cancer affects the whole family, not merely the patient. Professionals are often dealing with a family under great strain because of the cancer diagnosis. Research has shown that families of women with breast cancer have important informational needs that may be ignored by professionals (Rees et al 1998). If the patient is the main source of information it can lead to mixed messages and frustration among family members, who can in turn feel ostracised as the patient becomes the focus of all support. It is the family who provide care for the patient in the absence of health care professionals. For this reason they need to be as well informed as the patient. Indeed, information and good communication have been shown to ease stress among family members (Northouse & Northouse 1987). Whilst there is a confidentiality issue around giving information without the patient's consent, it is important for professionals to assess family dynamics and provide holistic support where possible. This can be supplemented by specialist support nurses or counsellors if necessary and their expertise should be referred to in difficult situations. Professionals should be aware that family dynamics can be a minefield, so it is advisable to try and work to bring families together, without being wholly influenced by either side. Misguided collusion with patients or family members by well-meaning professionals can be counterproductive (Faulkner & Maguire 1994). Family support teams are often an integral part of local palliative care services and these may serve as a resource for the isolated professional dealing with difficult family dynamics.

Written information

All the literature indicates that if verbal information is backed up by written, it is more likely to be understood, improving patient/professional partnerships and compliance with treatment (Ley 1982, Arthur 1995). There are already a huge number of leaflets and publications produced for the public about breast disease. In community care and hospitals, professionals are creating more written material to explain procedures and treatments to their patients. This is a positive step and fulfils the requirements of the Patient's Charter (DOH 1991) and the Calman–Hine Report on Cancer Services (DOH 1994). However, it is important to ensure that written information is understood and used by its target audience. Research indicates that medical material written for public consumption often exceeds the reading abilities of those it is produced for (Ley 1982). A recent study in the USA found that the mean reading level of US citizens was age 13, whilst most written material was written for an audience of age 15 or above (Foltz 1998).

It is also useful to remember that the shock and numbness produced by a cancer diagnosis, as well as the unfamiliar medical terminology involved, cause regression in patients' cognitive abilities. Thus, although simple language and short sentences may appear to patronise the average adult, they are essential to help the majority understand written material about their health at a time of personal crisis.

There are various readability tests that can be applied to written material. These include the frequency of gobbledegook (FOG) (North 1996) and the Rapid Estimation of Adult Literacy in Medicine (REALM) (Foltz 1998). Some computer packages such as MicrosoftWord, have the facility to test readability. It is generally recommended in the literature that either the readers or the written material are assessed, but this may not always be practical in the working environment.

The following general advice may be helpful:

- Keep sentences clear and concise – avoid saying in one sentence what could be said in two or three, but don't use too many sentences
- Keep words short where possible, i.e. two syllables rather than three or more
- Use correct medical words rather than abbreviations, e.g. ductal carcinoma in situ, rather than DCIS
- Avoid jargon, but beware of simplifying the medical facts so much that they lose their meaning (Coulter 1998)
- Consider text size – 10 point is too small but 16 point is too large
- Consider layout and the use of illustration to break up the text and hold the reader's attention
- If the information is long, use an index so the reader can choose where to start
- Always look at similar examples of the leaflet you wish to create. This will give an idea of best practice and avoid re-invention of the wheel
- Consider public focus groups to find out whether what you are providing is what is wanted
- Ask several people, lay and professional, to comment on the information before it is printed
- Written information should be audited or evaluated at least yearly to ensure relevance
- Audio-visual aids may be a suitable alternative for the non-reader
- Finally, it is important to remember that written information is '… a supplement, not a substitute for good communication between the health professional and the patient.' (Weinman 1990).

For more information on readability tests or producing patient information, contact:

The Basic Skills Agency
PO Box 3
1/19 New Oxford Street
Stockport SK12 4QP

Plain English Campaign
Commonwealth House
New Mills
London WC1A INY

Centre for Health information Quality (CHiQ)
Highcroft
Romsey Road
Winchester
Hampshire SO22 5DH

CONCLUSION

The material discussed in this section highlights the importance of informing and educating the public about breast disease. Increased awareness about their breasts will enable women to be more discerning about consulting a doctor and more persistent in asking to see a specialist. However, health professionals may have found that informing and educating are not always rewarding tasks. Many women only presenting when their cancer is advanced are not ignorant of the significance of breast lumps (Baum et al 1995), and sometimes it must seem as though our best efforts are falling on deaf ears. The public have a responsibility for their own health, but unfortunately, studied patterns of health behaviour dictate that people disregard information, for example, those who continue smoking in spite of government health warnings. Nevertheless, health professionals have a responsibility for health promotion and must keep trying. The media fanning the flames of the cancer myth may act as a trigger, motivating people to seek advice. This advice must be available, in the form of leaflets, posters, nursing and medical support. It must be easily accessible, readable and current. If people have surfed the Internet, health professionals must be willing to help explain the terminology and take away the mystery. The incidence of cancer is predicted to rise over the next decade and it is vital that the general public are made aware of relevant signs and symptoms. If health professionals can consistently provide written information and accurate advice about breast disease, both benign and malignant, then we are rising to the challenge of providing the best care for an increasingly proactive, concerned public.

HELPFUL NATIONAL ORGANISATIONS

N.B. More local support groups can usually be obtained via national organisations or local hospitals.

Breast awareness

Breast Care Campaign
Blythe Hall
100 Blythe Road
London W14 0HB
Tel: 0171 3711510

Dedicated to raising awareness of benign breast disorders. Leaflets available to public and health professionals free of charge.

The Women's Nationwide Cancer Control Campaign
(WNCCC)
Suna House
128 Curtain Road
London EC2A 3AR
Tel: 0171 729 2229
0171 729 4688

Encourages the provision of facilities for the early diagnosis of cancer in women. Written material, videos and mobile screening units.

Breast Cancer

Breast Cancer Care Kiln House, 210 New Kings Road London SW6 4NZ Tel: 0500 245345 0171 384 2984	National charity. Telephone support and leaflets.
Breakthrough Breast Cancer 6th Floor Kingsway House 103 Kingsway London WC2B 6QX Tel: 0171 405 5111	National charity committed to fighting breast cancer through research. Works in partnership with the Institute of Cancer Research in London.
The UK National Breast Cancer Coalition (UKBCC) P O Box 8554 London SW8 2ZB Tel: 0171 720 0945	A voluntary network founded in 1995 by women with personal experience of breast cancer. Works to improve access to the best treatments for all women with breast cancer and to help women take a full and influential role in decision making.

General cancer

BACUP 3 Bath Place Rivington Street London EC2A 3JR Tel: 0800 181199 0171 613 2121 Website – see Internet list	London- and Glasgow-based charity. Booklets and factsheets on cancer and its treatment (free to patients and relatives). Operated by cancer nurses. Good source for up-to-date information on research.
Cancerlink 11–21 Northdown Street London N1 9BN Tel: 0800 132905 (General helpline) 0800 591028 (Young people with cancer helpline) 0800 590415 (Asian information helpline) 0171 8332818 (Administration)	London-based charity. Booklets and fact sheets on cancer and its treatment. Good source for written information in Asian languages. Good source for advice and training in setting up support groups for health professionals or patients and families.
Macmillan Cancer Relief Anchor House 15–19 Britten Street London SW3 3TZ Tel: 0845 6016161 (Information line) 0171 351 7811 (Administration)	National charity. Financial support for building projects, health professionals providing cancer care for patients with cancer.

National Cancer Alliance
PO Box 579
Oxford OX4 1LB
Tel: 01865 793566

An alliance of patients and health professionals working together to improve the treatment and care of all cancer patients. Publications include a directory of cancer specialists in the UK.

Cancer Research Campaign
Cambridge House
10 Cambridge Terrace
London NW1 4JL
Tel: 0171 224 1333

National charity. Publishes regular research updates on all cancers. Produces some leaflets.

Winston's Wish
Gloucestershire Royal Hospital
Great Western Rd.
Gloucester, GL1 3NN

Support for bereaved children who have experienced the death of a mum, dad, brother or sister. Also has a national development programme that provides training and advice for people wanting to set up services in their local communities.

INTERNET SITES REGARDING BREAST DISEASE

General breast disease sites

- *http://www.obgyn.net/women/conditions/hc-breast.htm*
- *http://www.breastdiseases.com/*
- *http://www.womens-med-grp.com/fibro-breast.htm*
- *http://www.breastsurgeon.clara.net*

Cancer awareness and oncology-related sites

- *http://www.easynet.co.uk/aware/*
- *http://www.breakthrough.org.uk/* *(Breakthrough Breast Cancer)
- *http://www.breastcancercare.org.uk/* *(Breast Cancer Care)
- *http://www.cancerbacup.org.uk/* *(Cancerbacup)
- *http://www.macmillan.org.uk/* *(Macmillan Cancer Relief)
- *http://www.crc.org.uk/* *(Cancer Research Campaign – UK)
- *http://www.ons.org* (Oncology Nursing Society – USA)
- *http://arclx.reston.carsoninc.com/database/Cancernet/english/patient* (National Cancer Institute – USA)
- *http://www.ucl.ac.uk/oncology* (University College London – UK)

Male breast cancer

- *http://interact.withus.com/interact/mbc*

Complementary therapy in breast cancer

- *http://www.flyingcameraco.demon.co.uk/swallows.htm* (Swallows)

REFERENCED BOOKS, REPORTS AND FACTSHEETS

BACUP 1995 The Right to Know Summary. BACUP Publications, London

Baum M, Saunders C, Meredith S. 1995. Breast Cancer – A guide for every woman. Oxford Medical Publications, Oxford University Press, Oxford

Cancer Research Campaign (CRC) 1996 Factsheet 6.1.1996. Breast Cancer – UK

Department of Health 1991 The Patient's Charter. DOH, London

Department of Health (DOH) 1994 A Policy Framework for Commissioning Cancer Services – The Calman–Hine Report. DOH, London

Department of Health 1997 White Paper – The New NHS. DOH, London

Faulkner A, Maguire P 1994 Talking to cancer patients and their relatives. Oxford Medical Publications, Oxford University Press, Oxford

Guex P 1994 An Introduction to Psycho-Oncology. Routledge, London

Hall G, Patel P, Protheroe A 1998 Key Topics in Oncology. BIOS Scientific Publishers, Oxford

Jencks M 1995 A view from the Front Line and Constitution for a Cancer Caring Centre. Maggie's Centre, Edinburgh

Maher J et al 1996 Breaking Bad News. King's Fund Publications, London

National Cancer Alliance 1996 Patient-centred Cancer Services? What Patients Say. NCA, Oxford

Royal College of Radiologists 1995 Adult Patient Consent and Information. RCR, London BFCO(95) 3

Sheldon T 1996 Effective Healthcare. The Management of Primary Breast Cancer. Vol. 2 No: 6 ISSN: 0965–0288. Effective Health Care Bulletins, Churchill Livingstone.

REFERENCES

Arthur A 1995 Written patient information: a review of the literature. Journal of Advanced Nursing. 21: 1081–1086

Austoker J 1994 Cancer prevention in primary care; screening and self examination for breast cancer. BMJ 309: 168–173

Bilodeau B, Degner L 1996 Information needs, sources of information and decisional roles in women with breast cancer. Oncology Nursing Forum 23(4): 691–696

Buckman R 1996 Talking to patients about cancer. No excuse for not doing it. BMJ 313: 699–700

Clarke E 1998 Benign? Assessing breast disorders in post-menopausal women. Geriatric Medicine Oct. 1998: 53–56

Clement Jones V 1985 Cancer and beyond: The formation of BACUP. BMJ 291: 1021–1023

Coulter A 1998 Evidence based patient information. BMJ 317: 225–226

Degner L, Sloan J 1992 Decision making during serious illness: what role do patients really want to play? Journal of Clinical Epidemiology 45: 944–950

Denmark Friedman 1980 Coping with cancer: a guide for healthcare professionals. Cancer Nursing April: 105–109

Fallowfield L 1994 Improving the quality of communication and quality of life in cancer care. Cancer Forum 19(2): 129–131

Foltz A 1998 Get real: clinical testing of patients' reading abilities. Cancer Nursing 21(3): 162–166

Grahn G 1996 Patient Information as a necessary therapeutic intervention. European Journal of Cancer Care, Vol 5, Supplement 1: 1–8

Hagopian G 1993 Cognitive strategies used in adapting to a cancer diagnosis. Oncology Nursing Forum 20(5): 759–763

Healy B 1997 Editorial: breast cancer in the news: the rise of consumer power in medical care. Journal of Women's Health 6(2): 141–142

Koopmeiners L et al 1997 How healthcare professionals contribute to hope in patients with cancer. Oncology Nursing Forum 24(9): 1507–1513
Leino-Kilpi H 1993 Client and information: a literature review. Journal of Clinical Nursing 2: 331–340
Ley P 1982 Satisfaction, compliance and communication. British Journal of Clinical Psychology 21: 241–251
Liberati et al 1998 Do specialists do it better? The impact of specialisation on the process and outcome of care for cancer patients. Annals of Oncology 9(4): 365–374
Maguire P 1994 ABC of Breast Diseases. Psychological Aspects. BMJ 309: 1649–1652
Mead M 1997 Common conditions: breast lumps. Practice Nurse 21.02.97 156–157
Meredith L et al 1996 Information needs of cancer patients in west Scotland: cross sectional survey of patients' views. BMJ 313: 724–726
North G 1996 Guidelines for producing patient information literature. Nursing Standard 10(47): 46–48
Northouse P, Northouse L 1987 Communication and cancer: issues confronting patients, health professionals and family members. Journal of Psychosocial Oncology 5(3): 17–45
Paraskevopoulou D 1996 Dora's Story. European Journal of Cancer Care 5 (Supplement 1): 1–8
Rees C et al 1998 The information concerns of spouses of women with breast cancer: patients' and spouses' perspectives. Journal of Advanced Nursing 28(6): 1249–1258
Slevin M et al 1996 Emotional support for cancer patients: what do patients really want? British Journal of Cancer 74: 1275–1279
Solodky M et al 1986 Nurses' prognosis for oncology and coronary heart disease patients. Cancer Nursing 9(5): 243–247
Watts E 1995 Doctor/patient communication and the consumer's voice – who really knows what they want. Clinician in Management 4(4): 11–13
Weinman J 1990 Providing written information for patients: psychological considerations. Journal of the Royal Society of Medicine 83: 303–305

PART 2

PSYCHOLOGICAL SUPPORT

Siobhan Carroll

INTRODUCTION

In this part of the chapter, an overview of psychological aspects of women with breast cancer and of women with breast disease are presented. Incidence of psychological/emotional problems, assessment, aetiology and interventions on a number of levels, are outlined.

The aims of the chapter are to:

- Outline the incidence and nature of psychological problems associated with breast disease
- Outline the process of adaptation to a diagnosis of breast cancer and to highlight abnormal or problematic adaptation processes
- Give guidance on how to deal with these aspects in terms of communication, information and counselling
- Give guidance on when and who to refer on to
- Outline the specialist nurse's role in psychological support and liaison.

INCIDENCE OF PSYCHOLOGICAL MORBIDITY

The emotional responses of women with breast cancer differ widely and can range from little apparent disruption of mood to clinically significant states of anxiety and depression (Pinder et al 1994). It must be recognised that a crisis such as a diagnosis of breast cancer, requires a period of adjustment and adaptation, after which there is usually a return to normal functioning (Budin 1998). However, about 20–30% of patients with early breast cancer experience anxiety, depression, sexual dysfunction and low self-esteem at any one time in the year after diagnosis (Ramirez et al 1995). These figures vary of course, depending on the method and timing of assessments. This morbidity can continue long after the diagnosis is known and treatment is completed and is more common among younger patients (Watson 1991). Other factors that contribute to increased psychological problems are outlined in Box 7.1 (Burton & Watson 1998).

The period of time whereby the woman undergoes diagnostic investigations for symptoms of breast disease evidently constitutes a stressful period, and the existence of perceived and actual induced distress has been deduced by Scott (1983), Shaw et al (1994), and Northouse et al (1995). The significance of the 'waiting duration' in terms of distress experienced by women has not been investigated (Poole 1997). However, anecdotally, a long and ambiguous period

BOX 7.1 ***Patients at risk of psychological problems***

- A previous psychiatric history
- A lack of support from family and friends
- An inability to accept the physical changes associated with breast cancer or its treatments
- A lack of involvement in satisfying activities
- A prior adverse experience of cancer in the family
- Low expectations regarding the effectiveness of treatment
- Pre-existing marital problems
- A younger age at diagnosis

Adapted from Burton & Watson (1998).

of waiting for a confirmed diagnosis and treatment plan can lead to increased anxiety and diminished confidence in the health care team, with possible projection of problems into the treatment phase.

The advent of the screening programme has led to research into the psychological differences between those women with screen-detected disease and those with symptomatic disease (Farmer et al 1995). These authors found that women with screen-detected breast cancer showed a low incidence of psychological morbidity and saw their condition as early, curable disease. This may be due to the perceived rationale for a screening programme (See Ch. 3 on the breast screening programme).

Changes in treatment techniques impact on the incidence and changes in the types of problems breast cancer patients now experience. Two seminal papers published in the 1950s by Renneker & Culter (1992) and Bard & Sutherland (1995) described the psychological sequelae following mastectomy, almost the only treatment available at that time. However, while breast conservation can offer a similar survival advantage to mastectomy, there is little evidence to suggest that breast conservation confers a clean bill of psychological health (Fallowfield & Clark 1992).

Many women can now be offered a choice regarding the extent of their surgery and can be more involved in decision-making regarding their care. While it could be supposed that offering patients a choice in their treatment might improve psychological adjustment, it can also cause distress in some women who would prefer the doctor to choose for them (Carroll 1998).

Breast reconstruction is now offered to many women undergoing a mastectomy (King's Fund Forum 1986). Significantly, although studies indicate the benefits in terms of freedom of dress and body image, studies also show that psychological problems such as anxiety and depression continue to be experienced (Dean et al 1983; Gilboa et al 1990). Researchers have further broadened their scope from reaction to diagnosis and surgery, to include investigation of the impact of chemotherapy and radiotherapy (Rabinowitz 1997). In the literature, those women receiving chemotherapy had significantly more adjustment difficulties and reported more symptom distress (Rabinowitz 1997). Treatment effects can be far-reaching because treatment for breast cancer can often extend for up to a year and effects such as fatigue may last for some months, even when treatment is completed (Carroll 1998).

Many women with breast cancer will be survivors (Ferrans 1994). Breast cancer patients often talk about a shift in emotions once treatment has been completed, the dominant issues being fears of recurrence, feelings of loss, anger and depression and redefinition of self (Harber 1997). These feelings may be related to ongoing or chronic problems due to treatment effects such as menopausal symptoms, sexual problems, body image problems, chronic pain syndromes and lymphoedema (Ferrans 1994).

Research into the incidence of psychological problems when breast cancer recurs has been sparse, with mixed reports (Weisman & Worden 1986; Jenkins et al 1991). However, a recent 3-year prospective study found that patients with recurrence of their breast cancer are significantly more likely to experience psychiatric morbidity than women who are disease free (Hall et al 1996).

Similarly, in contrast to the large volume of research reporting psychological morbidity in early breast cancer, there has been surprisingly little work looking at the specific problems of those with advanced breast cancer (Fallowfield & Clark 1992) However, depression, sadness and despair seem to dominate as symptoms of psychological distress (Hopwood et al 1993, Koopman et al 1998). This may be related to increased pain, levels of dependency and disability (Koopman et al 1998).

One of the most common themes when talking to women with breast cancer at any stage is uncertainty about the future and the effectiveness of treatments; much support is often needed in accepting this uncertainty (Robinson 1994).

Studies also highlight that psychological and emotional problems are experienced by partners and families of patients with breast disease (Sheppard & Markby 1995, Northouse et al 1998).

Women at increased risk because of a family history of breast cancer may bear a heavy emotional burden and a recent evaluation of genetic counselling services suggested 27% of clinic attenders had levels of distress consistent with the need for psychological support (Kash et al 1992). Results from a population-based study of high-risk women indicate that over one-third suffer from significant levels of breast-cancer-related worry (Lerman et al 1993). However, while there may be psychological benefits in reducing uncertainty and doubts through BRCA (breast cancer susceptibility) genetic testing, empirical studies should be performed to examine the psycho-social aspects of undergoing testing (Bredart et al 1998). Genetic counselling is very important for these women.

Although the incidence of psychological morbidity in women with benign breast disease has not been recorded, many articles refer to the anxieties induced by breast symptoms such as pain and nodularity (Hirst 1984, Miers 1991, Galea 1993). In educating women to be alert to the signs of malignant breast disease, we may prompt unnecessary worry about breast symptoms that derive from normal processes, but can appear similar to signs of disease. It is not therefore surprising that women seek help to relieve both their anxieties and their symptoms (Miers 1991). Although many women who suffer breast pain and tenderness do not seek medical advice, fear of underlying malignancy or the disruptive effects pain can have on sleep, work and intimate relationships encourage some women to seek reassurance or treatment (Hughes et al 1989).

In conclusion, the incidence of psychological morbidity in women with breast disease is variable. It may be that some patients actually ‘fall through the net’ and are not identified as having unmet psychological needs. The evidence in Payne & Endall’s study (1998) suggests that the greatest barrier to effective identification of psychological problems in a breast clinic is the time constraint placed on consultations. Psychological morbidity is only discovered through good communication and indeed good communication can help to alleviate or prevent psychological distress in patients with breast disease.

EMOTIONAL PROBLEMS IN BREAST CARE

Assessment and measurement strategies

There are many important reasons why nurses should assess patients for signs of distress, anxiety or depression. Among these are:

- Effective intervention for depression and anxiety can have hugely beneficial consequences for patients and their families. However, such intervention cannot be offered without knowledgeable assessment
- Some studies have shown that women who adopt a hopeless/helpless or distressed/depressed attitude to their illness may have a poorer survival (Watson et al 1999). Identification of these women could lead to interventions to improve this situation. However, it is worth noting that in the same study a 'fighting spirit response' in patients with breast cancer did not improve survival. Therefore women should not be pressurised to adapt this response so that they can 'beat their disease and live longer'
- Assessment enables nurses to identify those patients for whom therapeutic nursing interventions are appropriate
- Assessment ensures early identification of those patients who need pharmacological, psychiatric or psychotherapeutic interventions.

However, a mere acceptance of these facts does not facilitate prompt identification of problems, when the reality for most nurses is that they feel ill-equipped to disentangle the 'normal' from the 'clinical'. One of the main problems associated with detection of anxiety or depression in cancer patients is disentangling symptoms associated with these states from symptoms of the disease or treatment, e.g. fatigue, poor appetite.

The other main issue is that most people experience grief reactions or a period of anger or fearful depression soon after a diagnosis of cancer. This may be an adjustment period before adapting to their situation. It is important to support patients during this time and acknowledge their distress. Also it is important to detect those not returning to normal functioning so that appropriate help can be offered and initiated (Watson 1991).

There is plenty of research evidence to show that emotional problems among cancer patients often go unrecognised unless they are specifically sought out, either through personal interviews or by means of a formal questionnaire such as the HAD (Hospital Anxiety and Depression) Scale (Bottomley 1998). Because emotional problems can arise at any time during the course of an illness, such screening should ideally be repeated at regular intervals for each patient. Whether or not a formal screening programme is in place, it is important that all patients are asked from time to time how they are coping with the emotional side of their illness, and given frequent opportunities to discuss their current concerns. In every encounter with a patient or family member, an opportunity exists for psycho-social assessment. This may include relationships, coping skills or self-esteem. Patients often choose to raise difficult issues during the night; existential issues, questions of spirituality or sexuality are commonly raised with night nurses. Most nursing documentation, particularly admission assessment data sheets include a section on worries and concerns, coping etc. This is a good time to elicit emotional problems and discuss referrals with the patient.

Many nurses lack confidence in their ability to elicit psycho-social problems. An assessment interview should be of optimal use both to the patient and professional carer. Some principles should therefore be adhered to:

- Setting the scene: seeing the patient alone is preferable. Patients often deliberately withhold important information if they are first seen with a partner, relative or friend. The patient may wish to protect their companion from the reality of their prognosis, suffering and fears, or may not usually confide problems to that person
- When time is short, establish which problem the patient most wants help with. Try to elicit its nature and severity and how the patient perceives and feels about the problem. Explain that you will attend to any other problems later
- Time limits should be negotiated
- Taking notes will avoid your forgetting important cues about possible problem areas. Noting key data tells patients that you are taking their problem seriously. It should not hinder disclosure
- Eliciting problems is easier if the professional carer does not interrupt the patient in the middle of a sentence or paragraph. Summarising the problems makes it clear to the patient that you have been listening and enables you to check if the list is correct
- Exploring each problem is necessary to understand it fully and to see how the patient perceives it and has reacted to it
- Most distressed patients will want their distress acknowledged and help to explain why they feel this way. If a patient states that a problem is too painful to discuss, this should be respected (O'Toole 1999).

As previously mentioned, Burton & Watson (1988) have identified a number of factors that have been associated with an increased risk of psychological problems among women with breast cancer (Box 7.1); it may be useful to bear these in mind during the assessment process. They also suggest that the key areas to explore are as follows:

- Patient's own view of her diagnosis and treatment
- Previous experiences of breast cancer within family and friends
- Recent stressful events (bereavement, divorce, redundancy) or chronic difficulties (financial, estranged family member)
- Key relationships: what aspects are important (practical, emotional, physical), how are they affected, is there open discussion/communication within the family?
- Satisfaction with employment, hobbies, interests
- Satisfaction with body image, sexuality, impact of treatment/diagnosis on these areas
- Importance of spirituality/faith
- History of anxiety/depression
- Recurring thoughts, concentration, mood, sleep patterns, fatigue, feelings of panic/tension

- View of the future/outlook
- Coping abilities/strategies.

Studies have shown that psychological distress is underestimated at outpatient clinics (Payne & Endall 1998). The evidence in this study suggests that the greatest barrier to effective identification of psychological problems in a breast clinic is the time constraint placed on consultations. With only a short time to spend with each patient, the surgeon is forced to focus on physical problems. None of the surgeons interviewed reported directly enquiring about psychological problems. They expected patients to volunteer that they were anxious or depressed. Nurses have a special role in being aware of the psychological distress that the surgeon may miss. Moreover, clinic nurses can offer follow-up to patients, a continuity of care that junior medical staff are unable to provide. This also applies to patients coming to GP practices or clinics, including those women with benign breast disease or those who are being monitored due to a strong family history of breast disease.

Formal measurements

Self-reporting measures should only be seen as an aid to assessment. Some patients may not admit to negative feelings on questionnaires. It is essential that any patient identified as having a level of symptomatology following self-assessment is followed up with a clinical interview by a clinical nurse specialist, psychologist or psychotherapist. Two assessment tools are:

1. Hospital Anxiety and Depression (HAD) scale. This is a self-assessment scale developed by Zigmond and Snaith (1983) for detecting anxiety and depression. It is quick and easy to complete and does not present a significant intrusion for patients. The HAD scale allows careful differentiation of anxiety and depression via two seven-item sub-scales. Scores indicate the severity of anxiety and depression during the preceding week using a scale of 0–21 (see Fig. 7.1). Summed scores of 0–7 are considered fine, 8–10 borderline, and 11–21 a case for further discussion and possible referral for specialist help.
2. Beck Depression Inventory (Beck et al 1961), is a self-report scale composed of 21 items, each comprised of four statements reflecting gradations in the intensity of a particular depressive symptom. The respondent chooses the statement that best corresponds to the way he has felt for the past week. The scale is intended for use as a screening instrument and as a measure of the symptom-severity of depressed mood (see Fig. 7.2).

There are other instruments such as the Cancer Locus of Control Scale (Watson 1990), which measures the degree to which patients feel control over their illness and the Mental Adjustment to Cancer Scale (Watson et al 1988), to elicit coping strategies. It is important that the chosen instrument is used consistently and confidently. Otherwise, measurements will not be accurate.

In conclusion, the best way to identify distress is through spending time in privacy with the patient and allowing an opportunity for venting of feelings through use of open-ended specific questions. Where time is short the use of such instruments referred to may also be of use.

HAD Scale

Name: Date:

Doctors are aware that emotions play an important part in most illnesses. If your doctor knows about these feelings he will be able to help you more. This questionnaire is designed to help your doctor to know how you feel. Read each item and place a firm tick in the box opposite the reply which comes closest to how you have been feeling in the past week. Don't take too long over your replies: your immediate reaction to each item will probably be more accurate than a long thought-out response.

Tick only one box in each section

I feel tense or 'wound up':

Most of the time ☐
A lot of the time ☐
Time to time, occasionally ☐
Not at all ☐

I still enjoy the things I used to enjoy:

Definitely as much ☐
Not quite so much ☐
Only a little ☐
Hardly at all ☐

I get a sort of frightened feeling as if something awful is about to happen:

Very definitely and quite badly ☐
Yes, but not too badly ☐
A little, but it doesn't worry me ☐
Not at all ☐

I can laugh and see the funny side of things:

As much as I always could ☐
Not quite so much now ☐
Definitely not so much now ☐
Not at all ☐

Worrying thoughts go through my mind:

A great deal of the time ☐
A lot of the time ☐
From time to time but not too often ☐
Only occasionally ☐

I feel cheerful:

Not at all ☐
Not often ☐
Sometimes ☐
Most of the time ☐

I can sit at ease and relaxed:

Definitely ☐
Usually ☐
Not often ☐
Not at all ☐

I feel as if I'm slowed down:

Nearly all of the time ☐
Very often ☐
Sometimes ☐
Not at all ☐

I get a sort of frightened feeling like 'butterflies' in the stomach:

Not at all ☐
Occasionally ☐
Quite often ☐
Very often ☐

I've lost interest in my appearance:

Definitely ☐
I don't take so much care as I should ☐
I may not take quite as much care ☐
I take just as much care as ever ☐

I feel restless as if I have to be on the move:

Very much indeed ☐
Quite a lot ☐
Not very much ☐
Not at all ☐

I look forward with enjoyment to things:

As much as I ever did ☐
Rather less than I used to ☐
Definitely less than I used to ☐
Hardly at all ☐

I get sudden feelings of panic:

Very often indeed ☐
Quite often ☐
Not very often ☐
Not at all ☐

I can enjoy a good book or radio or TV programme:

Often ☐
Sometimes ☐
Not often ☐
Very seldom ☐

FIGURE 7.1 HAD scale.

Beck Inventory

Name: ______________________ Date: ______________________

On this questionnaire are groups of statements. Please read each group of statements carefully. Then pick out the one statement in each group which best describes the way you have been feeling the PAST WEEK, INCLUDING TODAY! Circle the number beside the statement you picked. If several statements in the group seem to apply equally well, circle each one. Be sure to read all the statements in each group before making your choice.

1
- 0 I do not feel sad.
- 1 I feel sad.
- 2 I am sad all the time and I can't snap out of it.
- 3 I am so sad and unhappy that I can't stand it.

2
- 0 I am not particularly discouraged about the future.
- 1 I feel discouraged about the future.
- 2 I feel I have nothing to look forward to.
- 3 I feel that the future is hopeless and that things cannot improve.

3
- 0 I do not feel like a failure.
- 1 I feel I have failed more than the average person.
- 2 As I look back on my life, all I can see is a lot of failures.
- 3 I feel I am a complete failure as a person.

4
- 0 I get as much satisfaction out of things as I used to.
- 1 I don't enjoy things the way I used to.
- 2 I don't get satisfaction out of anything anymore.
- 3 I am dissatisfied or bored with everything.

5
- 0 I don't feel particularly guilty.
- 1 I feel guilty a good part of the time.
- 2 I feel quite guilty most of the time.
- 3 I feel guilty most of the time.

6
- 0 I don't feel I am being punished.
- 1 I feel I may be punished.
- 2 I expect to be punished.
- 3 I feel I am being punished.

7
- 0 I don't feel disappointed in myself.
- 1 I am disappointed in myself.
- 2 I am disgusted with myself.
- 3 I hate myself.

8
- 0 I don't feel I am worse than anybody else.
- 1 I am critical of myself for my weaknesses or mistakes.
- 2 I blame myself all the time for my faults.
- 3 I blame myself for everything bad that happens.

9
- 0 I don't have any thoughts of killing myself.
- 1 I have thoughts of killing myself, but I would not carry them out.
- 2 I would like to kill myself.
- 3 I would like to kill myself if I had the chance.

10
- 0 I don't cry any more than usual.
- 1 I cry more now than I used to.
- 2 I cry all the time now.
- 3 I used to be able to cry, but now I can't cry even though I want to.

11
- 0 I am no more irritated now than I ever am.
- 1 I get annoyed or irritated now more easily than I used to.
- 2 I feel irritated all the time now.
- 3 I don't get irritated at all by the things that used to irritate me.

12
- 0 I have not lost interest in other people.
- 1 I am less interested in other people than I used to be.
- 2 I have lost most of my interest in other people.
- 3 I have lost all of my interest in other people.

13
- 0 I make decisions about as well as I ever could.
- 1 I put off making decisions more than I used to.
- 2 I have greater difficulty in making decisions than before.
- 3 I can't make decisions at all anymore.

14
- 0 I don't feel I look any worse than I used to.
- 1 I am worried that I am looking old and unattractive.
- 2 I feel that there are permanent changes in my appearance that make me look unattractive.
- 3 I believe that I look ugly.

15
- 0 I can work about as well as before.
- 1 It takes an extra effort to get started at doing something.
- 2 I have to push myself hard to do anything.
- 3 I can't do anything at all.

16
- 0 I can sleep as well as usual.
- 1 I don't sleep as well as I used to.
- 2 I wake up 1–2 hours earlier than usual and find it hard to get back to sleep.
- 3 I wake up several hours earlier than I used to and cannot get back to sleep.

17
- 0 I don't get more tired than usual.
- 1 I get more tired than usual.
- 2 I get tired from doing almost anything.
- 3 I am too tired to do anything

18
- 0 My appetite is no worse than usual.
- 1 My appetite is not as good as it used to be.
- 2 My appetite is much worse now.
- 3 I have no appetite at all anymore.

19
- 0 I haven't lost much weight, if any, lately.
- 1 I have lost more than 5 pounds.
- 2 I have lost more than 10 pounds.
- 3 I have lost more than 15 pounds.

20
- 0 I am no more worried about my health than usual.
- 1 I am worried about physical problems such as aches and pains or upset stomach: or constipation.
- 2 I am very worried about physical problems and it's hard to think about much else.
- 3 I am so worried about my physical problems that I cannot think about anything else.

I am purposely trying to lose weight by eating less. Yes_____ No_____

21
- 0 I have not noticed any recent change in my interest in sex.
- 1 I am less interested in sex than I used to be.
- 2 I am much less interested in sex now.
- 3 I have lost interest in sex completely.

FIGURE 7.2 Beck inventory.

DEPRESSION

Depression is among the most frequently identified emotional problems in breast cancer patients, and it is important because it can often be treated successfully. Surveys show that up to 50% of patients at any one time report depressive symptoms, with 10–20% having a full-blown depressive illness (Barraclough 1994). Depression in any cancer patient can be difficult to diagnose and is easily missed.

Depressed mood is a frequent response to unpleasant life situations, especially those that involve a loss. Many patients diagnosed with breast cancer, though not all, go through a period of feeling depressed after first learning their diagnosis, or in reaction to disease progression or relapse. This is often an appropriate stage in the adjustment process, and some experts actually consider it a desirable one that will ultimately help to promote realistic acceptance. 'Sadness' would perhaps be a better term than 'depression'. This appropriate normal reaction may merge into the pathological forms of depression (clinical depression; depressive illness) which is more severe and prolonged.

As mentioned previously, depression cannot always be put down simply to the psychological stress of having breast cancer. Some patients may be depressed in response to unrelated life events and difficulties, for example a bereavement or a marital problem (although many patients would attribute the cause of their breast cancer to such events and some research would support this way of thinking (Bleiker & van der Ploeg 1999). Some patients have a constitutional vulnerability to depression, as shown by a past history or family history of this condition. In others biological complications of the cancer or its treatment are contributing factors, for example nausea, hypercalcaemia or cerebral metastases. Side-effects of drugs must be considered, including cytotoxics and steroids. Usually in any one patient a combination of several contributory factors is present.

Symptoms

Depression is a disorder in which mood and vitality are lowered to the point of despair. Patients report that life is meaningless and experience feelings of misery and hopelessness. Symptoms may include:

- Reduced activity, slow response to questions, non-expressive speech
- Sad and careworn facial expressions
- Lack of interest in appearance, with clothing and hair unkempt
- Withdrawn behaviour, lack of interest in social activities
- Lack of interest or pleasure in life (anhedonia)
- Inability to concentrate
- Feeling a burden to others
- Feelings of guilt, hopelessness, helplessness
- Diurnal mood variation, i.e. feeling worse at different times of the day
- Dysphoric mood, i.e. sad, anxious, tearful
- Feeling inconsolably negative about disease outcome when there is a realistic chance of 'cure'
- Suicidal thoughts.

Somatic (physical) manifestations are less helpful in assessing for depression as many of them may be caused by the disease or its treatment and are especially complicated by advanced disease. These signs include:

- Aches and pains, palpitations, headache
- Fatigue
- Insomnia
- Decreased libido
- Weight loss and loss of appetite
- Constipation.

Depressed patients may consider themselves too worthless to merit help; therefore they do not complain about the symptoms of their depression or those of their cancer. Physically they tend to look worse than they are and often investigations are ordered to rule out advancement of disease or complications of treatment.

There are a few guidelines for helping decide when a psychiatric referral is needed but Massie and Holland (1990) offer the following advice as criteria:

- Mild depressive symptoms are common with cancer, severe ones are not
- Symptoms of hopelessness, dysphoria, insomnia, isolation and suicidal thoughts (in combination) are representative of major depression. Evidence of threat to self or others, altered or unusual behaviour (often evidence of underlying delirium) or intolerable anxiety, may also be suggestive of the need for psychiatric support.

However, ideally patients should be referred for psychological support before the situation becomes this acute and good assessment through sensitive discussion with the patient or indeed the family should facilitate this.

Treatment

Depressed or unhappy patients should first be offered an opportunity to express their feelings of sadness or anger about their losses of the illness and how unfair it all seems. Many patients benefit greatly from a sympathetic acknowledgment of their distress. This can often be achieved through just one or two long periods of time spent with the patient, which will often include some tears as well as talking. Patients need to know that depression is a perfectly acceptable response to having cancer, and that open expression of negative feelings – as opposed to bottling them up – can actually help. After all, there is much that a woman with breast cancer might well be depressed about – coping with a mastectomy, hair loss, nausea, lifestyle changes, changes in libido. Many depressed patients say that they have not been given enough information about their diagnosis, treatment or prognosis. Whether information has been genuinely lacking or whether patients themselves have been unable to take it in, this aspect may require more attention.

If depression persists more than a few weeks, and does not respond to simple discussion of facts and ventilation of feelings, more specialised treatment in the form of a particular counselling approach such as cognitive behavioural therapy (Greer et al 1992), or interpersonal psychotherapy (Doris et al 1999) should be pursued. Antidepressants are very effective in the treatment of depressive symptoms and are reported to be effective in 70–80% of the depressed population

(Lovejoy & Matteis 1996). Treatment should continue for at least 2 weeks before suppression of symptoms can be expected. It should be maintained at the optimum dose for at least another month before any attempt at dose reduction is made. By informing patients of this anticipated delay, considerable distress may be avoided, and compliance with therapy is more likely. For some patients maintenance therapy may be needed for several months to prevent relapse (Doris et al 1999). The most commonly prescribed antidepressants in cancer care are the tricyclics such as amitriptyline or the serotonin re-uptake inhibitors (SSRIs) such as Prozac. Unfortunately side-effects may include headaches, nausea, insomnia, sexual dysfunction, anxiety, tremors and restlessness. Once a decision has been made to prescribe antidepressants, the patient should be monitored by a GP, psychiatrist, psychologist or specialist nurse, or indeed a nurse who is in constant contact with the patient in the community or hospital (see Case Study 1).

The woman in the following case study had a good response to treatments, feeling much more able to cope with life.

ANXIETY

Almost everyone is familiar with anxiety. Most people feel anxious in a situation that is unfamiliar, uncertain or frankly dangerous. Some degree of anxiety among patients with breast symptoms or breast cancer is therefore understandable and does not require psychiatric labels or treatments.

Around the time of the initial diagnosis, most, though not all patients feel anxiety. Paradoxical as it may seem, many express relief when the diagnosis is confirmed – knowing the truth is easier than fearing the unknown. As the illness progresses, anxiety may be rekindled by further points of uncertainty – waiting to begin a new treatment, being admitted to hospital for the first time, waiting for the results of diagnostic tests for suspected relapse, long periods at home between follow-up visits. Some patients suffer more anxiety than they need to at such times, because they are harbouring ungrounded fears about their illness or its treatment and are too frightened to mention these to the staff looking after them. Accurate factual information may dispel such fears. At the opposite extreme, some anxious patients seek out more information than they can cope with, for example reading up on possible side-effects of the proposed treatment and worrying that they will develop them all.

When anxiety develops for no apparent reason, or persists in a disabling form long after its initial cause has passed, an anxiety disorder may be diagnosed. This happens for some patients with breast cancer and for some patients with benign disease who worry they may develop cancer. They remain disabled by anxiety about their illness, even if from a physical point of view they appear to be doing well (Barraclough 1994).

Clinical types of anxiety and their effect on treatments

Anxiety may be present continuously, most of the time, or in acute bouts (panic attacks). A distinction can often be made between 'trait' anxiety, which has been present throughout life as an integral feature of the personality, and 'state' anxiety, which has arisen anew in reaction to stressful circumstances. These panic attacks

CASE STUDY 1

Letter to GP from Department of Psychological Medicine:

Dear Doctor,

Re: Mrs Jill Peters, etc.

I reviewed this woman today at the request of the nurse specialist in breast care. As you will be aware, she has had a further occurrence of a breast tumour (this time on the left side) a few months ago. This has apparently been treated successfully and she tells me there is no evidence of any spread, which reassures her considerably. Rather oddly, she says that following the previous tumour on the right side, 6 years ago, this has not come entirely as a shock and that in some way, she was almost prepared for it. Nonetheless, she agrees that this has been rather traumatic and has constituted yet another adverse life event in a catalogue of recent difficulties. As you may be aware, this includes the death last year of her mother, from breast cancer, as well as deaths in recent years of her elder brother from a myeloma and her father from prostate cancer.

Given her own longstanding difficulties with low self-esteem and anxiety and her historical background in what sounds a very dysfunctional family probably contributing to this, it is perhaps no surprise that recent events have led again to her feeling rather depressed. She feels in addition, that she cannot really confide in people beyond her husband and that somehow the 'real me' has never really been revealed to the world; she agrees that much of this anxiety probably relates to her difficult childhood. However, her husband has commented recently that she appears very tense, anxious and often quite irritable. This they both agree is really quite a significant change and I think these comments coming from her husband, who is normally very supportive of her, have partly contributed to her agreement to coming along to see us.

As you may know, she attended for some time here about 6 years ago for psychological support from Dr Green, at the time of the initial tumour. Reviewing the situation today, we agreed that although some psychological work in the past and present might still be helpful in working on her difficulties, the situation had got to the point where perhaps we ought to think about trying one of the new antidepressants with some anti-anxiety effect, such as venlafaxine. Mrs Peters was very open to this and agreed that things had got rather 'stuck'. Accordingly, I have issued her with a prescription for venlafaxine 37.5 mg bd and have arranged to review her in 3 weeks' time to check on her progress. Hopefully, this will improve her mental state to the extent that she will be able to cope herself and I shall keep you informed of her progress. In the meantime, I have advised her that you would be able to continue the prescription for her, assuming there are no adverse side-effects.

Yours sincerely

cc nurse specialist, breast care

may last for about 20 minutes and leave individuals fearful of the next attack, which leads them to isolate themselves from their social network. Phobic anxiety is that provoked by a specific stimulus; common examples in breast cancer patients are i.v. injections or being left alone in the radiotherapy room. Staff should be sensitive to these patients' needs. Other patients suffer from generalised or free floating anxiety, which they cannot relate to any particular cause, though in someone with breast cancer it is often a reasonable supposition that such anxiety is due to unexpressed fear of progressive disease and death.

Manifestations of anxiety

The following manifestations of anxiety were identified by Massie (1990):

- Restlessness
- Insomnia and nightmares
- Shortness of breath
- Irritability
- Worry
- Nausea and anorexia
- Diarrhoea
- Sweating
- Palpitations
- Headaches
- Flushed face
- Smoking
- Poor concentration and memory
- Weakness
- Exhaustion
- Fine tremor
- Elevated blood pressure
- Hyperventilation
- Menstrual changes
- Urinary frequency.

Management of anxiety

With so many potential sources and manifestations of anxiety (see Fig. 7.3) how can nurses help patients manage their worries?

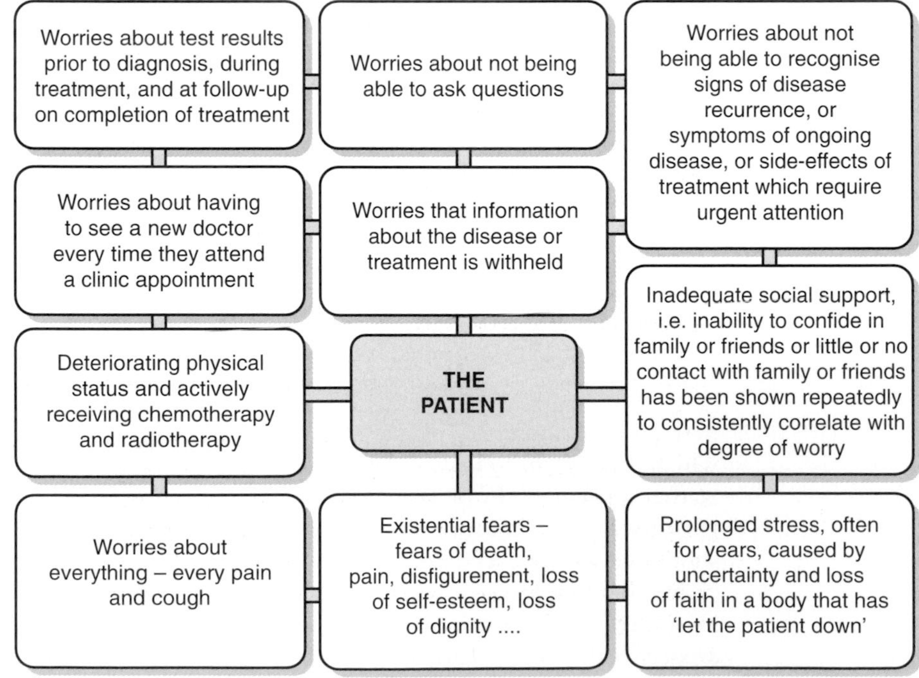

FIGURE 7.3

Patients at risk of psychological problems. Adapted from Burton and Watson 1998 Counselling People with Cancer. John Wiley and Sons, West Sussex.

Anxiety can be minimised by the sympathetic organisation of treatment services, for example:

1. Letting patients know the results of tests as soon as these come through, rather than making them wait days or weeks for their next outpatient visit
2. Providing continuity of care from familiar doctors and nurses
3. Trying to give the right amount of information for each individual case.

The ability to help individuals to disentangle fears and physical symptoms may be the most effective means that nurses have of working with patients and their families to manage anxiety. Explaining and exploring the origin of physical symptoms may help, for example, headaches may become less severe if the patient can be convinced they are not due to a brain tumour. Physical treatments such as massage and relaxation therapy can be especially helpful when physical symptoms are prominent. A referral to a psychologist or counsellor for behavioural (relaxation, distraction, hypnosis) and cognitive techniques are most useful for phobic anxiety. Drugs used for anxiety include benzodiazepines, antidepressants and beta-blockers. Recognising crisis points throughout the breast cancer continuum as referred to earlier such as diagnosis and recurrence, can help nurses intervene more effectively at these critical points (Burton & Watson 1998).

The following case illustrates the common combination of anxiety with depression

CASE STUDY 2

Excerpt from letter from local community health team to nurse counsellor at treating hospital

Re: Mrs Pat Smart:

The meeting was with her alone, and although she was clearly giving a direct honest account, it may be that her perspective on some areas is affected by her intense distress. The meeting was in the framework of her having attended the outpatient clinic at your hospital, the previous day, when it was confirmed that she would be admitted for mastectomy the following Sunday. She confirmed your account to me, that she had been told that she had a good 10-year prognosis.

Her level of distress and her feelings at times of an overwhelming need to escape had raised the question of inpatient treatment in our psychiatric unit in her mind. However, the likelihood that she would be likely to bring much of her distress with her made me doubtful that she would get the profound sense of relief from 'giving up' that is a powerful part of effective inpatient care.

She should continue diazepam at a dose of 2 mg/three times/day, having experienced some relief in her anxiety. At this moderate dose she is able to relax to some extent both in her mind and body, although symptoms in both areas recur when she is ruminating and fearful. The main evidence of depression lies in the length and level of her distress and impairment, rather than specific symptoms (since fearfulness and anxiety dominate her mood). Since the discovery of her breast lump and diagnosis, she has been progressively impaired to the point where she is now doing little of her usual routine and not leaving the house. Her appetite is decreased, but sleep remains possible (and is clearly a period of relief for her). On balance, I think that the evidence is sufficient to justify a change from trazadone to venlafaxine.

CASE STUDY 2 (contd)

She did seek reassurance from me several times, but my sense was that this was very briefly effective. Her earlier period of psychological difficulty, and brief contact with the psychiatric services, indicates overall that this earlier episode, which also focused on fear of a fatal illness (a brain tumour) was an anxiety disorder rather than a period of depression. Mrs Smart says that she has been said to take after her father in being vulnerable to anxiety.

In fact, Mrs Smart continued to be extremely tearful and anxious throughout her treatment regimes, continually worrying that she would die despite continual reassurance from the medical team, her specialist breast care nurse and nurse counsellor. The nurse counsellor, who engaged Mrs Smart in cognitive behavioural techniques, found her incredibly resistant to challenging her perception of her own condition and discontinued their sessions after some weeks. Mrs Smart had continued contact with the breast care nurse specialist, and over some months gradually she came to a calmer state, and accepted that at least in the short term, she would live to plan another year.

COPING STYLES

Coping with breast cancer or indeed symptoms of breast cancer, or being at increased risk of breast cancer, is defined by the cognitive, emotional and behavioural responses people give to the situation. It is important to understand the ways in which people cope with stressful situations such as receiving a diagnosis of breast cancer. In Watson et al's (1999) recent study on the influence of psychological response on survival in breast cancer, the main issue appeared to be the maintenance of hope as a method of improving survival. This may be because the woman is better able to mobilise resources such as complementary therapies, counselling, family support etc., which would have an influence on compliance and coping with treatments etc. This point is important for us as nurses to bear in mind – how do we instill hope in our patients and are we even aware of it? (Carroll 1999). We have already covered helplessness/hopelessness and anxious preoccupation as responses. The two other main styles that should be mentioned as common responses are denial and anger.

Denial

Perhaps the best-known of the ego defence mechanisms involves an unconscious refusal to acknowledge certain distressing aspects of reality (Greer 1992). Most people use denial to protect themselves against anxiety and unpleasantness in daily life – they 'turn a blind eye' to things they prefer to not know about. The term 'denial' is often used in relation to patients with cancer who apparently fail to realise their diagnosis or the gravity of the prognosis. Denial is also seen where the apparently educated woman with a large breast lump presents to her doctor saying 'I thought everyone had lumps like this'.

Many patients are in fact well aware of the truth about their illness but prefer not to think or talk about it. Many patients would be overwhelmed by facing up to the full implications of such bad news all at once, whereas letting it sink in gradually is more bearable. Transient denial at crisis points in the illness is a natural means of self-protection.

When deciding how to deal with denial as a staff member, it is important to establish what the patient has actually been told. The patient cannot avoid or deny things for which they have no knowledge in the first place. There is a good argument for leaving well enough alone unless patients give some indication that they are not sustaining the positive effects of that coping strategy. Collusion therefore involves going along with the patient's self-deception, an approach that many staff feel uncomfortable with. It is most often a family member or member of the nursing team who requests counselling for the patient because they themselves feel uncomfortable with the denial response. Denial is such a powerful psychological response. that it can be difficult to challenge. How different staff members choose to handle denial depends on their intuitive feel for the patient concerned. However, a good solution is to give patients ample opportunity to question the situation but never forcing unwanted information upon them (Greer 1992, Barraclough 1994).

Anger

Anger in the period after receiving a diagnosis of breast cancer is described as a normal phase in the adjustment process. Some patients can obtain a welcome release through spontaneous free expression of their anger – 'Why me?' and then become able to move on towards emotional acceptance. In other patients, anger becomes persistently ingrained, in which case it usually has destructive consequences for all concerned.

Being the target of patients' anger is one of the most difficult situations nurses have to deal with. Not surprisingly, the first reaction is to defend ourselves, but a good first principle is to try not to do this as a defensive attitude can cause us to become sucked into the conflict. Instead, it helps to acknowledge the anger, to give the patient the opportunity to make their points, and then to look at what can be done about it. Often this is cathartic and the patient becomes more rational. Done in the right way, it is possible to move from being the patient's adversary to being their ally (Burton & Watson 1998).

FAMILY ISSUES

Stress on family members may be as great, or greater, than that experienced by the patient, and increasing emotional pressures can put a tremendous strain on close relationships (Given et al 1993, Harrison et al 1995, Northouse et al 1998).

The family of a woman with breast cancer is often conceptualised in terms of a married couple or partner (Budin 1998). Marital status has been regarded as a measure of social support; however, not all individuals who are married perceive their support to be adequate, and not all individuals who are single, separated, divorced or widowed are lacking in social support (Budin 1998).

Northouse et al (1998) concluded that their research provides compelling evidence that breast cancer affects the emotional well-being of couples, resulting in a continuation of their elevated emotional distress levels and role problems following diagnosis. Partners of the patient with breast cancer can suffer a range of somatic and emotional problems: sleep disturbance, loss of appetite, concentration problems, headache, worry and fatigue. They may have their own health problems and feel ill-placed to provide the practical support needed. Partners often describe a feeling of helplessness and inadequacy in attempting to be a support for their loved one. It may help to give reassurance and positive feedback to them that sometimes just 'being there' is enough by taking in the information, asking questions and noting important dates etc. (Northouse et al 1998). Making sure to include the partner as far as possible, with the patient's permission, in any discussions on treatments and their side-effects etc. and possible common emotional reactions, may help to open communication channels between them. Providing opportunities for patients and partners to discuss their worries and concerns about the other and their family is also therapeutic. Too often, the partner is forgotten in the whole scenario (Zahlis & Shands 1993). It may be that a partner would like to pursue counselling or the couple together may benefit from counselling. Sometimes there are substantial differences between the patient's and the partner's psychological reactions that prevent them from acknowledging feelings. I am often asked by the patient to discuss their concerns with their partner in a way that conceals the fact that they asked me to in the first place! On the other hand, coping styles may be complementary. For example, Tessa is 35 years old with two young children; her immediate and lasting response to finding a breast lump and subsequent diagnosis was complete devastation and hopelessness. Her husband on the other hand, was reassuring and positive, listening to what the consultant had to say and reinforcing that to Tessa on a constant basis. Tessa explained to me weeks later that she needed her husband to be like that for her and that was how it normally was for them, him being an optimist and Tessa always seeing the negative side.

Children

Relationships between parents and children bring special problems. The communication difficulty tends to relate specifically to the issue of what to tell the children about the diagnosis and treatment of breast cancer, especially when they are not mature enough to fully understand. The desire is often to protect children and prevent them from becoming unnecessarily distressed. Sometimes a mother has strong ideas about what she wants to tell the children and this has to be respected. However, sometimes mothers will ask advice about what to tell their children. For young children, the fantasy is often worse than the reality. Explanations given in a way that the child can understand and from the security of the family may well be preferable to constructing an elaborate fabrication (Burton & Watson 1998). An important guideline is to listen carefully to what the child is asking and to reply as clearly and truthfully as possible. Children of ill parents may have difficulties at school, experience sleep and eating disturbances, show increased aggression, and exhibit anti-social behaviour. The disruption and change the parent's cancer has on their lives and the extent to which they worry about Mummy dying may be accountable for this behaviour. It is important that school teachers are made aware of the situation so that they can deal sensitively with the situation. The children may benefit from talking to a staff member whom they have met on a couple of occasions, for example the breast care nurse specialist. One family encountered recently had a difficult situation in that the parents although still living together, were estranged. The mother had breast cancer and was soon to be admitted for mastectomy. The father left the house and family 2 weeks prior to the event and the children became unmanageable for the mother. Talking to the children revealed their absolute fears about both Dad and Mum never coming back. A counsellor in the hospital spoke to the children at length and in the interim period Dad came back to live in the house. Thus they felt some security once again, but their problems are ongoing.

Families with single parents may be at particular risk and may need the offer of social service intervention in a sensitive manner. It is important to establish at the outset the extent of practical and emotional support the patient derives from family and friends.

A mother with breast cancer was particularly worried about her teenage daughter, who was withdrawn and was overeating. Through referral to the child and adolescent psychology service, Julie was able to identify patterns that were occurring in her life. This included feelings of sadness, emptiness and boredom that made her turn to food for feelings of comfort and warmth. Working on anxiety management skills, keeping a diary and challenging areas of her life where control was lacking helped Julie to feel more positive about herself and to communicate more with her mother about her worries.

In the event of death, families should always be offered information about bereavement services. Frequently the family will visit the ward team where their loved one died some weeks or months after the death. This is a good opportunity to provide that information.

PSYCHO-SEXUAL PROBLEMS

Throughout treatment sexual consequences should be considered and discussed with the patient and if possible the partner. At least five sexual problem areas arise in breast cancer treatment:

1. The alteration in body image as a result of the disease, surgery or treatment – painful scars, hair loss, weight alteration, premature menopause, loss of role function at work or in the family
2. The inability to have sexual intercourse, usually as a result of physical and psychological aspects of surgery or treatment. Chemotherapy causes loss of ovarian functioning, decreased oestrogen, difficulty with vaginal lubrication and decreased androgen levels causing decreased libido. Hormonal treatments such as tamoxifen also influence menstrual pattern and vaginal discharge and treatments generally may cause profound fatigue and sometimes nausea (Rabinowitz 1998)
3. Psychological and emotional responses in coming to terms with the diagnosis and prognosis – the woman and indeed the partner may be emotionally exhausted. If there are difficulties in talking to each other about basic feelings, it may be difficult to resume a sexual relationship (Rabinowitz 1997)
4. Infertility secondary to cancer treatments such as chemotherapy. If having children was a life goal, then it will be difficult for a couple or woman to

come to terms with the potential reality that having children may not be a possibility. On the other hand, a woman or couple may be told by their consultant that subsequent pregnancies may be detrimental to the chances of a recurrence. Contraception then becomes an issue; the contraceptive pill is generally advised against and barrier methods are the alternative, which does not suit every couple's sexual relationship. The woman may put pressure on her partner to have a vasectomy and this may further compound relationship difficulties

5. Fears of abandonment by one's partner.

Understanding sexual difficulties for the patient with breast cancer may be complicated because they are frequently multifactorial. The diagnosis, emotional reactions and treatment effects can interact in a way that reduces sexual feelings. Sexual problems may not arise until some months after diagnosis (Burton & Watson 1998).

Nurses or doctors who feel uncomfortable or underconfident in raising these issues might need to consider referral to a specialist nurse or counsellor (Waterhouse & Metcalfe 1991). Patients too may be uncomfortable about raising such issues or having them raised even by a professional. Sensitive and supportive listening, allowing women to express their fears and experiences, along with sound information on possible causes and advice on symptom control such as lubricating creams and advice on other avenues for specialised help, may do much to help women cope (Topping 1996). The following case illustrates how intertwined psychological, physical, emotional and sexual problems can be.

CASE STUDY 3

Letter to nurse specialist from clinical psychologist

Re: Mrs Sally Waters

Thank you for asking us to review this patient. Sally says she is experiencing anxiety and panic attacks since her mastectomy and reconstruction. She has also been finding it difficult to get off to sleep and frequently wakes up following nightmares, the theme of which is usually her cancer recurring. There was however, no evidence of clinical depression.

It appears that Sally's anxiety has been compounded by her husband's health problems. Following Sally's breast cancer and her husband Dan's second heart operation, they have both had to adjust to rather a dramatic change of lifestyle. In particular, since retiring from his own job, Dan has become involved in Sally's retail business, which has led to increased tension between them. Sally also mentioned concerns over their decreased sexual intimacy. They appeared to be coping differently with their health problems and this may have increased her tension, so that communication between them has become an issue needing to be addressed. I have offered Sally six further appointments, to focus on her anxiety management and problem-solving strategies.

Yours Sincerely

MULTIDISCIPLINARY TEAM – WHEN TO REFER, WHO TO REFER TO

Patients' ability to deal with the demands placed upon them at a time of crisis is dependent on the availability and utilisation of support services. Supportive care and interventions aimed at minimising the psycho-social impact of cancer improves quality of life and is an essential part of cancer treatment (Montazeri et al 1997). A number of outcomes have been associated with the utilisation of psycho-social support services, including positive adjustment to a diagnosis of cancer (Breitbart 1995), less emotional distress and longer life (Spiegel et al 1989) and improved coping methods (Marchioro et al 1996).

Supportive interventions cover a wide range of services:

- Information
- Support from health care professionals such as stress management and relaxation techniques
- Social services offer financial support and advice on practical services such as home-help; some offer counselling skills support
- Psychological and psychiatric interventions such as individual psychotherapy, psychoanalysis, cognitive therapy and family therapy
- Counselling
- Support and self-help groups (listed in at the end of this section)
- Complimentary therapies such as massage and aromatherapy
- 'Drop-in' centres that offer a wide range of complementary therapies, individual and group counselling and social support.

Not all of these services may be available at every hospital where a patient is treated for breast cancer. However, all professionals involved in the care of the patient have an opportunity to provide support. Nurses are in a key position to offer support and offer basic communication skills to identify needs and concerns. Some nurses may not feel adequately skilled and may therefore avoid talking to patients about their feelings (Maguire et al 1993). These nurses should endeavour to receive training in communication skills and should access a senior colleague to talk to a patient who is obviously in need of a sensitive listener. The degree of experience and education a nurse has in the field of cancer will influence how comfortable they feel in that situation. It is likely that if a nurse feels 'out of her depth' or if it is apparent that the patient has specific problems, such as those mentioned, that she/he will then refer on to the breast care nurse specialist, if available. It may also be that lack of time is a real issue for ward nurses. Most centres undertaking the primary management of patients with breast cancer now have specifically designated nurses who provide practical advice and support, and who may also have a community focus to their role (McArdle et al 1996).

Role of the specialist breast care nurse in providing psycho-social support

The breast care nurse specialist meets the patient at diagnosis and offers them a contact number. Patients can phone if they are worried and concerned about any aspect of their treatment and diagnosis. A meeting with the patient and a significant other if desired is usually set soon after diagnosis to allow the patient an opportunity to discuss all treatment options and to determine how the patient is coping. Sometimes this requires a number of meetings before any treatment is commenced. Informational support forms a significant component of the role and facilitating decision making for treatment choices (Carroll 1998).

Routine visits are made to the patient whilst in hospital for surgery (the most common primary treatment) and at the postoperative clinic when histology results are being explained and subsequent treatment planned. The breast care nurse specialist will see the patient a number of times throughout her treatments and follow-up care. Obviously some patients require more support than others. Studies since the 1980s have focused on evaluating the effectiveness of the role, which provides continuity of care, enables close monitoring of psycho-social adjustment to diagnosis and treatment, provides practical support, counselling or use of counselling skills and/or referral to an appropriate counsellor and support groups, and an open access system (Watson et al 1988, Wilkinson et al 1988, McArdle et al 1996).

Usually, the specialist nurse has close links with voluntary support groups, social workers, psychological medicine/counselling departments of the hospital (if available!) and community teams. They may also have been instrumental in setting up and facilitating a support group. The specialist nurse also has an educational remit, providing education to staff where requested and acting as a resource where needed. Patients are now more informed about the availability of a specialist breast care nurse, but it is useful for nurses in hospitals and in the primary health care team to inform patients how such nurses can be of help to them (Alderson et al 1996).

Further intervention

Table 7.1 describes levels of intervention and who might be expected to perform them. There may be confusion, particularly in a large general hospital about who to refer on to – psychologist? psychiatrist? counsellor?

The answer to this depends to some extent on what is available. The breast care nurse specialist usually has developed links in the available area and should be able to offer advice, if not intervention. The specialist nurse is a good first port of call before activating further intervention.

A psychologist generally offers skills in problem identification, a range of techniques in assisting the woman to cope with her cancer, help to dispel any maladaptive processes acquired, specific problem intervention, family and couple therapy. A counsellor may do the same or may have a specific mode of counselling, such as the use of Gestalt therapy.

A psychiatrist may also have skills in these areas, but their main focus would be on physical, chemical and neurological causes of mental illness; psychiatrists are experts in the prescription of medication for problems such as depression and anxiety. The patient may also perceive some stigma associated with a referral to a psychiatrist, whereas they may accept a referral more readily, for example to a nurse specialist in psychological support (if available).

It is evident therefore that the prevention and management of psycho-social distress is based on a multidisciplinary approach. This can be seen from the

TABLE 7.1 ***Psychological interventions***

Level of intervention	Staff performing intervention
Level 1: Basic communication and assessment skills	Department/ward based staff
• Providing information	
• Interviewing, listening and empathic skills	
• Representing psychological needs to others	
• Knowing when to refer a problem on	
• Support and advice regarding psychological assessment	Breast care nurse specialist Counsellor/psychologist/nurse specialist Psychological support
Level 2: Routine preventive psychological care	Senior staff
• Ability to cope with others' distress	Breast care nurse specialist
• Establishing rapport	
• Facilitating emotional expression	
• Knowing when to refer a problem on	
• Support with psychological component of assessment	Breast care nurse specialist Counsellor/psychologist/nurse specialist
• Support/supervision of psychological interventions	Psychological support
Level 3: Specific psychological interventions	Senior staff
• Problem-solving based on theoretical model/skills training	Breast care nurse specialist
• Supervised short-term work	
• Comprehensive mental health assessment support/supervision of psychological interventions	Counsellor/psychologist/nurse specialist Psychological support
• Specific psychological interventions	
Level 4: Specific psychological interventions/therapy	Counsellor/psychologist/nurse specialist
• Provision of recognised appropriate form of psychological therapy e.g. cognitive therapy, psychotherapy	Psychological support/psychiatrist

Adapted from Tunmore (1990b).

letters outlined as case examples in this chapter and ideally team meetings would facilitate discussion of patients experiencing particular problems (Edwards 1999).

Benign breast disease

It is important to recognise that women with benign breast problems may have psychological difficulties or situations may arise where a referral to a breast care nurse specialist and/or psychologist is advocated. For example, a woman I encountered had 20 years' experience of benign lumps appearing in her breasts. She also had multiple bilateral cysts, which were very tender and impossible to aspirate. Mammograms were increasingly painful for her and she was extremely distressed because she was afraid that a breast cancer diagnosis could be missed due to her breast problems. She wanted to have a bilateral mastectomy. The consultant was willing to do this and asked me to see her as breast care nurse specialist. I first wanted to establish her understanding of her situation, her family support and psychological history and then I explained what such surgery would involve, the possible complications and risks etc. I also introduced the idea of reconstruction. I then referred her to the clinical psychologist as would be necessary in such a situation, who examined her psychological soundness for making decisions, coping skills and social support. This woman went on to see the plastic surgeon and subsequently had the operation. She is very happy physically and psychologically as a result. This case is certainly rare, but it does illustrate the importance of a multidisciplinary approach to the psycho-social aspects of breast disease. Similarly, women contemplating prophylactic mastectomy for proven increased risk of breast cancer due to genetic causes and strong family history would need such an approach.

METHODS OF SUPPORT

Communication

Communication can be defined as an 'interchange of thoughts, feelings and opinions among individuals' and is effective when it satisfies basic desires for recognition, participation and self-realisation by direct personal contact between persons (Wilkinson 1992). As far back as 1975, Cassee suggested that effective communication is achieved when open two-way communication takes place and patients are informed about the nature of their illness and treatment, and are encouraged to express their anxieties and emotions. Examples of basic communication skills are listening and clarifying:

> 'You say that a lot of things are bothering you. What kinds of things?'

Another skill is sympathising, i.e. saying

> 'This must be very difficult for you.'

Perhaps these statements should be followed by an open question:

> 'Would you like to talk about it?' or 'Would you like some more information about treatments?'

and finally gentle probing can be used:

> 'So you're feeling very scared at the moment?'

Communication skills are also non-verbal and include establishing eye contact, sitting facing the patient, adopting an open posture and focusing attention on the patient (Egan 1994). These skills are not special skills peculiar to nursing. Rather, they are extensions of the kind of skills all of us need in our everyday interpersonal transactions.

However, although communication is one of the most important aspects of nursing, moreover breast care/cancer nursing, evidence suggests that nurses experience communication difficulties and frequently block patients from divulging their worries or concerns (Wilkinson 1991). Many nurses in this study felt that they did not want to get involved in talking to patients in such depth and did not feel confident in communicating with them beyond a certain point. However, in a study of women's experiences of breast cancer care, relationships with nurses were amongst the most highly valued and were cited as valuable alliances, aiding in the communication and understanding of the treatment and disease process (Bottomley & Jones 1997). Patient satisfaction studies indicate that good communication skills are important to patients and the quality of the skills influences how satisfied patients feel (National Cancer Alliance 1996). As a consequence of many of these studies, there is now more emphasis on training courses to enhance or teach these skills (Wilkinson et al 1998).

In the National Cancer Alliance (1996) study, communication skills were seen as particularly important at the time of diagnosis. Work up to diagnosis and the imparting of the diagnosis itself often sets the scene for how the patient will perceive care and treatment (NHS Executive 1996, Bottomley & Jones 1997). Much is written on the importance of communication when breaking 'bad news' and this is referred to in more detail in Part 1 of this chapter. Open communication, avoiding the use of euphemisms, ensures that the patient is clear about the aim of treatment and is the means by which the confidence and cooperation of the patient are secured (Wilkinson 1991). Importantly, Wilkinson (1991) also points out that failure of adequate communication can lead to ignorance or misunderstanding, which may later become the basis of complaint.

Good communication takes account of and perhaps elicits the fact that patients may be distressed, sometimes needing this acknowledged and even normalised, before being able to communicate further (Maguire et al 1993). This acknowledges that emotions may block or inhibit communication about issues surrounding diagnosis and treatment, such as fear of death, prognosis, and effects of treatment. Furthermore, communication is essential to ascertain where the diagnosis fits in the context of the patient's life, e.g. recent divorce, redundancy, bereavement etc. (Burton & Watson 1998).

Effective communication results in the early identification of needs and allows the professional to refer the patient to other health care professionals who provide a variety of supports (Payne & Endall 1998). For example, a distressed single, young mother, currently experiencing anticipatory nausea, who is worried about the effects of chemotherapy on her ability to perform at work, on her presentation or image for work and for her two young children, seriously considers not pursuing the rest of her chemotherapy regime. A skilled communicator will pick up on the non-verbal cues of distressed behaviour and ask some open-ended questions that will give the patient an opportunity to express her concerns and fears. Referrals to specialist nurses for extra support, discussion of problems and monitoring, appliance officers for a wig, a social worker for financial aspects, possibly complementary therapists for relaxation and/or aromatherapy to help in general coping, and a possible referral to the psychologist for cognitive behavioural therapy to help with anticipatory nausea would then be facilitated.

Finally, the need for skilled communication of information to patients is a common theme in studies of patients with breast cancer/disease (Smyth et al 1996). The point being that even when the professional does not possess the necessary information to impart to the patient, skilled communication can identify the informational gaps and needs and facilitate referral or direction in the appropriate path. Informational issues will not be covered in this section as this has been covered in depth in Part 1 of this chapter. Suffice to say that good information giving adhering to the principles outlined in the chapter will do much to reduce anxiety and distress.

Counselling

The British Association of Counselling (BAC) defines counselling as an interaction in which the counsellor offers or agrees explicitly to offer another person or persons temporarily in the role of client, the time, attention and respect necessary to explore, discover and clarify ways of living more resourcefully, and to his or her greater well-being (Chaytor 1997). Although there is considerable consensus about the core content of a counselling course, there are still clear varieties of methods of counselling. Some counsellors may identify strongly with a particular theory or school, for example Gestalt or cognitive–behavioural, and consider others inadequate, and other counsellors may adapt a more open, eclectic stance. This can lead to great confusion amongst the public but while terminology and methods or skills may differ, there is crucial common ground between the various schools, which appears to help people in distress (Sutton 1998):

- There is a relationship of warmth and trust in which the counsellor attempts to understand the person and to convey this understanding and respect for the person
- The person is offered support by the counsellor: this may be support in coping with a distressing or crisis situation, support in terms of acceptance and respect as an individual, or support in facing past events or traumas
- The person experiences a release of tension or reduction in anxiety, which allows him or her to face or talk about a particular problem or problems
- The adaptive responses of the person are reinforced. In learning to understand more about themselves and any self-defeating patterns of thought or behaviour, the person is given an opportunity of solving particular problems, improving relationships, etc. The counsellor shares any knowledge or skills that may be appropriate.

The popular image of a counsellor is that of one person sitting with another in a room and agreeing a series of meetings. In some cases, however, counsellors work with couples, families or groups of people, for example support groups.

There is a danger that counselling might be viewed as the panacea to all problems, and as such, education about the role of counselling is essential to public and professionals alike. It is also necessary to be aware that counsellors should adhere to certain guidelines, codes of practice and ethics, laid down by professional bodies, such as the BAC. A BAC accreditation scheme for counsellors and the United Kingdom Register for Counsellors are voluntary schemes for registration (Woolfe 1998). This is important to bear in mind when referring a patient for counselling or when suggesting to them that counselling may be an appropriate route to follow, to help deal with their difficulties or problems.

OVERVIEW OF SPECIFIC THERAPEUTIC APPROACHES IN COUNSELLING

Cognitive–behavioural therapy

This was first described by Beck (1976) and Meichenbaum (1977) and developed by Moorey & Greer (1989). This model is based on the idea that thoughts contribute in an important way to how we feel. In this respect, thinking is causal: changing the way we think about something may change the way we feel (Burton & Watson 1998). Negative automatic thoughts are thoughts that spring to mind automatically, without much awareness and little effort to control them. Sometimes these negative thoughts become distorted and do not represent reality. The process involves patients in learning how to monitor their negative automatic thoughts – that is they need to be able to identify beliefs that are irrational, for example thinking that every ache or pain means that the cancer has returned. This model shares with other models the need to encourage patients to ventilate and share their worries. However at this point it diverges and takes a more specific path. It is a short-term intervention lasting usually between four and eight sessions; it is problem orientated and driven by patients' agendas. It is collaborative and educational in that the patient is taught coping strategies; it makes use of homework assignments and forms the basis of a self-help programme.

Behavioural techniques can be helpful initially because they bring rapid relief in terms of depression and anxiety. One of the most useful ways of helping patients plan how they can live an ordinary life is through the use of activity scheduling. Making a list of daily activities helps people to focus on the structure of their day, examines the nature and number of activities they engage in and looks at how much pleasure and sense of control they are able to achieve within those activities. This model has been found in large trials to be of benefit in reducing anxiety and depression (Moorey et al 1994).

Anticipatory nausea and vomiting, whereby the patient associates seeing the hospital, staff and even thinking about coming in for the next treatment with nausea and vomiting is amenable to behavioural therapy and relaxation therapy (Watson 1991). It is important that these patients are recognised and offered this treatment if at all possible.

Psychodynamic model

The psychodynamic life narrative is a statement that places the physical illness in the context of the person's 'life trajectory'. In listening to the patient's story, it is often possible to begin to place the illness in the context of the patient's life history and current situation (Viederman & Perry 1980). It also offers a clarity and logic to their emotional responses at a time when they may be struggling with hopelessness and a loss of control, and it communicates understanding. From a relatively brief intervention, there is the potential therapeutic impact of feeling understood.

Psychodynamic therapists make links between early childhood experiences and the patient's current character structure and symptoms. The patient's emotional response to the therapist (transference) and the therapist's emotional response to the patient (countertransference) are also sources of learning. Psychodynamic psychotherapy may be conducted over short- or long-term periods. There are some criteria for its use for example, the client must not be currently heavily dependent on drugs or alcohol, and should be able to work with the 'transference' approach.

Gestalt therapy

The German word 'gestalt' means 'form, figure or shape'. Gestalt therapy arose in the early 1950s from the interactions of Fritz Perls, a psychoanalyst, Laura Perls, a Gestalt psychologist and dance therapist and their collaborators in New York and California, USA (Oldham et al 1988). Both these people were interested in how we create meaningful wholes out of the quantity of disparate sense data we receive from our world. The central concept of Gestalt therapy is that awareness, by and of itself, initiates therapeutic change. Most of us at some points in our lives, have learned to avoid awareness of certain parts of ourselves and of our experience, often in an effort to avoid frightening or unpleasant feelings. Gestalt therapy uses an experimental approach to creating awareness in the lived moment; it proposes that something must be experienced rather than talked about. The client, therefore must be willing to take an active role in sessions with a Gestalt therapist.

Client-centered counselling

Carl Rogers' impact on counselling has been enormous, through his copious writings, the school of counselling and psychotherapy that he founded, and through the indirect influence of his work on many areas of professional activity where the quality of human relationships is essential (Thorne 1993). Having considered the different types of therapy that he had worked with, Rogers concluded that to some extent, they converged in the attitude of the therapist. He went on to identify four basic attributes of the therapist:

1. Objectivity, in which he included a 'capacity for sympathy which will not be overdone, a genuinely receptive and interested attitude, a deep understanding which will find it impossible to pass moral judgements or be shocked and horrified' (unconditional positive regard, empathy)
2. A respect for the individual (unconditional, positive regard, congruence)
3. Understanding of the self, to which he allied the therapist's ability to be self-accepting as well as self-aware (congruence)
4. Psychological knowledge, by which he meant a 'thorough basis of human behaviour and of its physical, social and psychological determinants' (Rogers 1951).

It is significant that for Rogers the first three of these attributes far outweighed the fourth in importance. The concepts of empathy, unconditional positive regard and congruence are Rogers' most important and radical contributions to the understanding of helping relationships. Rogers had many critics in scientific circles, but in countless self-help groups, in counselling skills courses in colleges, churches and evening institutes, in human relations programmes within educational and institutional settings, it will often be the work of Rogers that underpins the enterprise.

In practice, many psychologists and counsellors working with women with breast problems and breast cancer may use an eclectic approach, that is using a variety of models and techniques, depending on what suits the individual patient at the time.

Support groups

Support groups are facilitated by trained health care professionals. The role of the facilitator is to promote open discussion among patients about emotional, practical and physical problems they have encountered and on how to cope with the illness. A diagnosis of cancer can create a sense of alienation for both patient and family members. Participation in support groups has been associated with improved methods of coping and adjustment (Spiegel et al 1989, Watson et al 1996).

Support groups can be structured, whereby a particular therapeutic model is used, for example, psycho-educational groups that extend over a 6–8-week period and focus on coping methods, relaxation, stress reduction, and health education (Watson et al 1996). They may also be unstructured, whereby the participants set the agenda and they may run over a non-specified length of time.

Self-help groups are generally established by former patients who found that their psycho-social needs were not being met within the conventional care setting, for example the Lymphoedema Support Network. They are self-governing and self-regulating and the emphasis is often on participation in the group as opposed to how the individual would benefit from the intervention. Health care professionals may be involved by offering support, advice and delivering talks to members.

Complementary therapies

Complementary and alternative therapies are those that generally lie outside the realm of conventional mainstream care. Studies estimate that between 7–72% of cancer patients use complementary or alternative cancer therapies (Ernst & Cassileth 1998). Cassileth (1999) defines complementary therapies as those that are applied in conjunction with conventional medicine. They aim to improve symptom control and quality of life. Alternative therapies are defined as products and regimes promoted for use instead of mainstream cancer care. Such therapies are unproven and are often invasive and costly.

Therapies such as aromatherapy and massage, relaxation therapy, acupuncture and some homoeopathic regimes have been associated with a number of positive outcomes including reducing stress, anxiety, improving symptom control and improving quality of life (Cassileth 1999). For this reason it is optimal if some of these therapies can be offered within the hospital setting. Otherwise patients need to pay for these treatments, in which case care should be taken to ensure the practitioner has proper training and is certified with a regulating body. Should patients enquire about the use of treatments such as massage, they may certainly be informed about the psychological benefits.

PROFESSIONAL ISSUES

Benefits and risks of involvement

Talking to patients about their feelings can be valuable in all stages of breast care: in screening and prevention programmes, at diagnosis and treatment and also when no further active treatment is possible (Moorey et al 1998). Emotional care is within the remit of every nurse and should be promoted and undertaken.

Becoming 'involved' with patients' emotional distress can be very satisfying and rewarding, in terms of it becoming apparent that the patient is deriving support and benefit from the process. This may be ascertained from patient feedback, psychological evaluation, using scales, e.g. the HAD scale or by the patient becoming visibly more relaxed and possibly happier as a result. Compliance with treatment may be enhanced by this therapeutic process (Burton & Watson 1998).

There are however some pitfalls. Egan (1994, p. 11) states, 'helping is a powerful process that is all too easy to mismanage' and 'helping is not neutral; it is for better or worse'. Egan (1994) means that an unskilled, inexperienced nurse or counsellor may, in fact, do more harm than good. An inexperienced nurse or counsellor may actually lead the client down an avenue that may not be of benefit to them. Statements from the client may have been misinterpreted or expressions misread or translated into issues that may not actually exist. For example, a patient who is apprehensive about the process of 'being there' with someone who is going to listen to their emotional problems, may appear sullen and withdrawn. The nurse senses the patient's discomfort, but thinks that she is angry rather than scared. She says 'Jenny, I'm wondering what's making you so angry right now.' Since Jenny does not feel angry, she says nothing. She is startled by this and feels even more insecure. The nurse takes Jenny's silence as a confirmation of her anger. She tries to get her to talk about it. The nurse's perception is wrong and disrupts the process of the therapeutic relationship.

It may be possible for the nurse engaging in emotional care to become very upset by distress/anger/hostility expressed by the client. This is natural to some extent and is why supervision is needed. Furthermore, the patient may divulge something in confidence that is actually very difficult for the nurse to morally or ethically hold on to. The inexperienced nurse may find this situation very disturbing (Bond & Shea 1998).

Counselling usually needs a focus for goal setting. An inexperienced or unskilled nurse may lack the confidence to challenge and help the patient to set goals. In nursing there is consistent tension between caring and empowerment, that is, a tendency to listen well and comfort, but a reluctance to induce further emotional or psychological upset by challenging the behaviour and thoughts of the patient (Malin & Teasdale 1991, Fealy 1995).

In conclusion, talking to patients about their feelings and emotions is a human activity that attests to the willingness of one person to help another in their psychological life journey. The work is not easy. In entering into a relationship, the nurse opens him or herself to an empathic experience of the hopes, fears and doubts of the patient, the setbacks and the strivings, the joys and the sadness. The nurse puts at the service of the client this empathic understanding, a professional attitude, varying degrees of training and practical experience, and the insights of their own experience of living. However, it is possible for a nurse to offer a therapeutic relationship, without formal counselling, its effectiveness being enhanced through a sense of shared humanity with patients (Taylor 1992).

Setting limits

The nurses offering emotional care should work within their own limits; it is an indication of competence when it is recognised that referral to a more skilled and qualified person is the appropriate route (Motyka et al 1997). They should actively monitor the limitations of their own competence through counselling supervision/consultative support, and by seeking the views of their patients and peers.

Nurses have a responsibility to themselves and their patients to maintain their effectiveness, resilience and ability to help patients and clients. They are expected to monitor their own personal functioning and to seek help or withdraw from emotional care, whether temporary or permanently, when their personal resources are sufficiently depleted to require this (BAC 1998).

Confidentiality

The management of confidentiality is one of the most recurrent sources of ethical difficulty for nurses. In nursing, a code of practice exists that adds to this the code of professional conduct (UKCC 1992). Confidentiality is a high priority because it is both essential to respect patient autonomy and because assurances of confidentiality maximise personal frankness, which is so essential to emotional disclosure. However, nurses are sometimes faced with making difficult choices between confidentiality and other ethical or legal imperatives. The safest way to resolve these dilemmas is to involve the patient in the decision-making process and to obtain his/her consent to any disclosures. This can be difficult if the patient is too distressed to make autonomous decisions, or simply refuses consent. For example a patient, Sara, is being physically abused by her husband; her recent breast surgery wound is not healing well as a result and she is constantly in clinic due to breakdown of the wound. This is affecting her progression to starting chemotherapy. Although she has confided in the nurse about this, she has refused to tell any other authorities.

The challenges for individuals working within medical organisations are more complex because of the potential for conflicting obligations to the patient and to the organisation. For example, there may be an expectation from a referrer to receive a progress report on the patient or for the cancer counsellor to collaborate in multidisciplinary meetings on the patient's psychological state (Burton & Watson 1998).

If records, written and computerised, of discussion of any intimate details or issues, are kept, the patient should be made aware of this (BAC 1998).

Information should be given about access to these records, their availability to other people, and the degree of security with which they are kept.

For the purposes of supervision, patients' identities should be protected or kept anonymous.

Supervision

Clinical supervision in nursing draws some parallels with counselling supervision (Cowe 1998). Its development is advocated by the UKCC document 'Position Statement on Clinical Supervision' (UKCC 1996). Cowe (1998) suggests that there are three key objectives for supervision:

1. An educational function, achieved through sharing knowledge relevant to practice and through the enhancement of self-awareness
2. A normative or quality control function, accomplished through the detailed discussion of practice with knowledgeable colleagues, who are able to identify examples of poor practice and make suggestions for changes and improvements where appropriate
3. A restorative or supportive function, attained through a process of peer support and the sharing of anxieties with colleagues. Thinking through anxieties may also allow problem-solving skills to develop so that these stresses can be avoided in future.

Supervision may be on a group or one-to-one basis and ensure that the values or principles that govern the approach, confidentiality, effectiveness and developing contracts for working together are adhered to. Supervisors must be competent and ensure that their supervisees are aware of the distinction between emotional care, accountability to management, supervision and education and training.

Training and education

Professions are characterised by a specific body of knowledge and range of skills that are exclusive to them. At present, there are no legal qualifications necessary to practise counselling and this can lead to considerable confusion when students first begin to examine their options, as there are numerous training courses and many examining bodies validating courses. Courses vary from a brief 1 day introduction, to a one-term evening course, to 1 year or 2/3-year part-time course. Some training institutions award internal certificates that are often simply certificates of attendance, and other validations are of variable standard. It is wise to investigate the value of the award with the course organiser (Chaytor 1997).

Courses listed as 'counselling skills' are not usually designed to train the student as a counsellor. They will enhance basic skills that may be valuable in a 'caring' profession or setting. A counselling or counselling skills course requires commitment and offers personal, social and emotional learning as well as more academic study. It is important to note that training of counsellors and training people from a wide range of occupations to use counselling skills in their work are two distinct activities. A BAC code of practice and ethics for trainers in counselling and counselling skills exists, which makes reference to issues such as staff:student ratio, trainer competence, confidentiality and management of training work.

Currently, there is no statutory regulation for counsellors. BAC, together with a number of major counselling organisations has established the UK Register of Counsellors, which is voluntary, but means that a registered practising counsellor will be an accreditated member of BAC. BAC accreditation is very frequently a requirement of employers. Courses occasionally include in their publicity material a reference to BAC accreditation, which implies some formal link with BAC and/or automatic acceptance of the course towards the training criterion of the individual accreditation scheme. BAC can only vouch for BAC-recognised courses and they publish a directory of such courses on a yearly basis to guide the potential student (Chaytor, 1997).

Some courses are aimed at helping people develop counselling or helping skills in specialist areas such as bereavement, cancer, marital problems etc. Before undertaking one of these it is important to ascertain if it is designed for those who are already familiar with basic counselling skills – a 'top-up' course – or whether it is designed as an introduction to offering counselling help in that field.

Training is only one aspect of accreditation as a counsellor. This also requires evidence of a defined length of supervised counselling practice. The length of practice varies in proportion to the training received.

CONCLUSION

The psycho-social problems associated with a breast cancer diagnosis have a dramatic effect on patients' quality of life. They can be experienced at all stages of the illness – at time of diagnosis, during treatment, after discharge, during follow-up and on recurrence. A diagnosis of breast cancer can also have serious psycho-social consequences for the patient's family. Patients and their families must be educated in the importance of informing health care professionals about any emotional and social problems they encounter. The stigma associated with psycho-social problems may prevent patients from informing health care professionals about problems experienced. Psycho-social problems should be referred to as 'distress' rather than with terms such as 'psychological' or 'psycho-social'. Support services must be recognised as an important part of the care of patients with breast-cancer-related problems and their families and incorporated into routine care. Information is a vital form of support and is essential for patients' adaptation to the disease.

As treatment of breast cancer is multidisciplinary, support systems must also be multidisciplinary in nature. All heath care professionals involved in the care of patients have an opportunity to provide support. Health professionals should receive training on how to recognise patients experiencing high levels of distress and the possibilities for referral.

Nurses are increasingly being challenged to be open to the distress of patients and to take on the 'emotional labour' of being with patients. In this chapter, an overview of emotional problems in breast care and guidelines on their management have been presented. It is important for nurses to reflect on the psychological and emotional care they deliver to patients in their care, to find out what psycho-social resources are available in the hospital and community and perhaps to spend time with professionals such as the breast care nurse specialist to identify her role better.

It should also be remembered that while some patients will gladly accept permission to acknowledge their emotional distress, others will be hostile and defensive and may refuse to explore this aspect further. This, of course, should be respected.

REFERENCES

Alderson P, Madden M, Oakley A et al 1996 Women's Views of Breast Cancer Treatment and Research. Report of a Pilot Project. KKS Printing, London

BAC 1998 The British Association for Counselling Code of Ethics and Practice for Counsellors (Appendix 1, p 534–544). In: Palmer S, McMahon C (eds) Handbook of Counselling, 2nd edn. British Association of Counselling, London

Bard M, Sutherland A M 1995 Psychological impact of cancer and its treatment IV: adaptation to radical mastectomy. Cancer (8): 652–672

Barraclough J 1994 Cancer and Emotion: A Practical Guide to Psycho-Oncology, 2nd edn, Sobell Publications, Oxford

Beck A T 1976 Cognitive Therapy and the Emotional Disorders. International Universities Press, New York

Beck A T, Mendleson M, Mock J et al 1961 Inventory for measuring depression. Archives of General Psychiatry 4: 561–571

Bleiker M A, Van der Ploeg H M 1999 Psycho-social factors in the etiology of breast cancer: review of a popular link. Patient Education and Counselling 37: 201–214

Bond T, Shea C 1998 Professional issues in counselling. In: Palmer S, McMahon G (eds) Handbook of Counselling, 2nd edn. Routledge, London

Bottomley A 1998 Depression in cancer patients: a literature review. European Journal of Cancer Care 7: 181–191

Bottomley A, Jones L 1997 Breast cancer care: women's experience. European Journal of Cancer Care 6: 124–132

Bredart A, Autier P, Audisio R A, Geraghty J 1998 Psycho-social aspects of breast cancer susceptibility testing: a literature review. European Journal of Cancer Care 7: 174–180

Breitbart W 1995 Identifying patients at risk for and treatment of major psychiatric complications of cancer. Supportive Care in Cancer 3(1): 45–60

Budin W C 1998 Psychosocial adjustment of breast cancer in the unmarried woman. Research in Nursing and Health 21: 155–166

Burton M, Watson M 1998 Counselling People with Cancer. John Wiley and Sons, West Sussex

Calman K, Hine D 1995 A Policy Framework for Commissioning Cancer Services Guidance for Purchasers and Providers of Cancer Services. Department of Health, London

Carroll S 1998 Role of the breast clinical nurse specialist in facilitating decision-making for treatment choice: a practice profile. European Journal of Oncology Nursing 2(1): 34–42

Carroll S 1998 Breast cancer, Part 3: psychosocial care. Professional Nurse 13(12): 876–883

Carroll S 1999 Letter to Lancet re psychological response and survival in breast cancer: Lancet 355: 406

Cassee E 1975 Therapeutic behaviour, hospital culture and communication. In: Cox C, Mead A (eds) Sociology of Medical Practice. Collier-Macmillan, London

Cassileth B R 1999 Complementary therapies: overview and state of the art. Cancer Nursing 22(1): 85–90

Chaytor D 1997 Training in Counselling and Psychotherapy, 13th edn. BAC, Warwickshire

Cowe F 1998 Clinical supervision for specialist nurses. Professional Nurse 13(5): 284–286

Dean A, Chelty N, Forrest A P M 1983 Effects of immediate breast reconstruction on psychological morbidity after mastectomy. Lancet i: 459–462

Doris A, Ebmeier K, Shajahan P 1999 Depressive illness. Lancet 354: 1369–1375

Edwards M J 1999 Providing psychological support to cancer patients. Professional Nurse 15(1): 9–13

Egan G 1994 The Skilled Helper – a Problem-management Approach to Helping, 5th edn. Brooks/Cole Publishing Company, CA, USA

Ernst E, Cassileth B R 1998 The prevalence of complementary/alternative medicine in cancer? British Journal of Cancer 83(4): 777–782

Fallowfield L, Clark A 1992 Breast Cancer. Routledge, London

Farmer A, Payne S, Royle G 1995 A comparative study of psychological morbidity in women with screen detected and symptomatic breast cancer. In: Richardson A, Wilson-Barnett J (eds) Nursing Research in Cancer Care. Scutari Press, London

Fealy G M 1995 Professional caring: the moral dimension. Journal of Advanced Nursing 22: 1135–1140

Ferrans C E 1994 Quality of life through the eyes of survivors of breast cancer. Oncology Nursing Forum 21(10): 1645–1651

Galea M 1993 Medical management of benign breast disorders. Prescriber 5: 1–4

Gilboa D, Borenstein A, Floro S et al 1990 Emotional and psychological adjustment of women to breast reconstruction and detection of subgroups at risk for psychological morbidity. Annals of Plastic Surgery 25: 397–401

Given C, Stommel M, Given B et al 1993 The influence of cancer patients' symptoms and functional states on patients' depression and family caregiver's reaction and depression. Health Psychology 12(4): 277–285

Greer S 1989 Can psychological therapy improve the quality of life of patients with cancer? British Journal of Cancer 59: 149–151

Greer S 1992 The management of denial in cancer patients. Oncology 6: 39–40

Greer S, Moorey S, Baruch J D R et al 1992 Adjuvant psychological therapy for patients with cancer: a prospective randomised trial. British Medical Journal 304: 675–680

Hall A, Fallowfield L J, A'Mern R P 1996 When Breast Cancer recurs: A 3 year prospective study of psychological morbidity. The Breast 2(3): 197–203

Harber S 1997 Breast Cancer: A Psychological Treatment Manual. Free Association Books Ltd, London

Harrison J, Haddad P, Maguire P 1995 The impact of cancer on key relatives: a comparison of relative and patient concerns. European Journal of Cancer 31A: 1736–1740

Hirst S 1984 The significance of breast pain. Nursing Times Jan 25th: 34–35

Hopwood P, Howell A, Maguire P 1993 Eliciting the current problems of the patient with cancer – a flow diagram. British Journal of Cancer 64: 353–356

Hughes L E, Mansel R E, Webster D J T 1989 Benign Disorders and Disease of the Breast: Concepts and Clinical Management. Baillière Tindall, London

Jenkins P L, May V E, Hughes L E 1991 Psychological morbidity associated with local recurrence of breast cancer. International Journal of Psychiatry Medicine 21(2): 149–155

Kash K M, Holland J C, Halper M S, Miller D G 1992 Psychological distress and surveillance behaviours of women with a family history of breast cancer. Journal of the National Cancer Institute 84: 24–30

King's Fund Forum 1986 Consensus Development Conference: treatment of primary breast cancer. British Medical Journal 293: 946–947

Koopman C, Hermanson K, Diamond S, Angell K, Spiegel D 1998 Social support, life stresses, pain and emotional adjustment to advanced breast cancer. Psycho-Oncology 7: 101–111

Lavery J F, Clarke V A 1996 Causal attributions coping strategies, and adjustment to breast cancer. Cancer Nursing 19(1): 20–28

Lerman C, Daly M, Sands C et al 1993 Mammography adherence and psychological distress among women at risk for breast cancer. Journal of the National Cancer Institute 85: 1074–1080

Lovejoy N C, Matteis M 1996 Pharmacokinetics and pharmacodynamics of mood-altering drugs in patients with cancer. Cancer Nursing 19: 407–418

Maguire P, Faulkner A, Regnard C 1993 Eliciting the current problems of the patient with cancer – a flow diagram. Palliative Medicine 7: 151–156

Malin N, Teasdale K 1991 Caring versus empowerment: considerations for nursing practice. Journal of Advanced Nursing 16: 657–662

Marchioro G, Azzarello G, Checchin F et al 1996 The impact of a psychological intervention on quality of life in non-metastatic breast cancer. European Journal of Cancer 32a (9): 1612–1615

Massie M, Holland J 1990 Delirium and the cancer patient. Journal of Clinical Psychiatry 51: 12–17

McArdle J M C, George W D, McArdle C S et al 1996 Psychological support for patients undergoing breast cancer surgery: a randomised study. British Medical Journal 312: 812–816

Meichenbaum D 1977 Cognitive Behaviour Modification: An Integrative Approach. Plenum Press, New York

Miers M 1991 Benign breast disease and disorders. Nursing Standard 5(45): 30–33

Montazeri A, Gillis C R, McEwen J 1997 Tak tent. Studies conducted in a cancer support group. Support Cancer Care 5: 118–125

Moorey S, Greer S, Watson M et al 1994 Adjuvant psychological therapy for patients with cancer: one year follow-up of a randomised controlled trial. Psycho-Oncology 3: 39–46

Moorey S, Greer S, Bliss J, Law M 1998 Comparison of adjuvant psychological therapy and supportive counselling in patients with cancer. Psycho-Oncology 7: 218–228

Motyka M, Motyka H, Wsojek R 1997 Elements of psychological support in nursing care. Journal of Advanced Nursing 26: 909–912

National Cancer Alliance 1996 Patient-Centred Cancer Services? What Patients Say. NCA, Oxford

NHS Executive 1996 Guidance for Purchasers: Improving Outcomes in Breast Cancer. The Research Evidence. Health Literature Line, London

Northouse L, Templin T, Mood D, Oberst M 1998 Couples adjustment to breast cancer and benign breast disease: a longitudinal analysis. Psycho-Oncology 7: 37–48

Northouse L, Jeffs M, Cracchiolo-Caraway A, Lampman L, Dorris G 1995 Emotional distress reported by women and husbands prior to a breast biopsy. Nursing Research 44(4): 196–201

Oldham J, Key T, Starak I Y 1988 Risking Being Alive. Pit Publishing, Australia

O'Toole S 1999 The role of nursing in the psychological support of patients. Oncology Nurses Today 4(4): 10–12

Payne S, Endall M 1998 Detection of anxiety and depression by surgeons and significant others in females attending a breast clinic. European Journal of Oncology Nursing 2(1): 4–11

Pearce B 1998 Counselling skills in the context of professional and organisational growth. In: Palmer S, McMahon G (eds) Handbook of Counselling, 2nd edn. British Association of Counselling, London

Pinder K L, Ramirez A J, Richards M A, Gregory W M 1994 Cognitive responses and psychiatric disorder in women with operable breast cancer. Psycho-Oncology 3: 129–137

Poole K 1997 The emergence of the waiting game – a critical examination of the psychosocial issues in diagnosing breast cancer. Journal of Advanced Nursing 25: 273–281

Rabinowitz B F 1997 Two decades of psychosocial research: an overview for the practitioner In: Bonadonna G, Hortobagyi G, Gianni A M (eds) Textbook of Breast Diseases. Martin Dunitz, London

Ramirez A J, Richards A, Jarrett S R, Fentiman I S 1995 Can mood disorder in women with breast cancer be identified preoperatively? British Journal of Cancer 72: 1509–1572

Renneker R, Cutler M 1952 Psychological problems of adjustment to cancer of the breast. JAMA 148: 833–838

Robinson L 1994 The experience of cancer recurrence: a phenomenological study. MSC Thesis. King's College, London

Rogers C R 1951 Client Centered Therapy. Houghton Mifflin, Boston

Scott D 1983 Anxiety, critical thinking and information processing during and after breast biopsy. Nursing Research 32(1): 24–28

Shaw C, Wilson S, O'Brien M 1994 Information needs prior to breast biopsy. Clinical Nursing Research 3(2): 119–131

Sheppard C, Markby R 1995 The partner's experience of breast cancer: a phenomenological approach. International Journal of Palliative Medicine 1(3): 134–140

Smyth M, McCaughan E, Harrisson S 1996 Women's perceptions of their experiences with breast cancer: are their needs being addressed? European Journal of Cancer Care 4: 86–92

Spiegel D, Bloom J R, Kraener H C, Gottheil E 1989 Effect of psychosocial treatment on survival of patients with metastatic breast cancer. Lancet 2: 888–91

Sutton C 1998 Counselling in the personal social services. In: Palmer S, McMahon G (eds) Handbook of Counselling, 2nd edn. Routledge, London

Taylor B 1992 From helper to human: a reconceptualisation of the nurse as a person. Journal of Advanced Nursing 17: 1042–1049

Thorne B 1993 Carl Rogers. Sage Publications, London

Topping A 1996 Sexuality and breast cancer. In: Denton S (ed) Breast Cancer Nursing. Chapman and Hall, London

Tunmore R 1990 Setting the pace. Nursing Times 86(34): 29–31

UKCC 1992 Code of Professional Conduct for the Nurse, Midwife and Health Visitor. UKCC, London

UKCC 1996 Position Statement on Clinical Supervision for Nursing and Health Visiting. UKCC, London

Viederman M, Perry S W 1980 Use of a psychodynamic life narrative in the treatment of depression in the physically ill. General Hospital Psychiatry 3: 177–185

Waterhouse J, Metcalfe M 1991 Attitudes to nurses discussing sexual concerns with patients. Journal of Advanced Nursing 16(9): 1048–1054

Watson M, Denton S, Baum M, Greer S 1988 Counselling breast cancer patients: a specialist nurse service. Counselling Psychology Quarterly 1(1): 23–31

Watson M 1990 Cancer locus of control scale. Psychological Reports 66: 39–48

Watson M 1991 Cancer patient care. Psychosocial treatment methods. British Psychological Society, Cambridge

Watson M, Fenlon D, McVey G 1996 A support group for breast cancer patients: development of a cognitive-behavioural approach. Behavioural & Cognitive Psychotherapy 24: 73–81

Watson M, Haviland J S, Greer S et al 1999 Influence of psychological response on survival in breast cancer: a population-based cohort study. Lancet 354: 1331–1336

Weisman A D, Worden J W 1986 The emotional impact of recurrent cancer. Journal of Psychosocial Oncology 3(4): 5–16

Wilkinson S 1991 Factors which influence how nurses communicate with cancer patients. Journal of Advanced Nursing 16: 677–688

Wilkinson S 1992 Confusions and challenges. Nursing Times 88(35): 24–27

Wilkinson S, Roberts A, Aldridge J 1998 Nurse-patient communication in palliative care: an evaluation of a communication skills programme. Palliative Medicine 12: 13–22

Woolfe R 1998 Counselling in Britain: present position and future prospects. In: Palmer S, McMahon G (eds) Handbook of Counselling 2nd edn. Routledge, London

Zahlis E H, Shands M E 1993 The impact of breast cancer on the partner 18 months after diagnosis. Seminars in Oncology Nursing 9(2): 83–87

Zigmond A S, Snaith R P 1983 The hospital and anxiety depression scale. Acta Psychiatrica Scandinavica 67: 361–370

FURTHER READING

Burton M, Watson M 1998 Counselling People with Cancer. Wiley, London

This book is written by two of the world's outstanding psycho-social oncologists, and they bring a wealth of clinical and research experience to this important topic. Dr Watson particularly, whom I have been lucky to work with, has many years of experience in counselling women with breast cancer. The book gives an overview of emotional problems encountered in patients with cancer and a practical guide on how to deal with them.

Denton S 1996 Breast Cancer Nursing. Chapman and Hall, London

This was the first book to be published on breast cancer nursing, Sylvia Denton being one of the pioneering breast care nurses in England. It includes excellent contributors from a multidisciplinary team who provide an excellent overview of treatments for breast cancer and their effects on the patient. There is also a good chapter on psychological care by Ann Tait.

Fallowfield L, Clark A 1992 Breast Cancer. Routledge, London

This book, although written in 1992 is still a great book in the year 2000, offering valuable insight into the world of the patient diagnosed with breast cancer and an excellent review of research studies with comments from the authors. Dr Fallowfield has written many papers, including research write-ups about patients with breast cancer and their families and her experience in this area is invaluable.

Further useful addresses (see also Part 1 of this chapter)

British Association of Counselling
1 Regent Place
Rugby
Warwickshire CV21 2PJ

United Kingdom Council Psychotherapy
167–169 Great Portland Street
London W1N 5FB

8 Recurrent Breast Cancer

Jan Smith

After reading this chapter you should:

- Have a broad overview of recurrent breast cancer and its management
- Understand the likely sites and complications of metastatic breast cancer
- Understand the principles of palliative care and the place of palliative care in the care of the woman with metastatic breast cancer
- Recognise the need for an holistic approach to pain and symptom management
- Understand the psycho-social impact of disease on patients and their families.

INTRODUCTION

Of women with operable breast cancer, over half will develop recurrence. This may be local, loco-regional or systemic. Local recurrence may involve the remaining breast tissue after breast conserving surgery, or the chest wall, following mastectomy. Loco-regional recurrence would include the axillary and/or subclavicular and/or supraclavicular lymph nodes. Local recurrence is usually palpable and diagnosis is confirmed by fine needle aspiration or biopsy. Limited recurrence in the scar or breast tissue may be treated by surgery alone. For recurrence in several areas of the breast or where there is lymph node involvement, local radiotherapy may be possible if the maximum dose has not been given, or more radical surgical excision may be necessary. If surgical excision is not possible, hormone therapy or chemotherapy may be given. Recurrence in the contralateral breast may occur and is treated in the same way as the original breast tumour. Local recurrence can be curable but is thought to be indicative of systemic relapse in up to half of patients who present.

Systemic recurrence occurs when cancer cells enter the lymphatic system or the bloodstream and are disseminated to other parts of the body. In breast cancer common sites of spread include the skeletal system, brain, lung and liver. Survival after the development of systemic disease is estimated at 18–24 months but this may be longer in women with hormone-sensitive tumours or shorter in women who develop systemic disease shortly after their initial treatment.

PALLIATIVE CARE IN ADVANCED BREAST CANCER

Once breast cancer has recurred systemically further treatment is essentially palliative (Denton 1996). Quality of life becomes the therapeutic imperative and the possible benefits of prolonging survival must be weighed against the risks and side-effects of further treatment.

Palliative care is 'the active, total care of patients and their families by a multi-professional team when the patient's disease is no longer receptive to curative treatment.' (WHO 1990). The key principles are:

1. Focus on quality of life, which includes good symptom control
2. A whole-person approach taking into account the person's life experience and current situation
3. Care that encompasses both the dying person and those who matter to that person
4. Respect for patient autonomy and choice
5. Emphasis on open and sensitive communication, which extends to patients, informal carers and professional colleagues. (National Council for Hospice and Specialist Palliative Care Services (NCHSPCS) 1995)

The traditional model of illness has been a two-stage model focussing initially on 'cure', during which palliation is not considered appropriate, and then on palliation and 'terminal care' at some unspecified point identified by the health care professionals involved, e.g. 'when the person's prognosis suggests that he/she has between 3 and 6 months to live' (Jeffrey 1995, Lowden 1998, Clark & Seymour 1999). This model is problematic however. Fallowfield (1990) identified the major impact that psychological distress has on quality of life in cancer patients and suggests that the palliative care approach might be appropriate earlier in the illness. Also, the transitions between curative, palliative and terminal stages are not always clear, which may result in inappropriate treatment and late referral to palliative care services. Finally, to equate palliation with 'terminal' denies hope and perpetuates the myth that 'there is nothing more we can do' (see Fig. 8.1).

As Figure 8.1 illustrates, when managing potentially life-limiting illness, it is possible to offer potentially curative treatment simultaneously with a palliative care approach. This could allow a more seamless delivery of care and with its emphasis on open communication, it could facilitate a real partnership with patients and their carers (Jeffrey 1995).

The palliative care approach, i.e. good practice informed by the knowledge and practice of palliative care principles can and should be offered by all health care professionals. It includes, but is not restricted to, terminal care (Biswas 1993) since a patient may be receiving treatment aimed at controlling but not curing their illness for months or even years before entering the terminal phase of their illness (Ahmedzai 1996).

Specialist palliative care is needed by a minority of patients with complex needs or problems and may be offered indirectly to the patient's professional carers or directly to the patient and their family.

COMMON SYMPTOMS AND THEIR MANAGEMENT

Symptoms in advanced breast cancer may be due directly to metastatic disease, indirectly due to the systemic effects of disease, the result of treatment, a side-effect of drugs, related to general weakness and debility or due to other concurrent disease (Brooks and Ahmedzai 1996). The concept of total symptom

FIGURE 8.1

'Sheffield' theoretical model for palliative care

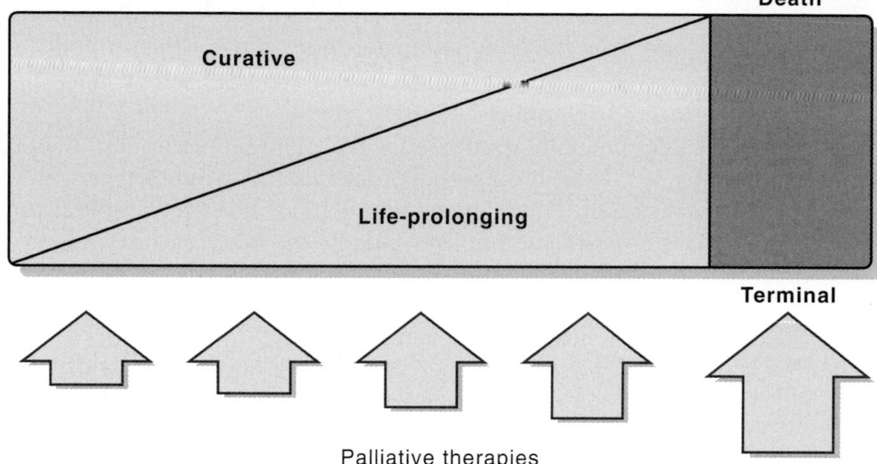

Sheffield theoretical model for palliative care. Reproduced with kind permission from Ahmedzai S 1996 Clark D, Seymour J (eds) 1999 Reflections on palliative care. Open University Press.

management should be applied since symptoms also comprise a totality of experience and it is the lived experience that needs to be understood in order to provide appropriate and effective individualised care (Campbell & Hately 2000). Thorough assessment and identification of the cause(s) is a prerequisite followed by explanation and involvement of the patient and family in management and in setting achievable and acceptable goals.

Pain

Central to the development of palliative care within the 20th century has been the concept of 'total pain' described by Saunders as:

> '... a complex of physical, emotional, social and spiritual elements. The whole experience for a patient includes anxiety, depression and fear, and concern for the family who will become bereaved, and often a need to find some meaning in the situation, some deeper reality in which to trust.' (Saunders 1996 p. 50)

To address total pain requires an approach that integrates nursing, pharmacological and medical assessment and intervention with awareness of the impact of social, psychological and spiritual factors on the illness experience. It attempts to implement a holistic model of care that acknowledges the patient as a person with an individual internal and external environment requiring an individualised assessment of their needs.

Pain management

Pain occurs in about 75% of patients with cancer. Successful pain management requires an understanding of the nature of pain, the likely causes and knowledge of appropriate intervention (Forbes & Faull 1998). An initial pain assessment is essential in order to provide a baseline against which the effectiveness of interventions may be evaluated.

Physiology of pain

The physiology of pain is complex and there is still much that is poorly understood. Pain may be classified as nociceptive or neuropathic (Twycross 1997).

Nociceptive pain

Nociceptors are specialised nerve endings present in skin, bone and muscle, connective tissue and internal organs that respond to chemical, thermal or mechanical stimuli. They synapse in the dorsal horn of the spinal cord with nerve fibres that cross to the opposite side of the body and ascend via the spino-thalamic tract to the thalamus and the sensory cortex within the brain, where pain becomes conscious. The transmission of pain depends on the balance of excitatory and inhibitory neurotransmission.

Nociceptive pathways contain two groups of fibres: all A fibres are myelinated, facilitating rapid transmission of stimuli. A-delta fibres are small diameter fibres responsible for pain perceived as fast and sharp. Large diameter A fibres respond to other stimuli such as touch or vibration (Hawthorn et al 1996). These also synapse in the dorsal horn and may have a role in inhibiting the transmission of painful stimuli to the thalamus and cortex or 'closing the gate' in terms of the gate control theory of pain perception. (Melzack & Wall 1965) (Fig. 8.2).

C fibres are thinner, non-myelinated fibres, slower conducting and responding to chemical, mechanical and thermal stimuli. They are responsible for dull, burning or aching pains. A simple example of theory in action is that of the stubbed toe. The immediate sharp pain is the result of rapid transmission of stimuli by large diameter myelinated A fibres; the severe throbbing pain occurring slightly later is the response to the slower conducting non-myelinated C fibres.

Connections between the thalamus, the cortex and the limbic system, which is involved with emotion, allow for the constant transmission of information. Information coming from the periphery can be modulated by the activity of the limbic system and also by neurotransmitters within the descending spino-thalamic tract, particularly serotonin and noradrenaline. This is the mechanism by which many adjuvant analgesics may work (Fig. 8.3).

Opioid receptors also occur throughout the brain and spinal cord and respond to the body's endogenous opiates. These have a similar pharmacological action to morphine and are reversed by naloxone, which explains the efficacy of opiate analgesia.

Neuropathic pain

Similar nociceptive pathways are activated in the experience of neuropathic pain but it occurs without external stimuli and results from damage to the peripheral or central nervous system. Damage may follow surgery (e.g. phantom limb pain) or in cancer patients, when peripheral or central nerve tissue is compressed or infiltrated by tumour, following radiotherapy, chemotherapy, or infection, particularly herpes zoster.

Neuropathic pain may present as superficial stinging/burning pain sometimes accompanied by stabbing/shooting pain (sometimes referred to as lancinating pain) with an underlying deep ache (Twycross 1997) and may also be associated with changes in sensation. It can be more difficult to treat than nociceptive pain, requiring adjuvant analgesia and persistence.

FIGURE 8.2

The nociceptive pathways. Reproduced from Melzack R, Wall P 1982 The challenge of pain. Penguin, London, with permission.

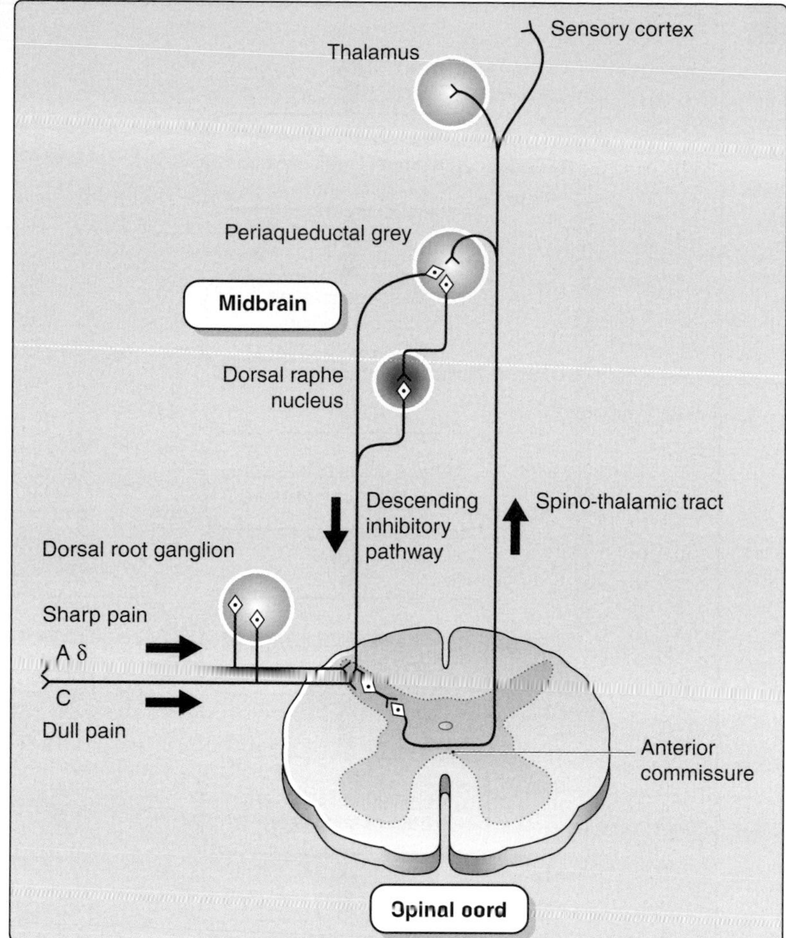

Pain perception

Pain is an isolating experience. In a subjective situation, it is not possible for other people to enter into the experience or understand it, except from descriptions given by the patient. Coping with pain absorbs energy and concentration, affecting relationships. When pain is perceived as 'intractable', friends and family may withdraw from the suffering of their loved one and professionals may shy away from constantly facing their failure, isolating the patient still further (Cleeland 1991). The perception of pain may be modified by many factors, hence the concept of 'total pain' (Saunders 1996).

Physical factors
Physical symptoms, particularly fatigue and/or sleep disturbance may lower the pain threshold and other symptoms, for example vomiting or persistent cough may aggravate pain.

Social factors
The distress caused to family members may be of acute concern to the patient, particularly if there are young children involved. Pre-existing family problems

FIGURE 8.3

Summary of events involved in the perception of pain. Reproduced from Melzack R, Wall P 1982 The challenge of pain. Penguin, London, with permission.

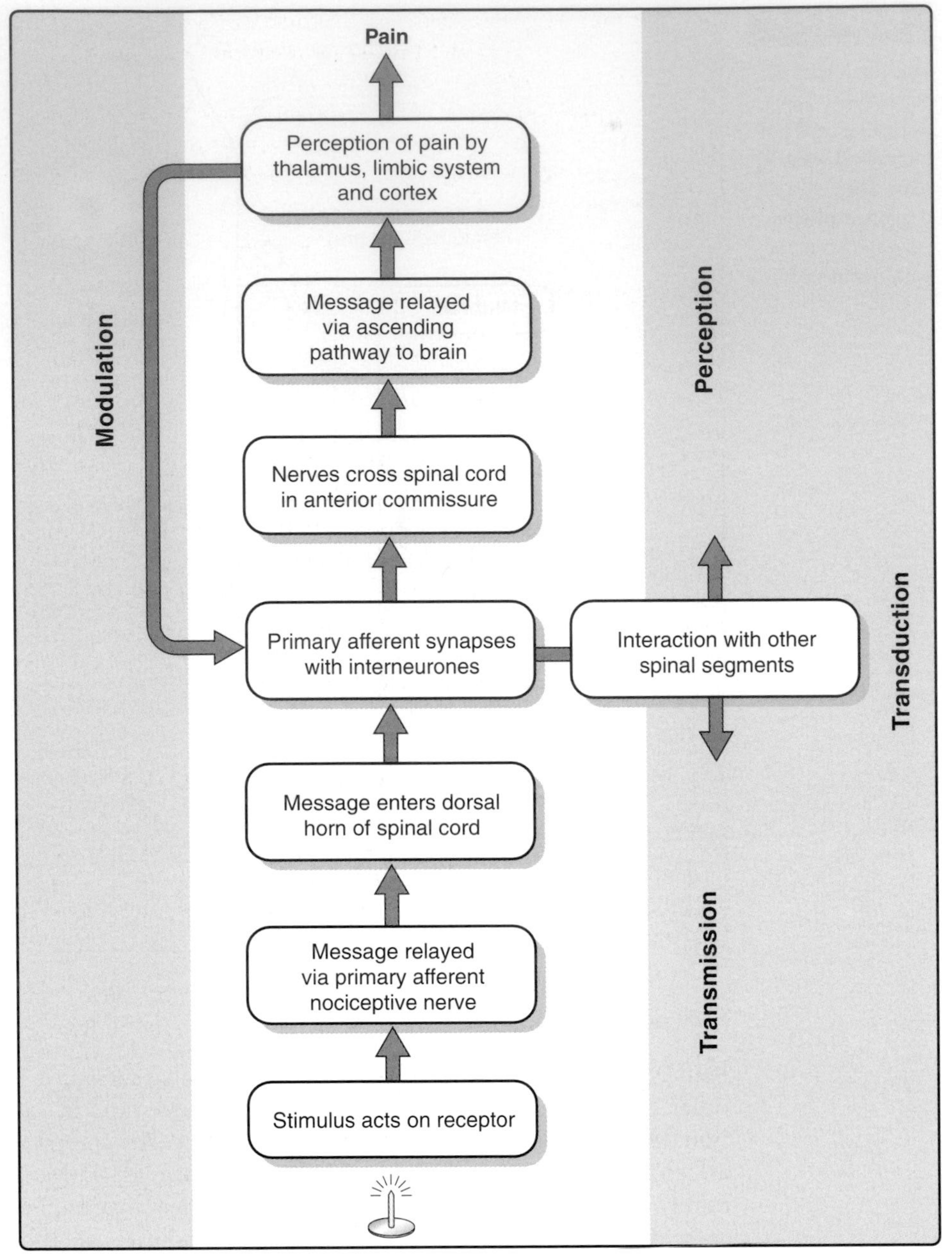

may be exacerbated by the patient's illness. There may be anxiety about how the remaining family members will cope practically when the patient becomes unable to continue their normal role and this may be a particular problem if there is little or no social support available from the extended family or friends. There may be financial concerns relating to loss of income, the need to make or change a Will, anxieties about life insurance and how family members will manage financially during the illness and following the death.

Cultural variations

These affect attitudes and beliefs about illness, death and dying and the extent to which these areas are discussed openly within the family. There are also variations in the ways in which pain and other symptoms are expressed both verbally and non-verbally (Bendelow 1993). Culturally insensitive care and language barriers that inhibit communication may exacerbate suffering. It is important for health care professionals to be aware of cultural variations and differences within cultures and to avoid cultural stereotyping.

Psychological factors

Psychological factors may be multiple. The patient is facing a series of losses:

- Health
- Normality
- Changes in domestic, occupational and social roles
- Changes due to treatment such as surgery or chemotherapy, resulting in altered body image and damage to their self concept
- Loss of the future and of the opportunity to see children grow up, get married and have children
- Loss of retirement years spent with a partner
- Loss of plans made for one's own future.

These losses will eventually culminate in the ultimate loss of life itself. The emotional responses to this may include:

- Anger
- Denial
- Anxiety
- Depression
- Anguish about the suffering caused to others
- Overwhelming fear of future suffering, dying and of death itself.

Spiritual factors

Spirituality has been described by Saunders as 'the whole area of thought concerning moral values throughout life' and within this context spiritual pain occurs when the individual desires ... 'to reach out to what is true and valuable ... and has feelings of being unable or unworthy to do' (1988, p. 30). Spirituality also encompasses the search for meaning to life, issues around unresolved guilt and regret, and the search for immortality, perhaps in the memories of others or in a continuation of individual existence. If health care professionals perceive spirituality as synonymous with religion then spiritual distress as a component of pain will not be recognised and the needs for spiritual care will not be addressed.

The meaning of pain in the experience of cancer patients may be related to their ability to control chronic pain (Arathuzik 1991). Twycross states that for cancer patients pain means 'I am incurable, I am going to die' (1997 p. 13) but this is perhaps an oversimplified view. Pain may also be seen as punishment, as a manifestation of weakness or a challenge to overcome (Copp 1974).

Assessing symptom distress

The profound biopsycho-social consequences of pain have been well documented (Arathuzik 1991). A thorough assessment of the person in pain will address the physical, psychological, social and spiritual components of pain and the concerns of the carers, and is essential if pain is to be managed effectively (Fordham & Dunn 1994, Woodruff 1997). The principles of holistic assessment are applicable and appropriate for any symptoms.

Assessment is an opportunity for the person to tell their story and this in itself may be therapeutic (Heiney 1995). It may be the first time that they have been heard and that the focus has been on their experience rather than on what the health care professional wants to know. It requires the nurse to:

- Give time and attention
- Be sensitive to non-verbal cues
- Hear both words and silences
- Affirm and validate what is being shared with her
- Understand and accurately interpret the information she receives
- Convey this information to other people.

It also requires her to act on the information she receives. An individual in pain is vulnerable; their normal coping mechanisms may be failing and they are dependent on health care professionals. The skills used in eliciting their story are open to abuse; we may encourage trust, facilitate disclosure of great distress and create vulnerability that becomes abusive if we do not then act to relieve their pain.

Pain assessment is completed by the negotiation of goals and interventions by which these goals may be achieved. Twycross suggests that goals should be progressive, aiming first that the patient should be pain-free at night, secondly when at rest during the day and finally on movement, adding the rider that this may be more difficult to achieve (Twycross 1997).

Rating scales

These enable the severity of the pain and the effectiveness of any intervention to be evaluated. There are many such scales in use and there is no one ideal version. They may be verbal, numerical or linear analogue scales and may be used in conjunction with a body outline (see Fig. 8.4, The Royal Marsden Pain Assessment Chart).

The advantages of rating scales are that:

(1) They are relatively easy to use
(2) They allow information to be shared with other members of staff
(3) They reveal patterns in the pain experience, which may provide useful information for management and
(4) They demonstrate the effect of intervention
(Fordham & Dunn 1994).

However, they are not suitable or appropriate for everyone; patients:

(1) May not understand or be capable of completing the scale
(2) May feel too ill or exhausted to do so
(3) Regard the scale as an unwelcome reminder of their pain, which interferes with their coping strategy.

Each pain must be charted separately, which may become confusing. Unless the chart is completed by the patient with minimal intervention by staff, it is possible that what is measured is the staff member's perception of the patient's pain rather than the patient's perception of their pain.

The Royal Marsden Hospital

Pain Assessment Chart

Surname: **Hospital no:**

First name: **Date:**

Initial Assessment

Patient's own description of the pain(s):

What helps relieve the pain?

What makes the pain worse?

Do you have pain

i) at night? Yes/No (comment if required)

ii) at rest? Yes/No (comment if required)

iii) on movement? Yes/No (comment if required)

Pain sites

Please draw on the body outlines below to show where you feel pain.
Label each site of pain with a letter A, B, C, etc.

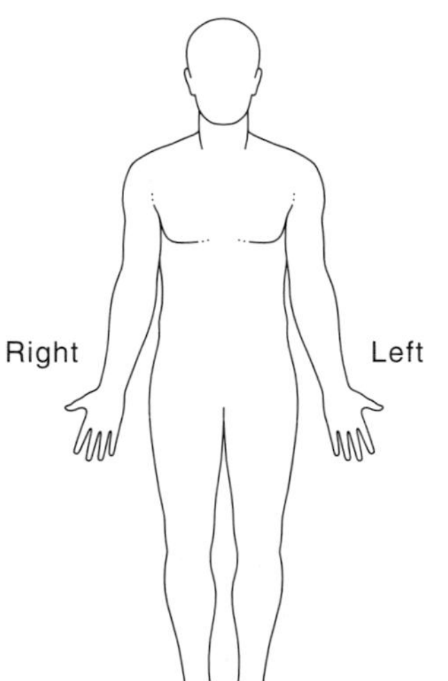

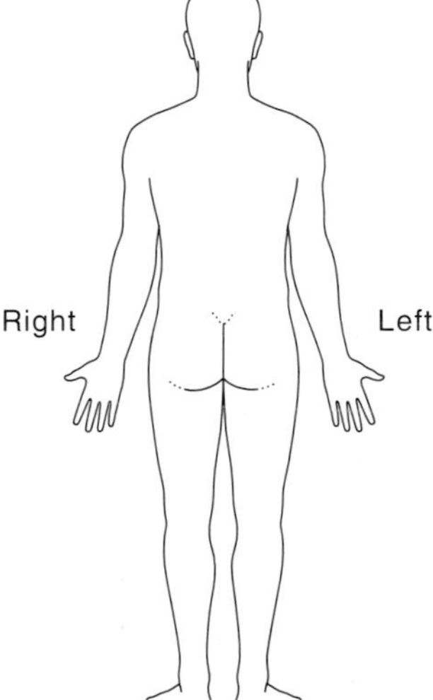

FIGURE 8.4 The Royal Marsden Pain Assessment Chart

Pain Assessment Chart

Key to pain intensity: **Continuation no:** ____________

0 = no pain
1 = mild pain
2 = moderate pain
3 = severe pain
4 = very severe pain
5 = intolerable/overwhelming pain

s = sleeping

It may be easier to determine the intensity of pain by looking at the pain scale below.

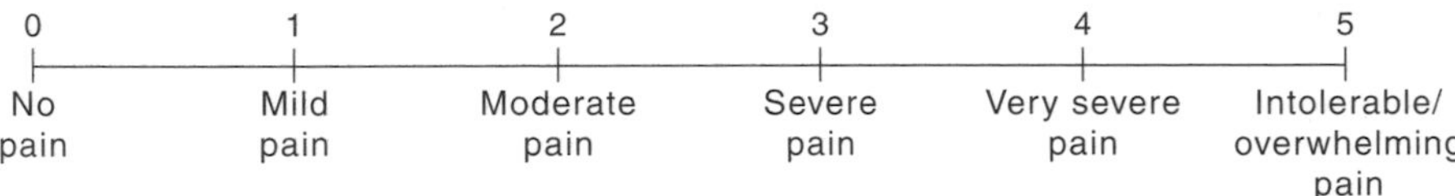

Date	Times	Pain sites								Analgesia name, route & dose	Patient activity and comments
		A	B	C	D	E	F	G	H		

FIGURE 8.4 Cont'd

Guidelines: Initial Assessment

Action	Rationale
1 Explain to the patient the purpose of using the chart.	To obtain the patient's consent and cooperation.
2 Where appropriate, encourage the patient to complete the pain chart himself/herself.	To encourage patient participation.
3 Where the nurse completes chart, record the patient's *own* description of his/her pain.	To reduce the risk of misrepresentation.
4 (a) Record any factors that influence the intensity of the pain, e.g. activities or interventions which reduce or increase the pain, such as distractions or a heat pad. (b) Record whether or not the patient is pain-free at night, at rest or on movement.	Ascertaining how and when the patient experiences pain enables the nurse to plan realistic goals. For example, relieving the patient's pain during the night and while he/she is at rest is usually easier to achieve than relief from pain on movement.

Guidelines: Pain sites

Action	Rationale
1 Encourage the patient, where appropriate, to identify pain sites himself/herself.	The body outline is ideally a vehicle for the patient to describe his/her own pain experience.
2 Index each site (A–H) in whatever way seems most appropriate, e.g. shading/colouring of areas or arrows to indicate shooting pains.	This enables individual pain sites to be located.

Guidelines: Monitoring pain intensity

Action	Rationale
1 Give each pain site a numerical value according to the key to pain intensity or to the pain scale and note time recorded.	To indicate the intensity of the pain at each site.
2 Record any analgesia given and note route and dose.	To monitor efficacy of prescribed analgesia.
3 Record any significant activities that are likely to influence the patient's pain.	Extra pharmacological or non-pharmacological interventions might be indicated.

Note: Fixed times for reviewing the pain have been intentionally omitted to allow for flexibility. It is suggested that initially the patient's pain be reviewed every 4 h. When the patient's level of pain has stabilised, recordings may be made less frequently, e.g. 12-hourly or daily. If a patient's pain becomes totally controlled the chart should be discontinued.

FIGURE 8.4 Cont'd

Domains of pain assessment

Pain can be considered using the following headings or 'domains':

Time:	When the pain began and under what circumstances How the pain changes throughout the day
Location:	Site(s)
Nature:	Descriptive terms Intensity
Variation:	Trigger factors Ameliorating factors
Effects:	On domestic, occupational and social roles On carers
Other symptoms:	e.g. Insomnia
Coping mechanisms:	
Treatment:	Previous treatment: pharmacological, surgical, complementary Current medication prescribed and being taken
Emotional:	Effect of pain on mood, e.g. increased irritability, depression
Goals:	Meaning ascribed to the pain.

INTERVENTION

Radiotherapy

Radiotherapy has a large part to play in the palliation of metastatic disease. External beam radiotherapy may be used in treating fungating lesions to shrink the lesion down. It gives partial or complete relief in 80% of patients with bone pain and can promote recalcification of bone, reducing the incidence of pathological fractures. Other analgesia should be used in the interim before it takes effect.

Radiation may be effective in nerve compression of the brachial plexus, lumbosacral plexus or cauda equina, and, in spinal cord compression in addition to relieving pain, it may prevent further loss of function. Brain metastases are normally treated by radiotherapy in a single high-dose treatment (known as radiosurgery) or in fractionated doses to the whole brain (Faull et al 1998). Radiotherapy is also the mainstay of treatment for superior vena cava obstruction. Any emergency treatment of radiotherapy will be given with steroids, which help to reduce localised swelling around the lesion. In any treatment modality, the costs in terms of side-effects and disruption to normal life must be weighed against the potential benefits.

Chemotherapy

Where tumours are sensitive to chemotherapy, it may have a role in pain management by treating the cause of the pain e.g. in reducing liver capsule pain by shrinking hepatic metastases (Woodruff 1997, Faull et al 1998). Again, the potential benefits must be balanced against side-effects and risks.

Hormone therapy

Corticosteroids are used as adjuvant analgesics and this will be discussed further in pharmacological interventions. Breast cancer may respond to a range of hormone manipulation and if the tumour is sensitive and reduces in size or activity, this may be an appropriate treatment modality for pain.

For further details on any of these treatment modalities, see Chapter 6.

Surgery

The role of surgery in metastatic breast cancer is limited. However it may be of value in specific circumstances and is most commonly used to stabilise fractures (usually fractured neck of the femur) when it will both minimise disability and alleviate pain, particularly incident pain.

Surgery may also be used in spinal cord compression where there is limited disease with good prognosis, if the spine is unstable and causing pain or where the tumour is radioresistant. It has a limited role in the treatment of brain metastases but may be appropriate when there is a solitary lesion in a patient with known metastatic disease but a reasonable prognosis (Faull et al 1998).

Analgesia

The principles of analgesic use are to give the right dose of the right drug at the right time intervals (Twycross 1997). In addition, drugs should be given:

- By mouth – as the preferred route
- By the clock – a regular regime will prevent pain from occurring rather than giving 'as required', which demands that the patient earn their analgesia by experiencing pain
- By the ladder – this is advocated by the World Health Organization (WHO) in an attempt to alleviate pain internationally (see Fig. 8.5).

FIGURE 8.5

The WHO analgesic ladder.

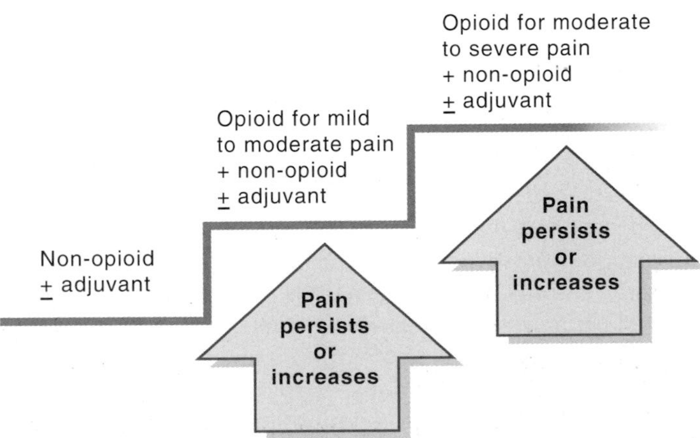

Non-opioids

These include aspirin, other non-steroidal anti-inflammatory drugs (NSAIDs) and paracetamol. Aspirin is rarely used because of the risk of damage to platelet function, gastric mucosa and possible tinnitus and deafness.

NSAIDs and paracetamol have an anti-inflammatory action that is particularly effective in bone and soft tissue pain. They may be given with strong opiates as adjuvant drugs.

Opioids for mild to moderate pain

The term 'opioids for mild to moderate pain' has replaced 'weak opioids' in recent revisions of the WHO analgesic ladder. Although there are many combination analgesics available in step 2, they are not all of equal value since they may have sub-therapeutic doses of either the opioid or the anti-inflammatory. Recommended drugs are co-codamol, dihydrocodeine and tramadol (Faull et al 1998). Tramadol has a role at the upper end of step 2 and the lower end of step 3 on the analgesic ladder. It has fewer adverse opioid side-effects than codeine or morphine but does lower the seizure threshold and should be used with caution. If pain is not relieved by regular use of a particular drug at its maximum dose, the next stage should be upwards rather than laterally.

Opioids for moderate to severe pain

This group of analgesics was previously known as 'strong opioids'. Within the UK oral morphine and parenteral diamorphine are the opioids of choice for the treatment of moderate to severe pain; however, others are becoming available and current research is examining the possible benefits of opioid rotation, i.e. changing from one of these opioids to another if the patient appears to be becoming tolerant.

Fears about opioid use are widespread. Patients may fear becoming addicted, heavily sedated or confused; they may feel that starting morphine signals 'the beginning of the end' and a sign that death is imminent. They may also fear that if they start morphine there will be 'nothing left' at the end and that pain will become intolerable. If morphine is started at the wrong dose resulting in over-sedation or uncontrolled pain, or if side-effects are not explained and prevented, the patient may lose confidence and refuse morphine, or complain that it did not work.

Unfortunately some of the patient's fears about morphine are shared by professionals who also have their own anxieties. These include the belief that morphine should be withheld until the patient is dying, that it causes respiratory depression and hastens death, that it results in tolerance and addiction, and that it causes side-effects that are intolerable.

Addiction is not a problem when morphine is given correctly for cancer pain. Physical dependence may occur in patients receiving regular morphine for weeks or months, but if their pain is relieved by other interventions they can be weaned off morphine by gradually reduced doses. Drowsiness may occur when morphine is started but wears off in a few days if the correct dose is prescribed. Confusion may occur initially, particularly in elderly patients or where morphine is used in combination with other drugs. It may be necessary to introduce morphine slowly and titrate with extra care. Morphine should not be left 'until the end'. Many patients are able to maintain a relatively normal lifestyle while taking morphine for months or even years.

There is no maximum dose, although if pain is poorly controlled on morphine doses in excess of 300 mg/day, specialist advice should be sought (Faull et al 1998).

Respiratory depression is a rare occurrence in patients with cancer pain if morphine is titrated against the patient's pain (Faull et al 1998), and Twycross suggests that this is because pain is a physiological antagonist to the central effects of morphine (Twycross 1997). It may occur if too high a dose is given, particularly to an opioid-naïve patient or in patients with renal failure, but is not normally a problem. See Table 8.1 for the analgesic equivalence to morphine.

Starting opiates

The starting dose of morphine depends on what analgesia the patient has previously been taking. Although morphine 5–10 mg 4 hourly may be an appropriate dose for a patient not previously receiving opioids, in some cases it may be less than the morphine equivalent of their previous analgesia, resulting in increased pain and loss of confidence. An immediate-release preparation of morphine prescribed 4 hourly should be used to control pain initially (Faull et al 1998), with the same dose prescribed hourly as required (prn) for breakthrough pain.

TABLE 8.1 ***Approximate oral analgesic equivalence to morphine***[a]

Analgesic	Potency ratio with morphine	Duration of action (h)[b]
Codeine Dihydrocodeine	1/10	3–5
Pethidine (meperidine USA)	1/8	2–3
Tramadol	1/5[c]	5–6
Dipipanone (in Diconal UK)	1/2	3–5
Papaveretum	2/3[d]	3–5
Oxycodone	1.5–2[c]	5–6
Dextromoramide	[2][e]	2–3
Levorphanol	5	6–8
Phenazocine	5	6–8
Methadone	5–10[f]	8–12
Hydromorphone	7.5	3–5
Buprenorphine (*sublingual*)	60	6–8
Fentanyl (*transdermal*)	150	72

a multiply dose of opioid by its potency ratio to determine the equivalent dose of morphine sulphate

b dependent in part on severity of pain and on dose; often longer lasting in very elderly and those with renal dysfunction

c tramadol and oxycodone are both relatively more potent by mouth because of high bioavailability; parenteral potency ratios with morphine are 1/10 and 3/4 respectively

d papaveretum (strong opium) is standardised to contain 50% morphine base; potency expressed in relation to morphine sulphate

e dextromoramide: a single 5 mg dose is equivalent to morphine 15 mg in terms of peak effect but is shorter acting; overall potency ratio adjusted accordingly

f methadone: a single 5 mg dose is equivalent to morphine 7.5 mg. Has a plasma half-life of 8–80 h which leads to cumulation in many patients when given repeatedly; overall potency ratio adjusted accordingly. Methadone also has a broader spectrum of receptor site affinities and may relieve pain which is responding poorly to very high doses of morphine (e.g. 1 g or more in 24 h) with relatively much smaller doses.

(Twycross 1997)

Rather than wake patients at night, Twycross suggests that giving a double dose at bedtime enables them to sleep through without waking in pain (Twycross 1997). Regular and frequent review is essential and the aim is to increase the regular medication until their pain is well controlled and breakthrough doses are rarely, if ever, required. When the patient is pain-free and their analgesic requirements are stable, it may then be preferable to change to a 12- or 24-hour slow-release preparation while maintaining an immediate release preparation for breakthrough pain.

Diamorphine

This is preferable to morphine for parenteral use because of its greater solubility. There is rarely a place for regular injections of diamorphine in palliative care and if these do become necessary, because of intractable vomiting, severe dysphagia or unconsciousness, a continuous s.c. infusion of diamorphine via syringe driver is indicated. Diamorphine by injection is more potent than morphine and as a general guide when converting from oral morphine to s.c. diamorphine, one-third of the oral dose should be given.

Other opioids for moderate to severe pain

Fentanyl is a synthetic opioid that has been used in anaesthesia for some time because of its short half-life. The development of transdermal patches (Durogesic) has resulted in it becoming increasingly popular in cancer pain management. It is no more effective than morphine and has similar side-effects but nausea, constipation and sedation may be much less severe. In addition, a drug delivery system that requires only that a patch is applied every 3 days allows patients more normality, freedom and distraction from their illness, and may be preferable. It is not appropriate for every patient; heat increases absorption and heavy perspiration may reduce adhesiveness, so management may be a problem in pyrexial patients. It does not allow rapid control of acute pain so the patient's pain must be opioid responsive, well-controlled and stable. Conversion from another opioid, particularly a sustained-release morphine preparation must be done with care, as must conversion to another opioid since a subcutaneous deposit of the drug remains for up to 24 h after a patch has been removed.

Other opioids are available for patients with impaired renal function or for patients for whom the side-effects of standard opiates are unacceptable. Also research is underway into the benefits of opioid rotation whereby patients may be changed from one preparation to another if they appear to be developing tolerance. Such preparations include hydromorphone, methadone, oxycodone and phenazocine. However, they should only be used following specialist advice.

Managing the side-effects of opiates

This involves careful preparation and explanation to patients and their carers; it is the unexpected and poorly understood that causes most anxiety and fear.

All patients should be prescribed a laxative with both softening and stimulant properties such as co-danthramer or co-danthrusate and these will need to be titrated against the patient's constipation as the analgesic requirement changes.

Rectal measures may be necessary if the patient becomes constipated, particularly if faecal impaction develops.

An anti-emetic should be available and if emesis is solely attributable to morphine; haloperidol 1.5–3 mg at night will relieve nausea as well as prevent vomiting. Haloperidol may also be useful for patients experiencing hallucinations, vivid dreams or nightmares.

Sweating may be part of the disease or be caused or exacerbated by morphine and can become very distressing and cause dehydration, fatigue and weakness. Provision of a fan may make patients feel more comfortable; they may need frequent washing and changes of nightwear and bed linen which at home may become burdensome for carers. They also need encouragement to take oral fluids.

Dry mouth (xerostomia) and changes in taste sensation may occur with opiates. Candidal infections are more likely and nursing care is central to management requiring regular assessment of the mouth and frequent and thorough oral hygiene using a soft toothbrush and toothpaste, cleaning of dentures, provision of accessible and acceptable drinks and/or ice to suck and appropriate treatment of infection.

Myoclonic jerks, or brief muscle spasms affecting one or more muscle groups can be frightening. Explanation and reassurance may be sufficient but if severe it may be necessary to review and reduce opiates or treat with benzodiazepines.

Adjuvant analgesia

The role of NSAIDs and paracetamol has already been discussed. Other adjuvant analgesic drugs include: antidepressants, anticonvulsants, anti-arrhythmics, corticosteroids, muscle relaxants and bisphosphonates. Each will be discussed in turn.

Antidepressants

These drugs are used in the management of neuropathic pain particularly for constant, burning, dysaesthetic pain (although they may have a role in lancinating pain). They relieve pain more quickly and at lower doses than when used for the treatment of depression and act directly on neurotransmission in the central nervous system. The lower doses given (amitriptyline may be started at 10–25 mg at night) mean that side-effects are not usually a problem. Tricyclics are said to be more effective in pain relief than the newer selective serotonin re-uptake inhibitors (Woodruff 1997, Faull et al 1998).

Anticonvulsants

These are also used in neuropathic pain, particularly lancinating (shooting or stabbing) pain and act by stabilising the cell membrane. The dose is similar to that used for anticonvulsant therapy and is increased until pain relief is obtained. Side-effects (drowsiness, nausea and vomiting, ataxia, confusion) may become intolerable, although it is suggested that gabapentin has fewer side-effects than the traditional drugs such as carbamazepine or sodium valproate.

Anti-arrhythmics

These also act as membrane stabilisers and include oral flecainide and mexiletine. They should only be used with specialist advice.

Corticosteroids

Steroids may have an anti-inflammatory analgesic effect, decreasing prostaglandin activity and nociception. They may also reduce oedema and relieve the pressure caused by tumour growth in cerebral metastases, in liver capsule pain and in nerve root compression. The risks and side-effects need to be considered carefully and appropriate measures taken to minimise these. For some patients the profound muscle wasting (which may seriously compromise mobility) and cushingoid side-effects become intolerable.

Muscle relaxants

These may be used to relax smooth muscle spasm, e.g. tenesmus or rectal spasm, intestinal colic or skeletal muscle spasm.

Bisphosphonates

Initially used for the treatment of hypercalcaemia these are used increasingly for the prevention and treatment of bone pain. I.V. infusions may be given initially followed by oral maintenance therapy but capsules are poorly absorbed orally and may be difficult for patients to swallow. Intravenous pamidronate may therefore be given regularly.

Interruption of pain pathways

Interruption of nerve pathways may be useful when pain is difficult to control with drugs or the side-effects are unacceptable, perhaps because very high doses are necessary or when pain appears to be very localised. A diagnostic block is usually performed to assess response and if this is effective, an injection of local anaesthetic plus steroid may be effective for several weeks. If pain recurs the procedure may be repeated or a more permanent block performed.

Local nerve blocks have in many cases been displaced by spinal analgesia, particularly for patients whose pain is in the lower part of the body. Spinal analgesics may be given epidurally or intrathecally. Patients need to be selected with care; if they are to remain at home, resources in the community are needed to support the patient and family and maintain the drug delivery system. It is also important for these patients that specialist advice be available round the clock. Side-effects such as sedation, respiratory depression, sensory changes or hypotension may occur and patients will need to be monitored initially. Breakthrough analgesia must still be prescribed.

Non-pharmacological methods

For pain due to advanced cancer non-pharmacological methods are rarely effective alone but are part of a holistic approach that addresses all the components of pain. Non-pharmacological methods tend to have fewer side-effects; they can be learnt and initiated by the patient and family, giving back some power and control and reducing dependence on professionals. These methods of pain relief can also enable the family to participate in care and reduce feelings of helplessness and failure (although family members should not be coerced into helping in this way).

Some methods fall within the scope of professional practice. Others are part of the growing range of complementary therapies, not all of which have been subject to thorough research and evaluation. Before such methods are offered consideration must be given to patient safety. This will include ensuring that: (1) the intervention is appropriate and safe, (2) the professional using the method is knowledgeable and skilled, (3) adequate and appropriate information is given to the patient and family without creating unrealistic expectations and (4) monitoring of both side-effects and the effectiveness of the intervention takes place.

Physical methods

Massage has been in use for thousands of years (Pietroni 1993) and is growing in popularity. The mechanisms by which it may relieve pain include increasing local blood flow, muscle relaxation, promoting release of endorphins or 'closing the gate' by stimulating large diameter nerve fibres. Massage can also be a powerful form of human contact, 'touching' both physically and emotionally and reducing isolation in the patient in pain. When only limited touch is acceptable or possible, for personal or cultural reasons or because of the disease process, hand or foot massage may be possible and is easily given by staff or family.

Massage is contraindicated or should be used with extreme caution in patients who have clotting disorders, in limbs affected by deep vein thrombosis, on areas of skin affected by radiotherapy or close to bone metastases. Aromatherapy oils may be used in massage but only by those qualified in their use. It is always worth checking with medical staff if massage is appropriate.

Local heat and cold

The mechanisms of heat are similar to those of massage, i.e. facilitating increased blood supply, stimulation of large diameter nerve fibres and muscle relaxation. Warmth may also enhance the sense of wellbeing and diminish the experience of pain. Heat may be applied using a local heat source, e.g. a heat pad or generally via a warm bath. The patient must be protected from burning or scalding and it is important to ensure that heat is appropriate and will not increase bleeding.

Cold is often less acceptable to patients because it does not have the association with comfort and relaxation (Fordham & Dunn 1994). Mechanisms by which it may work include 'closing the gate', reducing muscle spasm and decreasing the inflammatory process. Local applications include using ice or cold-packs.

Acupuncture involves the insertion of very fine, sterile needles in various sites. This may be done according to traditional Chinese medicine or using Western knowledge of nerve pathways. Mechanisms of action include stimulation of endorphins, release of serotonin (which affects mood), alteration in local blood supply and increased production of corticosteroids (Faull et al 1998). Acupressure and shiatsu are based on the same concepts but use manual pressure or massage.

Transcutaneous electrical nerve stimulation (TENS) uses electrical stimulation via electrodes placed on the skin either directly over the painful area or over nerves proximal to the area. A-beta fibres may be stimulated, reducing the input from unmyelinated C fibres thus 'closing the gate', or A-delta fibres may be stimulated increasing release of endorphins within the spinal cord.

Psychological interventions

Psychological interventions focus on enabling the patient to cope more effectively with their pain by changing the perception of pain or by providing strategies to deal with it. Such interventions affect the cognitive and emotional aspects of the pain experience. They require an effective therapeutic relationship (which in itself may help to modify the pain experience) and an individualised programme of care.

Basic to any intervention is the provision of adequate information (Hayward 1975) and ongoing support. Other interventions include:

1. *Progressive muscle relaxation*. This involves increasing the awareness of muscle tension and practising muscle relaxation techniques, which may break the cycle of anxiety–tension–pain:
2. *Distraction*. Involves the use of sensory stimuli to direct the attention away from the pain. Structured distraction may use audio or video tapes, conversation, music or art therapy. It may only be effective for short periods and so could be useful during painful procedures.
3. *Guided imagery*. May be used either to visualise a special place, e.g. a garden that produces feelings of peace, safety, tranquillity and deep relaxation or to visualise the pain as something concrete that can then be acted on by the body's resources or by medication.
4. *Hypnosis*. Increases suggestibility and may be used to modify pain perception or to divert attention from the pain. Self-hypnosis may enable the patient to maintain this experience in the absence of the therapist.

OTHER SYMPTOMS OF RECURRENT BREAST CANCER

Anorexia

Anorexia is common in advanced cancer and is a cause of major anxiety to relatives and friends. If it is associated with other symptoms such as nausea and vomiting, these should be addressed. Otherwise management includes explanation to patient and their carers that with reduced activity in advanced disease, little energy is being expended and appetite is often diminished. Advice can be given to offer small portions of favourite foods attractively presented on a smaller plate. The expert advice of a dietician may be supportive and dietary supplements may be recommended. Traditionally, corticosteroids have been used to increase appetite and promote a sense of wellbeing but recent research suggests that progestogenic drugs may increase appetite and promote some weight gain with minimum side-effects (Brooks & Ahmedzai 1996).

Nausea and vomiting

It is estimated that 40–70% of patients with advanced cancer experience nausea and vomiting that may cause more distress than pain (Fallon & Welsh 1998). Nausea and vomiting may be locally or centrally modulated. Within the gastrointestinal tract, mechanoreceptors respond to overdistension of the stomach or duodenum, or reduced gastric motility and chemoreceptors to gastric irritants or other toxic substances; stimuli are transmitted via the vagus nerve to the vomiting centre in the brain. Toxins within the systemic circulation or cerebrospinal fluid are detected by the chemoreceptor trigger zone (CTZ) in the fourth ventricle, which also activates the vomiting centre. Neurotransmitters involved in this process include dopamine, histamine, acetylcholine, gamma-amino butyric acid (GABA), 5 hydroxytryptophan (5HT) and anti-emetic therapy depends on identifying the cause, the pathway and the appropriate receptor antagonist.

Prokinetic anti-emetics (metoclopramide, cisapride) increase the rate of gastric emptying and may be used in gastric outflow obstruction. Dopamine antagonists, (metoclopramide, haloperidol and domperidone) and 5HT receptor antagonists, (ondansetron, granisetron and tropisetron) are used for nausea induced by drugs or when the CTZ has been stimulated by hypercalcaemia or toxins. Antihistamines (cyclizine) act on the vomiting centre and the vestibular system and can be used when there is raised intracranial pressure or meningeal involvement as can anticholinergics (hyoscine hydrobromide, hyoscine butylbromide).

In advanced breast cancer, the cause of nausea and vomiting may be multifactorial including effects of the disease or its treatment, drugs, infection and psychological factors. Disease-related causes may include hypercalcaemia due to bone metastases, hepatomegaly causing gastric outflow obstruction, liver failure, raised intracranial pressure or leptomeningeal disease. Chemotherapy is notorious for causing nausea and vomiting and nausea may persist even when vomiting has occurred or is controlled. Anticipatory vomiting may develop as a conditioned response to the sights, sounds, smells or emotional components related to the environment in which chemotherapy is administered. Other drugs causing nausea and vomiting include those with anticholinergic effects (e.g. tricyclic antidepressants), opiates and anticonvulsants.

Adjuvant treatment addresses the cause wherever possible, i.e. by relieving constipation, reversing hypercalcaemia, reducing tumour bulk or oedema with steroids and/or radiotherapy. Oral anti-emetics may not be absorbed and initially it may be necessary to set up a continuous s.c. infusion. Methotrimeprazine is often used in this way; it has a broad range of activity and is an effective anti-emetic, which at low doses does not cause sedation. Other drugs that may be given by this route are cyclizine, haloperidol, hyoscine butylbromide, hyoscine hydrobromide and metoclopramide and the subcutaneous route may be used for prolonged periods if necessary.

Nausea and vomiting are not easily hidden from relatives and friends, and patients may therefore become isolated or choose to isolate themselves because of embarrassment or the need to protect other people from witnessing their symptoms. Mealtimes can be significant and symbolic occasions within families, offering opportunities for family and social interaction. Inability to participate may increase family anxiety, and be perceived as 'giving up' or rejecting help. Nursing care involves helping carers to understand what is happening and find ways to cope more effectively. Other nursing measures include preserving privacy and dignity, maintaining oral hygiene and protecting from environmental triggers such as odours or sounds.

Complementary therapies that may help include relaxation, hypnosis and acupuncture (Zollman & Thompson 1998).

Constipation

Constipation may be defined as the passage of hard stools less frequently than is the patient's norm. Common causes include:

- Drugs – particularly opiates, drugs with anticholinergic activity and anti-emetics
- Hypercalcaemia
- Anorexia
- Dehydration
- Immobility and weakness
- Inability to reach the toilet/anxiety about lack of privacy
- Nerve damage.

Management will identify and treat the cause where possible, e.g. rehydration and the use of bisphosphonates to correct hypercalcaemia. Problems may be anticipated and prevented by prescribing appropriate laxatives for all patients requiring regular analgesia, reviewing regularly and titrating the laxative as analgesic requirements increase (this is discussed in relation to side-effects of opiates). The laxative prescribed must be acceptable to the patient. Bulk-forming laxatives are unpleasant to take and may prevent the patient eating or drinking more pleasant things; the sweet taste of some laxatives may not be well tolerated, particularly if changes in taste occur with advanced disease. Suppositories may be required to remove local blockage or if faecal impaction has developed, arachis oil or phosphate retention enemas may be necessary.

Measures may be taken to improve oral intake, to add fibre to the diet or to increase fluid intake but in advanced disease the focus is on maintaining comfort by less active management.

Patients need to be enabled to use normal toilet facilities as far as possible and privacy and dignity maintained.

Shortness of breath

Respiratory symptoms can be amongst the most distressing experienced by patients with advanced cancer and may adversely affect every aspect of daily life, provoking extreme anxiety. Patients may be particularly anxious about the manner of their death, fearing that they may choke or suffocate and their fear and anxiety exacerbate symptoms. Applying the theory of 'total symptom management' to assessment and intervention will help to elicit the meaning of the symptoms to the individual and the behavioural, psychological and social components, enabling these issues to be addressed. Figure 8.6 shows a chest X-ray of lung metastases caused by breast cancer.

The lung is a common site for metastases in breast cancer. When confined to lung tissue, secondaries may cause few symptoms (Fallowfield & Clark 1991) but secondaries invading the pleura reduce the elasticity of the lung and may cause the accumulation of large amounts of fluid (malignant pleural effusion) resulting in increasing breathlessness. Symptom management of respiratory symptoms involves treating reversible causes, pharmacological management and nursing interventions.

FIGURE 8.6

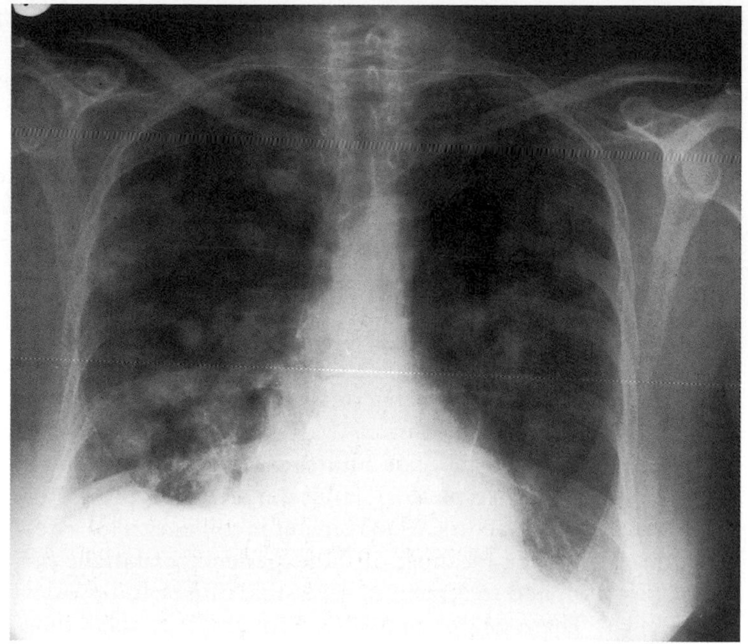

Chest X-ray showing lung metastases caused by breast cancer. Reproduced with permission from Addenbrooke's Hospital Photographic Department.

Treating the cause

Secondaries within lung tissue may respond to radiotherapy or chemotherapy.

Needle aspiration of pleural effusion may be useful for loculated fluid but is ineffective for large collections of fluid. Tube drainage may be sufficient to control pleural effusion alone or may be followed by pleuradhesis using talc, tetracycline or bleomycin. These procedures can be painful and adequate analgesia cover must be given. Surgical management via thoracotomy may be used but is rarely appropriate in advanced disease.

Pharmacological management

Corticosteroids may be useful for their anti-inflammatory effect and when breathlessness is caused by superior vena cava obstruction or carcinomatous lymphangitis but Wilcock suggests that there is little evidence to support their use (Wilcock 1998). Bronchodilators may be effective in airflow obstruction, otherwise opioids are the pharmacological mainstay of treatment. These act centrally and reduce ventilatory drive stimulated by hypercapnia or hypoxia. Small doses are used in opiate-naïve patients (2.5 mg/4-hourly) and titrated against symptoms. In patients already receiving opiates increasing the dose may be effective. There is still no clear evidence that nebulised opiates are more effective than using the oral or subcutaneous route.

Non-pharmacological interventions

Oxygen may be beneficial in hypoxic patients but must be used with care as psychological dependence may quickly develop without other evidence of benefit. Using an electric fan or giving easy access to an open window may be as effective and allow independence and mobility to be maintained. Acupuncture has also been shown to be of benefit (Zollman & Thompson 1998).

Research is currently underway into more active nursing management of breathlessness using nurse-led clinics at which patients are offered psycho-social support, taught relaxation and breathing training and are helped to develop adaptation and coping strategies. Initial results suggest that these interventions are effective in reducing levels of perceived breathlessness and increasing functional ability (Corner et al 1996, Bredin et al 1999).

Fatigue

Fatigue is increasingly being recognised by professionals as a problem for patients with advanced cancer (McPhail 1999). Fatigue may be multifactorial and causes include anorexia and cachexia, raised intracranial pressure, metabolic disturbance, respiratory failure, infection, sleep disturbance, over-activity or psychological factors. Management involves careful assessment that attempts to understand the meaning of the experience of fatigue for the individual, the identification and treatment of reversible causes and the development of coping strategies. These enable individuals to structure their time around periods of rest and activity and to maintain some quality of life by using their limited energy on the activities that are of most importance to them.

Fungating wound management

Breast cancer is the most commonly seen fungating wound and this occurs when cancer cells infiltrate epithelium, lymph nodes and blood vessels (Gowshall 1996). Local recurrence may present as a fungating wound but fungation may also be indicative of rapidly developing breast cancer, which may be unresponsive to treatment. Sadly because of fear, embarrassment or other psychological or social reasons, some women fail to seek help for developing disease until a fungating wound has developed.

Initially, the skin has an eczematous appearance with dry, red, itchy skin, which then begins to discharge. Excessive exudate is produced and areas of unhealing ulceration develop possibly with blood loss. There may be continual irritation of the skin, severe pain that may have a neuropathic component, and infection resulting in offensive odour.

The psycho-social sequelae of fungating wounds are enormous. The wound is an external manifestation of the cancer and a constant reminder that it is spreading. Body image and sexuality is almost certainly affected and the individuals often see themselves as unclean, unattractive and unacceptable, particularly if there is a malodorous discharge. This may result in isolation, loneliness and abandonment and feelings of anger, disgust or despair.

Treatment options include radiotherapy, chemotherapy, and endocrine therapy, depending on the responsiveness of the tumour. Palliative surgery using muscle and skin flaps to promote healing may be possible following radiotherapy or chemotherapy, but is a major undertaking and symptom control and wound care are the mainstays of treatment. Management requires a thorough assessment and an individualised approach to care. A holistic assessment will attempt to understand the psychological, spiritual, physical and social impact of the wound on the individual.

For a systematic approach to wound management, the reader is referred to Gowshall (1996) and Walding (1998). A clean, rather than aseptic technique may be sufficient for cleaning and dressings may be selected for their ability to control odour and/or bleeding without causing pain or further tissue damage either in their application or their removal.

Odour may be very distressing. It is constantly present for the patient, affecting appetite, causing nausea, creating feelings of uncleanness and embarrassment as its impact is seen on staff and visitors. Local or systemic metronidazole can help, although clindamycin may be more effective (Walding 1998). Charcoal dressings may help and complementary methods that include the use of essential oils in an electric burner can help to mask the offensive odour. An air conditioned or well ventilated room may help to reduce distress caused by the effect of the odour on staff or visitors.

Capillary bleeding may be controlled by direct gentle pressure; dressings should be non-adherent, should not be allowed to dry out and should be soaked off, in the shower if necessary. Alginate dressings and silver sulphadiazine may have haemostatic properties although little definitive research exists (silver sulphadiazine is contraindicated during radiotherapy). Topical application of adrenaline 1:1000 applied to the dressing pad may be helpful as may prophylactic tranexamic acid 1 g tds

Patients with fungating lesions will be cared for primarily in the community thus effective communication between health care professionals and the patient and family, a coordinated approach to care and skilled and knowledgeable nursing are essential.

Lymphoedema

Lymphoedema is the accumulation of a high protein fluid in the interstitial spaces between cells in the tissue of a limb or other area. It is the result of a defective mechanism of lymph drainage due to tissue fibrosis, disease, or a congenital disorder.

Approximately 25% of women with breast cancer will develop some degree of lymphoedema characterised by a swollen arm, often with some swelling of the adjacent chest and back. This condition can cause considerable physical and psychological distress.

Pathophysiology

Women with breast cancer who have axillary surgery to remove some of their lymph glands, those who receive radiotherapy to the axillary region, and those who develop metastatic disease in the axilla are at risk of developing lymphoedema in the affected arm. Scarring from these treatments or blockage of the lymph system due to tumour infiltration will result in the closure or narrowing of many lymph vessels and will reduce the efficiency of lymphatic drainage from the arm. The lymph drainage can remain adequate, and collateral vessels may develop to increase the pathways for drainage. However, lymphoedema may develop weeks, months or years after the original breast cancer

FIGURE 8.7

Lymphoedematous left arm. Reproduced with permission from Addenbrooke's Photographic Department.

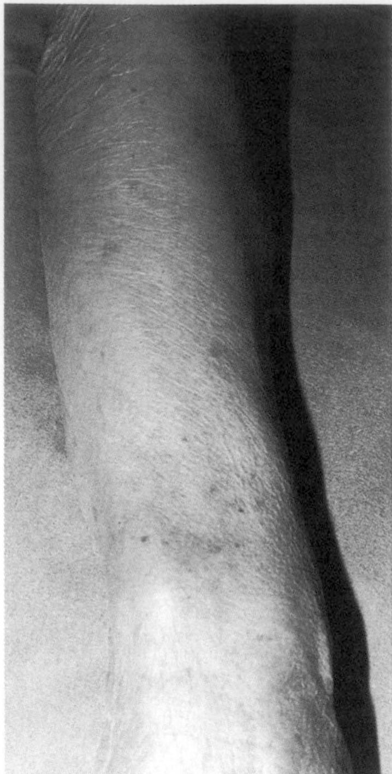

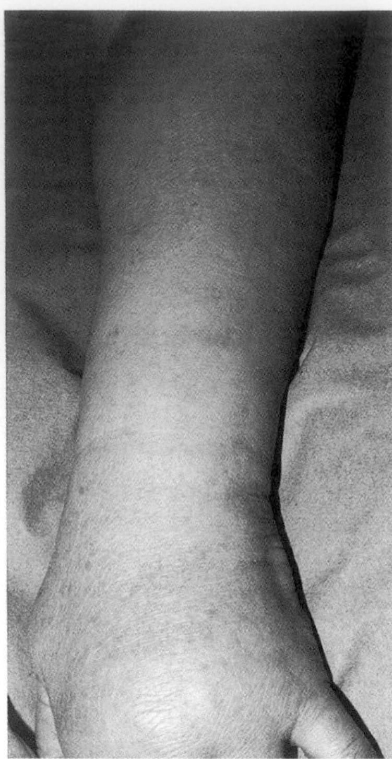

treatment; sometimes it may follow injury or infection, be an indication that the breast cancer has recurred in the axilla, or occasionally, appear when a woman presents with an advanced carcinoma of the breast. Figure 8.7 is a photograph of a lymphoedematous left arm compared to the patient's normal right arm. The swelling was due to recurrent breast cancer in the patient's left axilla.

Lymphoedema may remain mild, or gradually progress until the arm is so heavy that it is difficult to lift and impossible to use. Over time, fibrosis within the tissue of the arm may occur, causing hardness. There is also a higher risk of infection and cellulitis, as the high-protein lymph fluid is an ideal breeding ground for bacteria.

Medical management

The options for medical management are fairly limited. The choice of treatment depends on whether the lymphoedema has been caused by fibrosis or by axillary disease. Assessment may include computerised tomography (CT) scanning and colour Doppler ultrasound to determine the amount of scarring, venous obstruction or disease.

In the past, efforts to reduce the size and weight of the lymphoedematous arm by surgically removing a large amount of tissue had little success and frequently caused further problems with infection, swelling and pain, as well as extensive scarring. When axillary recurrence is present, surgery to remove as much of the cancer as possible may be of use by reducing the obstruction of lymph and venous flow. However, chemotherapy or endocrine therapies, which have the advantage of not causing the same disruption to normal structures as surgery, are more likely to be used (Burnet 2000).

Pain relief may be important, particularly if the the pain is due to brachial plexus damage by disease or radiotherapy. A range of drugs may be used and these should be used under the guidance of the palliative care team (Twycross 1997).

The risk of infection (cellulitis) in a swollen limb is likely. A small cut or insect bite may provide an entry point for infection and result in severe cellulitis, requiring treatment by antibiotics. If cellulitis is recurrent patients are often given a prescription of antibiotics they can keep at home so they may take them as soon as there are any signs of infection.

Nursing management

Nurses have made a great impact on lymphoedema care over the past decade. Any treatment aims to reduce the size and weight of the arm, and for most people this is possible. However, sometimes all that can be done is to increase the softness and movement of the arm, and to reduce the discomfort, but these improvements can represent a substantial increase in the quality of life for the patient.

When caring for the patient with lymphoedema the nurse needs to consider (1) assessment, (2) measurements, (3) nursing interventions, (4) exercise, (5) self-care, (6) compression sleeves, (7) compression bandaging and (8) massage. Each of these will be discussed in turn

Assessment

Any nursing interventions must be preceded by an assessment to identify the physical and psycho-social needs of the patient. The physical assessment should include:

- Medical history, particularly of any surgery or radiotherapy, or of axillary disease
- Condition of the skin of the arm
- Size of the arm
- Duration of oedema and any precipitating or aggravating factors
- Presence of oedema in the adjacent tissue of the chest wall
- Any previous treatment for lymphoedema
- The type and severity of any discomfort experienced
- The individual's range of shoulder movement and ability to use the arm in activities of daily living.

Measurements

The circumference of both arms should be measured at 4 cm intervals from a fixed point at the wrist to the root of the arm so that a comparison can be made between each limb and the severity of the oedema estimated to form a baseline for treatment. There is a special calculator available, which can work out the volume of lymphoedema from the 4 cm interval measurements around the arm and is used by many lymphoedema nurse specialists.

The psycho-social assessment should include:

- How the lymphoedema has affected the woman's self-esteem and body image and whether she has been able to wear the clothes she wishes
- How the lymphoedema has altered the woman's lifestyle, work and social role.

Nursing interventions

The aim of nursing interventions in the management of lymphoedema is to:

- reduce arm size
- improve the use of the arm
- improve the comfort of the arm
- improve the shape of the arm.

To achieve these aims bandaging, massage and exercises have become the treatments of choice. The aim of each treatment regime should be clearly explained to the woman and she should have realistic expectations of her treatment. Although therapy is aimed at control rather than cure, the patient who is given sufficient information and encouraged to participate in treatment is likely to take a more positive attitude toward her situation.

The main treatment methods are related to the degree of severity of the lymphoedema and the patient's wishes:

1. *Mild oedema*: Gentle exercise of the limb and positioning of the limb at rest
2. *Moderate oedema*: All of the above plus an elasticated compression sleeve
3. *Severe oedema, or if there is lymphorrhoea*: All of the above plus compression bandaging for 2–3 weeks, after which the patient wears a compression sleeve.

Exercise

Muscle contraction exercises and shoulder exercises can be taught to improve and maintain movement, and to encourage the return of lymph and venous fluid in the arm. Arm exercises include:

- Clenching and relaxing the hand
- Full circular movement of the wrist
- Extension and flexion of the elbow joint
- Clasping hands in front of the body and raising the arms, held straight, above the head.

A combination of these exercises should be performed for 5 min 4 times a day.

Self-care

Patients should be given advice on how to care for the skin of their arm, to reduce the risk of infection and to avoid straining the arm. This advice should be given to all women undergoing surgery or radiotherapy involving the axilla as this will help prevent lymphoedema occurring and encourage early detection where it does occur (see Ch. 6 on care of the arm following surgery to the axilla).

Compression sleeves

Compression sleeves are central to the treatment of lymphoedema and there are several ready-made varieties available, e.g. Medi, Pan-Med, Sigva. An effective compression sleeve needs to be fairly strong (around 40 mmHg) if it is to be effective. Supports such as Tubigrip are not adequate. Sleeves may be difficult to put on and should be eased onto the arm carefully, avoiding a shearing action, which could damage the skin. They should be supportive and comfortable enough to wear all day, and should not be allowed to form creases, as this will cause ridging in the swollen tissue. The patient will wear the sleeve for several months, during which time their condition must be assessed regularly. The patient should be warned that progress will be slow.

If the oedema is mild it may be possible for the arm to return to its normal size. The sleeve can be removed if the swelling has been significantly reduced, but the patient should be reminded that the oedema may return, in which case the sleeve should be reapplied.

Compression bandaging

For women with severe lymphoedema, lymphorrhoea (leakage of the lymph fluid from the tissues), skin problems or difficulty using a sleeve, compression bandaging is the treatment of choice. Low stretch bandages are used to bandage the fingers and hand before the arm is encased. The pressure applied should be graduated, more being applied at the lower end of the limb. The bandages should be reapplied daily and because of the size of the arm and the number of bandages required, this may need to be undertaken on an inpatient basis. This also provides an opportunity for the provision of physiotherapy, occupational therapy and psychological support if required. However, community nurses practised in this technique could undertake compression bandaging in the patient's home. This is particularly helpful for those patients who have advanced disease and are unwell. Bandaging of a large arm may provide great comfort and relief from pain, even if there is no hope of reducing arm size. Although this bandaging technique is not difficult once learned, it does require practice and guidance.

Massage

The type of massage used is light, aiming to stimulate the lymphatic vessels in the skin. The patient can be shown how to massage the affected limb and adjacent part of the chest and back, where some degree of swelling may also occur. Using the hand or an electric massager, the chest and back are massaged by applying light pressure in a direction away from the arm. Next, the arm should be massaged starting at the top of the arm and working down the arm, but always applying pressure upwards. It is a good idea to show relatives how to perform therapeutic massage.

Readers wishing to understand more about lymphoedema should refer to Regnard et al *Lymphoedema: Advice on management* (1988) and Woods *A hospital based service for lymphoedema management* (1993).

EMERGENCIES IN ADVANCED BREAST CANCER

Spinal cord compression

This must always be considered, particularly where there is known metastatic disease. Patients may complain of weakness and possible loss of sensation in the legs and may have back pain. Immediate admission for investigation and treatment is essential to prevent permanent neurological deficit. Treatment is usually with high-dose steroids and radiotherapy, although surgical decompression may be considered for fit patients with an otherwise good prognosis. Figure 8.8 shows a photograph of a magnetic resonance scan of a spinal cord compression due to metastatic breast cancer.

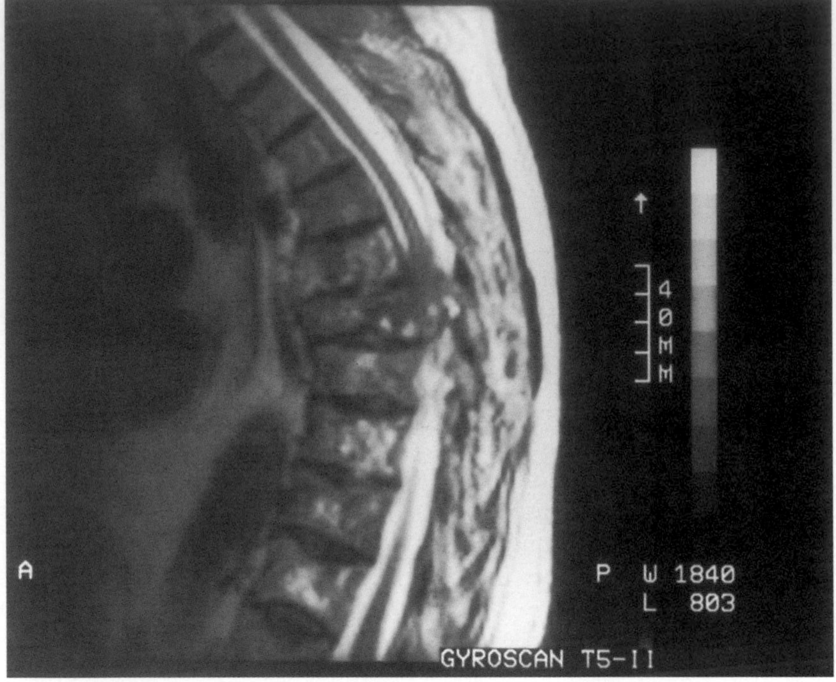

FIGURE 8.8

Magnetic resonance scan of a spinal compression. Reproduced with permission from Addenbrooke's Photographic Department.

Pathological fractures

Skeletal metastases are often the first to develop in breast disease and lytic lesions, particularly of long bones, may result in fractures. Bisphosphonates are becoming more widely used as evidence grows that they may reduce the incidence of bony metastases (Diel et al 1998). Fractures can be predicted by radiological changes and prevented by internal fixation followed by radiotherapy. This will avoid pain and complications and enable more rapid rehabilitation. Once a fracture has occurred internal fixation is the treatment of choice. If surgery is not possible, radiotherapy and immobilisation are indicated and pain on movement (incident-related pain) may require specialist management.

Superior vena cava obstruction

This may be due to direct pressure from the tumour or lymph nodes, or thrombosis. Symptoms include oedema of the face and arms, swelling of the neck, a feeling of tightness or fullness in the head, neck and chest, and shortness of breath.

Steroids may be given, although their effectiveness is unproven (Faull & Barton 1998). Radiotherapy is the mainstay of treatment although surgical stenting is increasingly becoming available in specialist centres.

Management involves bed-rest with the head of the bed elevated, pharmacological management of breathlessness and oxygen if it is helpful. Patients and their carers need careful explanation that although the symptoms are frightening they are not immediately life-threatening.

Pericardial tamponade

This is a rare complication of breast cancer. Symptoms include a feeling of fullness in the chest, possibly pain and breathlessness exacerbated by lying flat. As the pericardial effusion increases, symptoms of right heart failure develop. Once the diagnosis is confirmed, fluid is removed over 24–48 hours and a permanent window in the pericardium created if necessary. Again, this can be a terrifying event for the patient, both to experience the symptoms and to realise that an organ so crucial to life as the heart has been affected by disease. Clear explanations and ongoing support must be offered.

Hypercalcaemia

Hypercalcaemia in breast cancer is not directly related to bony metastases but to the release of tumour-excreted parathyroid hormone-related protein, which induces increased bone resorption and release of calcium into the circulation. Symptoms include constipation, anorexia, nausea and vomiting, thirst, dehydration, drowsiness, and confusion and pain. Management includes i.v. fluids and bisphosphonates by infusion.

It is not possible to address within this chapter all the needs of patients with advanced breast cancer. Essential texts may be identified from the references and practitioners are encouraged to obtain advice from their local hospice or specialist palliative care service. A comprehensive directory of such services may be obtained from St Christopher's Information Service.

PSYCHO-SOCIAL ISSUES

The psycho-social impact of recurrent and advanced cancer has not been well researched (Fallowfield & Clark 1991, Mahon & Casperson 1997, Burnet & Robinson 2000). Meyerowitz (cited by Rowland & Holland 1990) suggests three main categories in the psycho-social impact of recurrent breast cancer:

1. *Psychological discomfort* may include anxiety, depression and anger although for some women who have lived with the dread of recurrence for some time, the actual recurrence may come almost as a relief
2. *Changes in life patterns* relating to activities of daily living, independence, social and occupational roles and relationships and how these are affected by the illness
3. *Fears and concerns* may be about progress of the disease and how it will affect them. There may be fear of further treatment or fear of none being possible, fear of suffering and concern about family members.

Although the threat to femininity and self-esteem are seen as common to all women, other variables affecting adjustment and coping include the age at which the cancer occurs and what social tasks are disrupted. Other issues include:

- Sexual attractiveness and fertility, which may be particularly important in younger women, especially if they are childless or without a partner

- There may be anguish about leaving young children to grow up without their mother
- A woman may be the carer for elderly dependent parents
- In later life cancer may occur as one of a succession of losses.

Other factors include personality differences, coping style, previous psychological problems and social support from significant others (Rowland & Holland 1990). These continue to be significant as the individual faces advanced disease.

Spiritual or philosophical beliefs, the unique meaning of death to the individual, the presence of close emotional support and the physical ability of the family to give care are also of importance.

Impact on relatives

The diagnosis of advanced cancer may have a devastating impact on relatives. Studies have demonstrated a high incidence of anxiety and depression amongst relatives and a correlation between scores for mood disorder amongst patients and their next of kin (Cassileth et al 1985).

The genetic component of breast cancer is well known if poorly understood by the general public and female relatives may have fears about their own future. Children of women with breast cancer may demonstrate regressive behaviour and conflict with parents, particularly if the disease occurs during their adolescence. Daughters, in addition to coping with their own anxieties, are more likely to bear the burden of caring and to need support.

Younger children are a neglected group in that while there is acknowledgement of their need for information, preparation and support (Chochinov & Holland 1990), many health professionals feel unable to help. Childrens' informational needs are in many ways similar to those of adults. They need to be given information at a level they can understand in a sensitive and empathic manner; they need to have their questions answered honestly and gently without the imposition of facts for which they are not ready. They need to be able to express their feelings in a safe environment; families may need help and support in enabling them to do this. The instinctive need to protect children may result in lack of preparation and in children being excluded and isolated with their own fears and fantasies (Kissane et al 1994). The growth of such charities as Winston's Wish (see Ch. 7, p. 149) have heightened the awareness of health professionals about the needs of children and there are resources available that can be used with and by family members.

Facing death and finding hope

A diagnosis of cancer has been described as 'raising the spectre of death' (Colyer 1996, Mahon & Casperson 1997) and recurrence brings this spectre closer. Colyer goes on to suggest that while this existential crisis may be isolating and paralysing, there also exists the possibility of living creatively with dying and this is confirmed by Tierney (1996).

Hope has received increasing attention within the literature in recent years, particularly in relation to its persistence in patients receiving palliative care (Herth 1990, Flemming 1997).

Herth identifies the following factors as important in maintaining hope:

- Meaningful shared relationships with another person
- Attainable aims (which may change with the changing illness)
- Spiritual beliefs and practices
- Personal attributes such as determination, courage and serenity
- Light heartedness
- Positive reminiscences
- Affirmation of personal worth and value.

Factors that decreased hope included:

- Isolation and abandonment
- Uncontrolled pain
- Feeling devalued and worthless
- Uncertainty
- Loss of control (Krishnasamy 1996, Burnet & Robinson 2000).

Although the patients within Flemming's study still hoped for a cure or at least for their disease to remain stable, the role of professionals was still important: the maintenance of concern and 'being there'.

CONCLUSION

In caring for women with systemic breast disease our role as nurses is complex, central and challenging. In order to fulfil this role we need current and up-to-date knowledge and skills. In order to refer for specialist help and advice when necessary, we need to be knowledgeable about the disease and its management, be able to assess holistically, identify needs and appropriate interventions, offer skilled psychological support to patients and their families, act as advocates with other professionals when necessary and recognize our own limitations.

REFERENCES

Ahmedzai S 1993 The medicalization of dying: a doctor's view. In: Clark D (ed) The Future for Palliative care. Open University Press, Buckingham

Ahmedzai S 1996 Making a success out of life's failure. Progress in Palliative Care 4: 1–3

Arathuzik D 1991 Pain experience for metastatic breast cancer patients. Cancer Nursing 14(1): 41–48

Bendelow G 1993 Pain perceptions, emotions and gender. Sociology of Health and Illness 15: 273–294

Biswas B 1993 The medicalization of dying: a nurse's view. In: Clark D (ed) The future for Palliative Care. Open University Press, Buckingham

Bredin M, Corner J, Krishnasamy M, Plant H, Bailey C A, Hern R 1999 Multicentre randomised controlled trial of nursing intervention for breathlessness in patients with lung cancer. British Medical Journal 318: 901–904

Brooks D, Ahmedzai S 1996 Palliative care. In. Hancock B (ed.) Cancer Care in the Community. Radcliffe Medical Press, Oxford

Burnet K 2000 The reproductive systems and the breast. In: Alexander M, Fawcett J, Runciman P (eds) Nursing Practice, Hospital and Home, The Adult. Churchill Livingstone, Edinburgh (in press)

Burnet K, Robinson L 2000 Psycho-social impact of recurrent cancer. European Journal of Oncology Nursing 4(1): 29–38

Campbell T, Hately J 2000 The management of nausea and vomiting in advanced cancer. International Journal of Palliative Nursing 6(1): 18–25

Cassileth B R, Lusk E J, Strouse T B, Miller D S, Cross P A 1985 A psychological analysis of cancer patients and their next of kin. Cancer 55(10): 72–76
Chochinov H, Holland J 1990 Bereavement: a special issue in oncology. In: Holland J, Rowland J (eds) Handbook of Psycho-Oncology. Oxford University Press, New York
Clark D, Seymour J 1999 Reflections on Palliative Care. Open University Press, Buckingham
Cleeland C 1991 Research in cancer pain. Cancer 67(Suppl 1): 823–827
Colyer H 1996 Women's experience of living with cancer. Journal of Advanced Nursing 23: 496–501
Copp L A 1974 The spectrum of suffering. American Journal of Nursing 74(3): 491–495
Corner J, Plant H, A'Hern R, Bailey C 1996 Non-pharmacological intervention for breathlessness in lung cancer. Palliative Medicine 10(4): 299–305
Denton S 1996 Breast Cancer Nursing. Chapman and Hall, London
Department of Health 1994. A Policy Framework for Commissioning Cancer Services. The Calman–Hine Report. DOH, London
Diel I J, Solomayer E F, Costa S D, Gollan C et al 1998 Reduction in the new metastases in breast cancer with adjuvant clodronate treatment. New England Journal of Medicine 339: 3557–3562
Fallon M, Welsh J 1998 The management of gastrointestinal symptoms. In: Faull C, Carter Y, Woof R (eds) Handbook of Palliative Care. Blackwell Science, Oxford
Fallowfield L 1990 Quality of life. The missing measurement in health care. Souvenir Press, London
Fallowfield L, Clark A 1991 Breast Cancer. Routledge, London
Faull C, Carter Y, Woof R 1998 Handbook of Palliative Care. Blackwell Science, Oxford
Flemming K 1997 The meaning of hope to palliative care cancer patients. International Journal of Palliative Nursing 3(1): 14–18
Forbes K, Faull 1998 The principles of pain management. In: Faull C, Carter Y and Woof R Handbook of Palliative Care. Blackwell Science, Oxford
Fordham M, Dunn V 1994 Alongside the Person in Pain. Baillière Tindall, London
Gowshall K 1996 The nursing management of malignant fungating breast lesions. In: Denton S (ed) Breast Cancer Nursing. Chapman and Hall, London
Hawthorn J, Aranda S, Webb P 1996 Management of cancer pain. Glaxo Wellcome, Australia
Hayward J 1975 Information: A Prescription Against Pain. RCN, London
Heiney S 1995 The healing power of story. Oncology Nursing Forum 22(6): 899–904
Herth K 1990 Fostering hope in terminally-ill people. Journal of Advanced Nursing 15: 1250–1259
Jeffrey D 1995 Appropriate palliative care: when does it begin? European Journal of Palliative Care 4: 122–126
Kissane D, Bloch S, McKenzie D, Posterino M 1994 Psychological morbidity in the families of patients with cancer. Psycho-Oncology 3: 47–56
Krishnasamy M 1996 Social support and the patient with cancer: a consideration of the literature. Journal of Advanced Nursing 23: 757–762
Lowden B 1998 Introducing palliative care: health professionals' perceptions. International Journal of Palliative Nursing 4(3): 135–142
McPhail G 1999 Chemotherapy in palliative cancer care: changing perspectives. International Journal of Palliative Nursing 5(2): 81–86
Mahon S, Casperson D 1997 Exploring the psychosocial meaning of recurrent cancer: a descriptive study. Cancer Nursing 20(3): 178–186
Melzack R, Wall P 1965 Pain mechanisms. A new theory. Science 150: 971–979
Melzack R, Wall P 1982 The Challenge of Pain. Penguin, London
National Council for Hospice and Specialist Palliative Care Services 1995 Specialist Palliative Care: a Statement of Definitions. National Council for Hospice and Specialist Palliative Care Services, London
National Health Service White Paper 1998 'A First Class Service – Quality in the new NHS', London
Pietroni P 1993 Complementary medicine – its place in the care of dying people. In: Dickenson D, Johnson M. Death, Dying and Bereavement. Sage, London
Regnard C, Badger C, Mortimer P 1988 Lymphoedema: advice on treatment. Beaconsfield Publishers, Beaconsfield
Regnard C, Badger C, Mortimer P 1991 Lymphoedema: Advice on Management. Beaconsfield Publishers, Beaconsfield
Rowland J, Holland J 1990 Breast cancer. In: Holland J, Rowland J (eds) Handbook of Psycho-Oncology. Oxford University Press, New York
Saunders C 1988 Spiritual Pain. Journal of Palliative Care 4(3): 30
Saunders C 1996 A personal therapeutic journey. British Medical Journal 313: 274–275

Solodky M, Mikos K, Bordieri J, Modesitt R, Solodky M 1986 Nurses' prognosis for oncology and coronary heart disease patients. Cancer Nursing 9(5): 243–247

START Standardisation of Breast Radiotherapy Protocol 1998 A randomised comparison of fractionation Regimes after local excision or mastectomy in women with early stage breast cancer. START Trials Office, Institute of Cancer Research

Tierney K L (1996) The experiences of mothers who are diagnosed with recurrent breast cancer. MSc Dissertation. St. Georges Medical School, London University, London

Twycross R 1997 Symptom management in advanced cancer. 2nd edn. Radcliffe Medical Press, Oxford

Walding M 1998 Pressure area care and the management of fungating wounds. In: Faull C, Carter Y, Woof R Handbook of Palliative Care. Blackwell Science, Oxford

Wilcock A 1998 The management of respiratory symptoms. In: Faull C, Carter Y, Woof R Handbook of Palliative Care. Blackwell Science, Oxford

Woodruff R 1997 Cancer Pain. Asperula, Melbourne

Woods M 1993 A hospital-based service for lymphoedema management. European Journal of Cancer Care 2: 165–168

World Health Organization 1990 Expert Committee on Cancer Relief and Palliative Care. Technical Report Series No 804, WHO, Geneva

Zollman C, Thompson E 1998 Complementary approaches to palliative care. In: Faull C, Carter Y, Woof R. Handbook of Palliative Care. Blackwell Science, Oxford

Index